Social Aggression among Girls

Marion K. Underwood

Foreword by Eleanor Maccoby

THE GUILFORD PRESS
New York   London

© 2003 The Guilford Press
A Division of Guilford Publications, Inc.
72 Spring Street, New York, NY 10012
www.guilford.com

Printed in the United States of America

This book is printed on acid-free paper.

Last digit is print number: 9 8 7 6 5 4 3 2 1

Library of Congress Cataloging-in-Publication Data

Underwood, Marion K.
    Social aggression among girls / by Marion K. Underwood.
       p. cm. — (The Guilford series on social and emotional
development)
    Includes bibliographical references and index.
    ISBN 1-57230-866-4 (hardcover) — ISBN 1-57230-865-6 (pbk.)
    1. Aggressiveness in children. 2. Aggressiveness in adolescence.
    3. Girls—Psychology. I. Title. II. Series.
BF723.A35 U53 2003
302.5′4′08342—dc21

                                   2002152968

For Andrew, Louisa, and Sophia

About the Author

Marion K. Underwood earned her undergraduate degree from Wellesley College and her doctoral degree in clinical psychology from Duke University in 1991. She began her faculty career at Reed College in Portland, Oregon, where she was granted tenure, and moved to the University of Texas at Dallas in 1998, where she is Associate Professor of Psychology in the School of Human Development. Dr. Underwood's research examines anger, aggression, and gender, with special attention to the development of social aggression among girls. Her work has been published in numerous scientific journals, and her research program has been supported by the National Institute of Mental Health since 1995. She received the 2001 Chancellor's Council Outstanding Teacher of the Year Award.

Foreword

Social Aggression among Girls is a timely and much-needed book. Studies of aggression have focused for many years on physical aggression, and much of the emphasis has been on aggression in men and boys. This has been understandable in view of the fact that males are so much more likely than females to be involved in the kinds of aggressive and other antisocial behaviors that are a danger to society and call for social restraint.

Recently, however, there has been a growing interest in girls' aggression. No doubt this interest represents in part a reaction against the stereotype of girls being cloyingly sweet and kind. But it also fits in with a larger theme: that when it comes to reactions to frustration or stress, the two sexes may not be fundamentally different after all—that both experience anger, but that social pressures on girls to be feminine and ladylike cause them to deflect their anger and express it in indirect ways.

There is now a large and growing body of research on girls' aggression, particularly on indirect forms of aggression, but so far this work has been scattered and it has been difficult to see what it all adds up to. Now we have a scholarly book that brings together a wide range of pertinent work. It guides us through the thicket of competing terminologies. The distinction between direct and indirect forms of aggression is not new, but a new element is added with the use of the terms "relational aggression" and "social aggression," terms meant to imply that that the aggressor does *social* harm to another's friendships or social standing. Within this focus, a number of other distinctions are possible, that is, between social aggression that is overt or covert (behind the victim's back); verbal or gestural (rolling eyes, turning away); hot or cold (involving or not involving anger, feelings of hostility); planned or impulsive; and so forth. Underwood notes wisely that we are probably dealing with a fuzzy set here, where no specifiable set of criteria apply fully in each case, but where nonetheless some of the core attributes and processes are clear enough for study. She has adopted the term "social aggression" for this fuzzy set.

When aggression—either physical or social—occurs among children, it typically occurs between same-sex pairs or in larger, same-sex groups. This follows from the fact that through childhood and into adolescence, children choose to associate primarily with others of their own sex. This is especially true in contexts where children interact with their peers in situations only minimally structured by adults—the same contexts where aggression is more likely to occur. Thus, in naturally occurring situations, perpetrator and victim are usually matched in gender. And when researchers bring in pairs or groups of children for observation of peer interaction in a laboratory setting, they have typically studied same-sex pairs or groups. What this book tells us, then, is how social aggression fits in with the themes and processes that prevail in all-male or all-female pairs or groups.

The book has chapters on four successive age groups, helping the reader to trace the developmental trajectories of social aggression for the two sexes. There are gaps in the available quantitative evidence, but the author has made good use of ethnographic reports to fill in these gaps, and leaves the reader in no doubt that social aggression deserves its name: it does indeed hurt victims, sometimes in deep and lasting ways.

Most of the work on girls' aggression has had a comparative focus. It has asked, for example, whether girls are more or less aggressive than boys, whether sex differences are greater for physical than social aggression, and whether aggression in childhood is a better predictor of future adjustment problems in one sex than the other. Underwood tells us which of these questions can now be answered confidently, and which are still unresolved. She confirms, first of all, the well-established fact that boys are considerably more likely to engage in physical aggression than are girls. However, the situation is much less clear as to whether and how greatly the sexes differ with respect to social aggression. The answer appears to depend in no small degree on the measurements used and the age of the children being studied. Also unresolved is the question of how prevalent genuinely hurtful social aggression is among girls; it is not yet clearly known whether there is some level of this behavior that is widespread and normative at certain ages, or whether it is something more concentrated among a minority of "mean girls" for whom there will be maladaptive consequences.

Underwood seeks to understand the roots of girls' social aggression, looking, for example, for connections with girls' earlier relationships with their parents. She also considers whether there is something
distinctive about girls' friendships or social networks that foster social
aggression. It is interesting to see the development of Underwood's
own thinking about this matter as the book progresses. Early in the
book, she is skeptical about whether there are reliable quantitative
and/or qualitative differences between the sexes in the nature of their
social relationships. But later, as the author analyzes the nature of girls'
reactions to being the victims of social aggression, she notes that girls
seem to be more sensitive than boys to this kind of attack. She cites evidence that points to their being especially upset by social exclusion or
betrayal by a friend, and especially in need of being perceived by peers
as accepted within a social group. These reactions and feelings appear
to be particularly intense among girls in early adolescence, suggesting
that there must indeed be something distinctive about the nature or
functions of girls' friendships and social networks at this time. As the
book progresses, a picture of what these functions and processes might
be begins to emerge. These things appear to have little to do with the
relative frequency of social aggression in the two sexes, but rather reflect some distinctive elements in the quality of the cognitions, emotions, and relationships involved in girls' social aggression, and the mo-
tivations that underlie it. We are given an excellent account of some of
the features of the "culture" of girls' social groups. A striking example
is Underwood's discussion of the meaning of "popularity" for girls. Up
to now, we have had a much clearer understanding of what goes on in
boys' groups, especially where conflict and aggression are concerned,
than we have had for girls' groups, and Underwood's account is a very
welcome addition indeed.

We must be aware, of course, that this book of necessity tilts toward an emphasis on the negative side of interaction. Since it is a book
about aggression, it deals only tangentially the positive elements in
girls' social interactions, such as the importance they attach to being
"nice" and maintaining positive relationships, their collaborative discourse style, and their mutual empathy and responsiveness. There are
a number of places in the book where Underwood shows us some
conflict-mitigating effects of these aspects of girls' interactions. But no
doubt in later work, she or other researchers will give additional
thought to the balance between the prosocial and antisocial interactions among members of male and female groups.

In her analysis of the social processes and functions of social aggression among girls, Underwood deals with a number of important
questions: Do girls have a stronger need to have a secure position in a

social network than boys do? Does social status have a different meaning and function for boys and girls? Are girls' friendships indeed more "intimate" in some sense? Or is the meaning of intimacy somehow different for the two sexes? Despite the limited data, Underwood makes progress toward answering these questions, and does the reader a great service by bringing the questions into focus and locating the answers in social relationships and processes rather than merely in a personality trait labeled "social aggressiveness." She notes, too, that social "aggression"—that is, exclusion—can sometimes have positive functions and need not imply any sort of deficit or maladjustment in the perpetrator.

Underwood seeks to go beyond the comparative approach, noting that there are things about aggression among girls that need to be understood on their own terms, apart from the question of whether they are different from what occurs among boys. She gives us a detailed, qualitative picture of how social aggression is carried out among girls, and the changing functions it appears to serve at successive ages, as the nature of girls' friendships and cliques change. This is a refreshing perspective, and greatly adds to the depth of the book.

Finally, Underwood notes how much the research on social aggression has been shaped by the methods and concepts that have grown up in studies of physical aggression. This approach has seemed appropriate in view of the fact that the two kinds of aggression are often substantially correlated, occurring in the same children and thus presumably reflecting similar etiologies. Nevertheless, Underwood urges that we need to free ourselves from this constraint. The two types of aggression are different in crucial ways; for example, they typically have a different time course and often involve a different social configuration (i.e., "It only takes two to fight, but it takes three or more to gossip"; Xie, Cairns, & Cairns, in press). The developmental consequences of being either a perpetrator or a victim of social aggression in childhood may or may not be similar to the consequences of physical aggression, but Underwood urges that we need to look for some possibly different antecedents and outcomes. In other words, as she says, comparing physical and social aggression is a comparison between things that are sufficiently unlike that we need to study each "for its own sake." This point of view clearly offers a challenge to any simplistic ideas about social aggression being merely a displaced outlet for anger when direct expression is blocked. It also adds to a growing conviction among gender researchers that the question of which sex is the more aggressive is hardly a meaningful one.

A valuable feature of the book is its willingness to tackle the question of whether it might be justified to intervene with children and adolescents in an effort to reduce the incidence and harmful effects of social aggression. Underwood considers what kind of interventions might be effective and justified, and this chapter will be especially valuable to people raising children, teaching them, and/or working to mitigate their problems.

Underwood's topic is one of widespread interest and concern to developmental and social psychologists, to parents and teachers, and to professionals who seek to optimize children's life experiences. They will find in this clearly written, accessible book a host of new information and a wealth of ideas—sometimes competing ones—that will deepen the reader's understanding and stimulate fresh thinking. It is a fascinating read.

ELEANOR MACCOBY, PHD
Professor Emeritus of Psychology, Stanford University

Acknowledgments

*T*o whom much is given, much is expected, and I have been given a great deal to enable me to write this book. My deepest thanks go to the following people: My parents, Margaret Ann and Jim Underwood, provided me with boundless love and a spectacular education. My sisters, Andy McDowell and Beth Patterson, give me friendship, inspiration, and the comfort of knowing that I will never be truly alone. Jonathan Cheek, my mentor during my undergraduate years, showed me the joys of academic psychology. John Coie, my graduate school adviser, helped me learn to love research, strengthened my writing, and continues to serve as a stellar example of combining the highest possible intellectual standards with genuine care for relationships. My colleagues and students at Reed College stretched me intellectually and vastly improved my scholarship. Allen Neuringer took me seriously as a researcher and taught me how to teach. Britt Galen and Julie Paquette were students who became colleagues and friends, and from the start offered excellent insights about girls. Jennifer Hurley, Alyssa Schockner, Gretchen Bjornstad, and Victoria Cox served as outstanding research coordinators and carried out complex, sensitive projects with grace and aplomb.

It takes a village for a working mother of two preschool children to write a book, and I am forever grateful to many members of my current community. Dean Bert Moore and Associate Deans Duane Buhrmester and Bob Stillman guide our academic unit with wisdom, humor, and patience—they are sterling leaders. I appreciate the University of Texas at Dallas granting me a leave to work on this book. Many UTD students helped me gather materials and carry out research projects; special thanks go to my first doctoral students, Bertrina Moore and

Mikal Galperin. Talented administrative assistants supported the writing of this book and make me laugh daily, especially Kayety Rowlett, Bonnie Dougherty, and Kent Mecklenburg. My heartfelt thanks go to Doris Record for loving our Sophie like a mother, and to the excellent teachers at the Palisades Day School.

I have always been fortunate to do my academic work in settings rich with amazing women. Thanks especially to Avril Thorne and Claire Zimmerman of Wellesley College; Martha Putallaz and Carol Eckerman of Duke University; my academic sisters Julie Hubbard and Audrey Zakriski; Carol Creedon, Dell Rhodes, and Kathy Oleson of Reed College; and Melanie Spence, Margaret Owen, Susan Jerger, Virginia Marchman, and Karen Prager of the University of Texas at Dallas. Sisterhood really is powerful.

Steve Asher served as my editor for this work, and I am forever in his debt for his generosity with ideas and sage advice on matters large and small. I admire his formidable intellect, unfailing good humor, and careful attention to detail. Thanks also to Debra Pepler and Lisa Serbin for insightful, constructive reviews.

Most of all, I thank my husband and best friend, Andrew Liles, for his unending love and support of my professional life, and our daughters, Louisa and Sophia, for bringing us such joy.

Contents

PART II. Development

PART III. Clinical Implications

PART I

SETTING THE STAGE

Chapter 1

Girls' Anger and Aggression
The Bind between Feeling Angry and Being Nice

Three-year-old Chelsea moves around her preschool classroom, telling all of the other girls, "Samantha is a baby. Don't be her friend." She and the other girls start teasing Samantha, saying "Crybaby, crybaby." Then Chelsea announces, "You're such a baby you can't come to my birthday party." (The entire class had recently been invited to and most had attended Chelsea's third birthday celebration, so her next birthday party was a good 11 months away.)

Sarah, who is 10 years old and in the fourth grade, is upset because her best friend Amy is starting to spend time with a new girl at school, Tasha. She starts telling other girls in the class that Tasha stinks, and when Tasha tries to sit down with them at lunch, Sarah sneers and holds her nose and goads the other girls into doing the same. Tasha walks away, feeling desperate and left out.

Jennifer, Ashley, and Courtney are all seventh-grade cheerleaders, and because of their agility, balance, and short stature, they are "fliers," the girls who stand on top of pyramids (called "bases") and lead cheers while waving their arms in unison. Ashley and Courtney resent Jennifer because she has a new boyfriend whom they also like. At cheerleading camp, Ashley and Courtney decide to alter their arm motions on the night of the competition so it will appear that Jennifer is out of step. When the three girls are on top of their pyramids and Jennifer realizes that Ashley and Courtney are both doing different arm motions

3

than those they practiced, she almost falls while looking at them both frantically, trying to mimic their movements.

Among one group of ninth-grade girlfriends, conflicts develop because some girls invite a friend or two over to their homes informally and then other friends find out and feel excluded. The girls in the group tell everyone at school that one of their members, Susan, has become snobby and stuck up. Susan decides to address the situation using Instant Messenger (an online communication program), sending other members of the group a message apologizing for her part in the misunderstanding and requesting that they stop spreading rumors about her. Her friends respond with brief, hostile messages including "U R such a bitch" and "U R so gay." Susan dreads going to school for several days and avoids these girls, until one walks up to her and says, "Oh, we decided we're not mad at you anymore."

Rachel and Victoria are doctoral students in a small psychology graduate program. Victoria calls Rachel's home and asks to speak to Sam, Rachel's live-in boyfriend. Rachel replies that he is not there and asks if she can take a message. Victoria giggles and says, "Well, I don't think he wants you to know this, but he and I are going to hang out together tonight and smoke pot. Just let him know I called." Rachel is furious. She panics because she knows that Victoria has been romantically interested in Sam since they started the graduate program and that Sam used to like smoking marijuana. She finds Sam where he is playing soccer, calls him off the field, and demands an explanation on the spot. Sam claims to have no knowledge of any plans with Victoria and swears that she made the whole thing up to upset Rachel.

For a group of people reputed to be "everything nice," girls and women can be extraordinarily mean. When girls feel angry or resentful, they hurt one another sometimes by fighting physically, but more often by verbal insults, friendship manipulation, or nonverbal expressions of disgust or disdain. Girls attack each other with behaviors that might be less overt and obvious than boys' fighting but are no less hurtful or injurious. Girls hurt each other's feelings by social exclusion via sneers, verbal comments, nasty notes, gossip, and electronic mail. Girls hurt each other's friendships by spreading ugly rumors about those they do not like and by manipulating those they do like by saying, "I won't be your friend if you don't . . . [do what I say]." Sometimes, too, girls fight physically, and although these behaviors may be less common, they, too, are important to understand.

Girls' hurtful behaviors have been largely ignored by researchers and clinicians, perhaps because boys' physically aggressive behaviors are so dramatic and worrisome. Most previous research on mean behavior among peers has focused on physical aggression among boys (Fry & Gabriel, 1994). Although gender stereotypes dictate that anger and aggression are predominantly male domains, research does not support this claim (Kring, 2000). Recently, scholars have recognized that girls might express anger and contempt in subtler but still hurtful forms called social aggression (or relational aggression). Social aggression is behavior directed toward harming another's friendships, social status, or self-esteem, and may take direct forms such as social rejection and negative facial expressions or body movements, or indirect forms such as slanderous rumors, friendship manipulation, or social exclusion (Galen & Underwood, 1997).

Recently, there has been an explosion of research investigating these more subtle types of hurtful behaviors that may be more common among girls than physical aggression. We know that children view social aggression as hurtful. In one study, girls rated social and physical aggression as equally hurtful (Galen & Underwood, 1997); in another study when children were asked to describe personal experiences, both boys and girls said that being the victim of social aggression hurt worse than physical aggression did (Paquette & Underwood, 1999). Girls who are nominated by peers as highly socially aggressive are also nominated as disliked (Crick & Grotpeter, 1995). Research suggests that socially aggressive girls show biases in processing social information, in that they interpret ambiguous cues related to relationships as hostile (Crick, 1995; Crick, Grotpeter, & Bigbee, 2002). Research suggests that both social and physical aggression are relatively stable over time and predict later negative consequences (see Crick et al., 1999, for a review).

Some researchers have even gone so far as to argue that boys and girls are equally aggressive but that they aggress in different ways (Bjorkqvist, 1994; Crick et al., 1999). Even leaving aside the issue of whether this is an honor I would want to claim for girls, it is difficult to understand what it means to argue that girls are "as aggressive" as boys when physical and social aggression seem so different in form.

As researchers have begun examining subtle forms of aggression that might be more likely among girls than fighting, they have quite reasonably adopted some of the same frameworks and research questions that have been studied with respect to physical aggression among boys: links with peer rejection, relations to social information processing biases, and long-term negative consequences. However, as useful as it has been to borrow definitions and frameworks from research on physical aggression, it seems dangerous to rely only on these theoretical approaches. This book will argue that fully understanding aggression among girls and women might well require novel constructs and methods, more consideration of the emotions underlying the behavior, and attention to different social contexts. Social aggression is important to understand for its own sake and in its own right, regardless of whether it is similar to physical aggression in its forms, developmental functions, and harmful consequences. The most complete understanding of the phenomenon of social aggression requires that we carefully consider gender and emotion regulation.

EMOTION REGULATION: THE BIND AND WHY SOCIAL AGGRESSION MAY BE A WAY OUT

Strange as it seems, much research to date on aggression has ignored the role of emotions, as if aggression is somehow separate from affective experience. Research on physical aggression has only rarely considered the role of anger in these behaviors (Lemerise & Dodge, 2000). Early research on aggression among girls has followed this precedent (see Underwood, Galen, & Paquette, 2001, for a discussion). This book will attempt to understand aggression among girls as it relates to girls' emotions—not only anger, but also jealousy, shame, sadness, and fear.

All children in this culture must cope with conflicting messages about managing negative emotions: be honest, but if you want people to like you, refrain from expressing negative feelings openly (Saarni & von Salisch, 1993). How do girls respond to this dilemma when they feel furious? How might social aggression be a way for girls to resolve their desire to be overtly nice but somehow express their feelings of anger? What does girls' anger and aggression look like, from infancy to early childhood and beyond? How might parents respond differently to sons' and daughters' anger, and how might these differences lead girls to learn social aggression? How might young girls participate in their gender socialization by adjusting their behavior to fit the feminine role and by preferring to play with other girls? How early has social aggression been observed, and are there gender differences from the beginning? The answers to these questions will be a developmental story intimately intertwined with gender and with emotion regulation.

This developmental account is unlikely to be simple or straightforward. In commenting on research on gender and emotion, Deaux (2000) observed, "these two areas of study demand much of us" (p. 30). The study of emotions has long been fraught with definitional and conceptual problems (see Saarni, 1999, for a discussion of some of these). To observe gender differences in anything approaching an objective manner is difficult in the context of a popular culture so entranced with notions of dramatic gender differences that men and women are characterized as coming from different planets (Gray, 1992). Our strong beliefs about the existence of gender differences may make them seem larger than they really are (Deaux, 2000). Gender stereotypes about emotion expression are global, misleading, and possibly even deceptive, because they fail to consider the effects of emotional intensity, frequency, modality, and social contexts (Brody, 1997). For example, the stereotype that women rarely show anger ignores important subtleties such as the form of the emotional expression (physical, verbal, nonverbal, or completely "behind the back"), the woman's relationship with the target of her anger, and different social responses elicited by men's and women's anger. Gender stereotypes seem to shape how we perceive women's and men's emotional expressions; adults rate women's ambiguous angry/sad faces as more sad and men's ambiguous faces as more angry (Ashby-Plant, Hyde, Keltner, & Devine, 2000). When these challenges are added to the fact that anger is such a "coarse" emotion that it is taboo in social interaction (Scheff, 1984), it is really no wonder that until recently girls' and women's anger has been territory in which few have dared to tread.

Still, recent advances inspire hope that a more rich understanding of girls' anger and aggression is possible. Together, these bodies of work suggest that social aggression may be a way for girls to resolve the vexing dilemma of feeling angry and wanting to be honest while wanting to be nice.

First, emotions researchers have made great progress in defining emotions, emotion regulation, and what emotional competence might mean (see Saarni, 1999, for a thorough discussion). Emotion regulation is the "ability to manage one's subjective experience of emotion, especially its intensity and duration, and to manage strategically one's expression of emotion in communicative contexts" (Saarni, 1999, p. 200). Girls may limit their expressions of anger and contempt by refraining from overt aggression toward the target. One way that girls may cope with the subjective experience of fury is by taking consolation in the fact that later, behind the person's back, they can retaliate and make the other person pay for the transgression by harming his or her social relationships. But would this strategy be particularly emotionally competent? Saarni (1999) proposes that "we demonstrate emotional competence when we emerge from an emotion-eliciting encounter with a sense of having accomplished what we set out to do" (p. 3). If girls seek to maintain nice conduct but find some channel to express their anger or pursue their social goals in ways for which they may not be held accountable, social aggression might be emotionally competent indeed, at least in some immediate sense. However, the longer-term consequences may be more negative. Socially aggressive children must inevitably realize that they too are likely subject to malicious gossip and manipulative behavior, and therefore feel threatened and unable to trust in their peer relationships. What works as a short-term strategy for maintaining control may come at a considerable emotional price.

A second advance that will guide our understanding of anger and aggression among girls is that gender scholars have proposed provocative theories for why gender differences in social behaviors may emerge. This fascinating body of theory and research will be described more fully in Chapter 3. As examples of what these theories are like, researchers have proposed that girls are socialized (1) to value relationships more than boys (Block, 1983) and (2) to develop interdependent self-construals in which they define themselves on the basis of relationships, affiliations with groups, and maintaining harmony (Cross & Madson, 1997). If it is indeed the case that girls value relationships so dearly, it makes sense that when they feel furious, they might seek to harm others by damaging friendships and social standing (Crick & Grotpeter, 1995; Galen & Underwood, 1997). This book explores the evidence for these fascinating theories about gender and peer relations and the implications for girls' anger and aggression but avoids getting carried away and concluding that each gender specializes in only one type of aggression.

Third, recent research on how adult women manage anger fits with the idea that girls may use social aggression as a way of reconciling their feelings of anger with their desire to be overtly nice. Research by social psychologists suggests that women find provoking situations more aversive than do men. For example, women are more troubled by teasing than men are (Keltner, Young, Heery, Oenig, & Monarch, 1998). Women report feeling worse about themselves after behaving angrily than men do (Kring, 2000). An anthropologist, Lutz (1990), has argued that at least in the North American culture, women's anger is seen as something that must be managed and controlled. One way in which adult women might try to avoid or minimize their feelings of fury is by choosing to distract themselves when they feel angry (Rusting & Nolen-Hoeksema, 1998). Although in this book I plan to focus on how girls express anger and behave aggressively in their peer relationships, I also must acknowledge the impact of cultural pressures on adult women to contain their anger. After all, children witness these pressures as they observe their mothers and other female adults, and as these adult women socialize girls to express emotions in particular ways.

Girls as young as 2–3 years show reduced levels of physical fighting when they learn to label gender (Fagot, Leinbach, & Hagan, 1986), as if they might understand that physical fighting violates the rules about what sort of person they are supposed to become. It seems reasonable to suppose that when girls feel angry, they might resort to less overt ways of hurting others, behaviors that are perhaps less likely to be punished but highly effective in hurting what other girls most value.

In attempting to resolve the dilemma of feeling furious but wanting to behave nicely, girls may resort to social aggression. Although girls' expressions of anger and aggression may be less easily observed and less likely to leave gaping wounds and bloodied bodies than physical aggression, social aggression is important to understand on its own terms. Social aggression hurts girls and perhaps also boys, and it is time to examine carefully how these behaviors develop and what they become.

OVERVIEW OF THIS BOOK

This book examines how girls experience and express anger and aggression in their peer relationships from infancy through adolescence. This book integrates research on emotion regulation, aggression, gender, and peer relations to describe the forms and functions of girls' anger and aggression, developmental origins and consequences associated with girls' anger and aggression, and whether intervention is possible or desirable to reduce social aggression among girls. Moreover, the book emphasizes what we do and do not know about social aggression in girls, how social aggression might lead to physical violence among females, how important it is that we use observational as well as questionnaire methods to understand fully how social aggression unfolds among girls, and how social aggression may serve positive as well as negative developmental functions.

Although the focus of this book is girls, it seems important to caution against assuming that social aggression is the exclusive province of girls. Girls may engage in more social aggression than physical aggression, but it may not necessarily be true that they engage in more social aggression than boys do. That girls are more socially aggressive fits with many of our stereotypes of females as catty and manipulative, and with the provocative suggestion that girls can be just as mean and aggressive as boys can. However, the fact remains that the evidence for gender differences in social aggression is inconsistent and merits careful examination.

In Part I, the first three chapters of this book lay the groundwork for understanding how emotion regulation, definitions of aggression, and research on gender and peer relations relate to social aggression among girls. This first chapter has discussed how studying gender and emotion regulation might guide our efforts to examine how girls' anger and aggression develops from preschool through adolescence.

Thus far, I have used the terms *social aggression* and *relational aggression* as if they are interchangeable, but they are not. There are important differences between definitions and constructs, and these deserve close analysis. In Chapter 2, I describe the different categories of behavior that have been proposed to capture forms of aggression more likely among girls than physical fighting: indirect aggression, relational aggression, and social aggression. How can we best define anger and aggression in terms that capture girls' as well as boys' experiences? Chapter 2 considers issues of definitions and subtypes in relation to the abounding number of subtypes proposed for physical aggression. Chapter 2 also addresses how we might use research to determine which subtypes most accurately describe behaviors that occur together, share similar developmental origins, and have important developmental consequences.

Chapter 3 examines how gender differences in peer relationships more generally might help to explain why girls might express anger and aggression in particular ways. Chapter 3 also compares the dramatic gender differences in peer relationships proposed by gender scholars with the more modest differences found by peer relations researchers, and it discusses how gender theories could fruitfully guide research on social aggression.

In Part II, Chapters 4 through 7 offer a developmental analysis of girls' social aggression during the infant, preschool, middle childhood, and adolescent years. This analysis incorporates research on anger and aggression, but also on girls' experiences of empathy, guilt, and shame. As Zahn-Waxler (in press) has argued, "Understanding of cruelty and violence requires knowledge not just of emotions that facilitate harm doing (e.g., anger, hostility), but also of those moral emotions that mitigate against antisocial behavior" (p. 224). For each developmental period, Chapters 4–7 describe what we know about various forms of anger and aggression, with special attention to social aggression. Then, each chapter draws on related literatures to examine possible origins and explanations for girls' anger and aggression: temperamental and biological factors, emotion regulation, socialization by parents and teachers, gender segregation, gender stereotypes, social cognition more broadly, and peer relations and friendships. Because few investigations have directly examined developmental origins of social aggression, these sections may be more speculative but the clues from related research are too tantalizing to omit.

In Part III, the last three chapters of this book address clinical issues related to anger and aggression among girls. Chapter 8 examines the developmental consequences and clinical outcomes associated with girls' being socially and physically aggressive. Chapter 9 describes how prevention and intervention programs might reduce social aggression. Finally, Chapter 10 highlights similarities and differences between social and physical aggression, and the urgent need for a comprehensive developmental model of social aggression.

This book is organized around several large questions:

- What does research evidence suggest about how girls express anger and behave aggressively?
- How does social aggression unfold among girls, and might this differ from boys?
- Are there developmental differences in the forms and functions of social aggression?
- What are the developmental antecedents of social aggression among girls? How and why might girls come to express anger and aggression in this particular way?
- What are the developmental consequences of girls' anger and aggression?
- What does research on the processes involved in social aggression suggest for intervention?

In examining these questions, this book draws on diverse research literatures. Because it is clear that girls are far more socially than physically aggressive, the coverage of social aggression in this book is as comprehensive as it is possible to be for a field that is advancing so rapidly. This book also draws fairly heavily from research on girls' physical aggression, for practical and scientific reasons. Social aggression is likely involved in the rare occurrences of girls' fighting physically and social and physical aggression are positively correlated (Crick et al., 1999). A careful examination of the research on girls' physical aggression is also important because investigators have identified important conceptual and methodological issues that can guide research on social aggression. In my discussions of possible developmental origins of social aggression, reviews of related literatures are much more selective, highlighting the highest-quality empirical evidence in the search for antecedents and maybe even causes of social aggression.

The primary goal of this book is to explore how girls develop particular ways of expressing anger and aggression with peers. Girls are clearly more socially than physically aggressive. Why? What dispositional and socialization factors interact to result in girls so desperately needing and wanting close relationships, then using these to break each others' hearts?

In examining this question, it is necessary to discern what is and what is not distinctive about girls' anger and aggression. Therefore, particularly in the developmental chapters, the book reviews research on both genders and tracks whether gender differences in social aggression emerge consistently.

However, gender differences are not the most important issue to be examined here. Rather, this will be an account of what social aggression means for girls: how it unfolds in their peer groups, and what its developmental origins and consequences might be. I hope that this book will inspire even more basic research on social aggression; this is fertile terrain for diverse approaches and methods. I hope that understanding girls' anger and aggression will enhance our understanding of girls' development more broadly, their strengths and possible ways in which they have been misunderstood and underestimated. I hope this account may also guide the development of specific, focused interventions to reduce or even to prevent social aggression, so that girls can feel a sense of belonging and acceptance without having to exclude others.

Chapter 2

Childhood Aggression
Sticks and Stones and Social Exclusion

Whenever the day came for Elkanah to sacrifice, he would give portions of the meat to his wife Peninnah and to all her sons and daughters. But to Hannah he gave a double portion because he loved her, and the Lord had closed her womb. And because the Lord has closed her womb, her rival kept provoking her in order to irritate her. This went on year after year. Whenever Hannah went up to the house of the Lord, her rival provoked her till she wept and would not eat.

—1 SAMUEL 1:5–8

For I am afraid that when I come I may not find you as I want you to be, and you may not find me as you want me to be. I fear that there may be quarreling, jealousy, outbursts of anger, factions, slander, gossip, arrogance and disorder.

—2 CORINTHIANS 12:20

Women must likewise be dignified, not malicious gossips, but temperate, faithful in all things.

—1 TIMOTHY 3:11

At the same time they [referring to widows] also learn to be idle, as they go around from house to house; and not merely idle, but also gossips and busybodies, talking about things not proper to mention.

—1 TIMOTHY 5:13

Since biblical times, observers of human behavior have noted that although women are unlikely to incite persecution by hurling sticks and stones, they are capable of using their social influence to harm others. Somewhat surprisingly, psychologists have been rather slow to study systematically "quarreling, jealousy, outbursts of anger, factions, slander, gossip, arrogance and disorder" and reluctant to consider these behaviors to be aggressive.

13

For decades, most research on aggression has focused exclusively on physical aggression, behaviors that are much more common among boys and men than among girls and women (see Coie & Dodge, 1998). Although hitting would seem to be a behavior that is fairly obvious and overt and easy to identify, researchers have struggled to define even physical aggression.

Historically, definitions have focused on one or more of four features of aggression: topographic, antecedents, consequences, and social judgments (Coie & Dodge, 1998; Hartup & deWit, 1974; Parke & Slaby, 1983).

1. Topographic definitions focus on forms of aggressive behavior that can be observed without regard to preceding events, for example, the "beating movement" (Blurton-Jones, 1967). Topographic definitions have not been useful in the effort to understand human aggression because the range of our hurtful behavior is so broad that invariant behavioral components of aggression have been difficult to identify (Hartup & deWit, 1974).

2. Others have proposed definitions that focus on events preceding the aggressive behavior, for example, defining aggression as behavior that is intended to harm or as behavior that is driven by frustration or passion (Dollard, Doob, Miller, Mowrer, & Sears, 1939). Although this definition fits with most of our intuitive understanding of what the term "aggression" really means, it poses problems in that antecedents such as desire to harm cannot be observed and some forms of aggression seem more intent on achieving a particular outcome (getting a desired toy or demonstrating dominance or higher status) than they are fueled by anger or intended to be mean.

3. Other theorists have argued that the key feature of aggression is the outcome that another person is harmed (Parke & Slaby, 1983). The advantage of this approach is that outcomes are usually observable. However, challenges of focusing on outcomes include that sometimes harm is caused unintentionally and most of us are reluctant to call such accidental types of harm aggressive. Also, some forms of aggression miss their mark but still would be viewed as aggressive (firing a gun that misses the target, or spreading a vicious rumor that never gets back to the person being maligned but harms his or her social standing nonetheless). Last, focusing on outcomes does not take into consideration the role of emotions in aggression.

4. Yet other theorists have responded to the definitional challenges by proposing that deciding whether behavior is aggressive involves a complex social judgment (Walters & Parke, 1964), requiring the observer to consider precursors to the behavior, mediating factors,

the social context, the type and degree of harm, the identity and status of the perpetrator and victim, and cultural norms (Coie & Dodge, 1998). Although this definition is helpful in that it forces consideration of the context and norms, it is a bit unwieldy for research purposes.

All in all, investigators have proposed more than 200 definitions of physical aggression, but most of these share two common features: the behavior must be intended to harm and the victim must feel hurt (Harré & Lamb, 1983). These are the criteria that have most often been applied in determining which nonphysical behaviors deserve to be considered aggressive (Galen & Underwood, 1997). Still, it seems important to remember that, in most of our hearts, mean behavior that is intended to harm seems aggressive even if the behavior misses the mark and the target remains unaware.

As early as the 1960s, scholars began to recognize that the criteria of intent to harm and perceived harm might also apply to less overt behaviors that hurt others by harming their friendships or social status (A. H. Buss, 1961; Feshbach, 1969). Consider the following example:

> Jessica, age 13, was angry because another girl, Marla, had been flirting with her boyfriend. Jessica started telling all of her friends that Marla was pregnant. One of the girls got so excited by this rumor that she wrote this graffiti on the bathroom wall: "Marla is knocked up." Marla saw the writing and was devastated. She went to someone she thought was a friend, who told her that everyone knew it was true and that they had all been talking about it and wondering who the father might be.

In this example, the malicious rumor was certainly intended to harm its target. Because the rumor resulted in some obvious social behavior that Marla observed, she was badly hurt. Although most rumors do not get broadcast on bathroom walls, it seems likely that much nasty gossip becomes manifest in some kind of negative social behavior, if not being directly reported right back to the target. Worse yet, whereas targets of physical aggression at least know who has attacked them, victims of social aggression may not know who the perpetrator is and often must cope with their victimization with the sense that everyone else is involved and working against them.

Researchers have proposed several constructs to capture these forms of nonphysical aggression that may be more common among girls and women than is physical fighting. These categories have been called indirect aggression, social aggression, and relational aggression. Although these terms are sometimes used interchangeably, there are important differences among them (Underwood et al., 2001b).

To make progress toward the goal of understanding anger and aggression among girls, we must be as clear as possible about which behaviors belong in the type of aggression that we propose to be more common among females than physical fighting. If we define the category too broadly, then everything and everyone becomes aggressive and developmental origins and consequences will be difficult to discern. If we define the construct too narrowly, we might expend our resources studying only the most rare, extreme behaviors, and not attending to more common social exchanges that may hurt many girls but may also serve some positive developmental functions for the individual or the group.

This chapter explores how researchers have defined childhood aggression, with special attention paid to the categories proposed for types of aggressive behaviors that may be more common among girls than is physical fighting. Many theoretical models of aggression in girls begin by arguing that these behaviors serve similar functions as does physical fighting among boys (Bjorkqvist, Lagerspetz, & Kaukiainen, 1992; Crick & Grotpeter, 1995; Galen & Underwood, 1997). In seeking to apply some of the same criteria in defining aggression among girls, we have inherited the legacy of definitional problems from research on physical aggression and have similarly tried to respond to these challenges by proposing different subtypes.

The following sections begin with a general discussion of subtypes of aggression, with some consideration of which subtypes have been most helpful and generative for research on physical aggression. Then, I carefully examine the three constructs proposed to describe types of aggression that may be more characteristic of girls than is physical fighting: indirect, social, and relational aggression. Next, I consider how these constructs overlap and why working with competing constructs might facilitate or impede research progress. Then, I speculate about how we might design research to test the usefulness of the different constructs, and to help us work toward some consensus. Last, I explain why this book will use the term and the construct of social aggression.

SUBTYPES OF AGGRESSION

For decades scholars have proposed subtypes of aggression, and subtypes abound (Underwood et al., 2001b). A list that is by no means exhaustive includes the following: antisocial versus prosocial (Sears, 1961; Sears, Rau, & Alpert, 1965; as cited by Feshbach, 1969), physical versus verbal (A. H. Buss, 1961), indirect versus direct (Bjorkqvist, Osterman, & Kaukiainen, 1992; A. H. Buss, 1961; Feshbach, 1969; Frodi, Macualay, & Thome, 1977), targeted versus targetless (A. H. Buss, 1961), instrumental versus hostile (Feshbach, 1964), attack versus defense (Feshbach, 1964), expressive (Maccoby & Jacklin, 1974), reactive versus proactive (Dodge & Coie, 1987), institutional (Bjorkqvist & Niemela, 1992a), rational versus manipulative (Bjorkqvist, Osterman, & Kaukiainen, 1992), physical versus social (Cairns, Cairns, Neckerman, Ferguson, & Gariepy, 1989; Galen & Underwood, 1997; Paquette & Underwood, 1999), overt versus relational (Crick, 1996; Crick, Bigbee, & Howes, 1996; Crick & Grotpeter, 1995), and physical versus nonphysical (Rys & Bear, 1997). Why have researchers proposed such subtypes of aggression?

First, they may have proposed subtypes to reflect different factors that can cause aggression: different preceding events, different intentions, and different goals (Coie & Dodge, 1998). For example, reactive aggression is aggression that seems fueled by anger and the goal of retaliating against someone who has done you wrong, whereas proactive aggression is aggression that does not seem hostile but instead works to achieve the goal of gaining status or even access to a desired object (Dodge & Coie, 1987).

Second, and following the first reason, investigators have proposed subtypes to reconcile discrepant research findings. For example, the distinction between reactive and proactive aggression helps make sense of the observations that not all aggression seems angry (Averill, 1982) and that some aggressive behaviors seem more strongly related to being disliked by peers. At least for 5- to 6-year-olds, reactive aggression is more strongly related to peer rejection than is proactive aggression (Price & Dodge, 1989). Hitting or shoving someone to get a desired object may seem much more understandable and less threatening than trying to get along with someone who seems chronically angry and overreacts to perceived slights.

Third, and perhaps most important for our discussion here, researchers have proposed some of the newer subtypes of aggression because they argue that existing definitions of aggression such as those that restrict aggression to physical fighting leave out hurtful behaviors that may be more characteristic of girls and women. The subtypes proposed to describe aggressive behavior in girls are indirect, social, and relational aggression. We consider each in turn below.

Before examining definitions of indirect, social, and relational aggression, it seems important to note that constructs of this type have at least two types of definitions. Usually in the introductions of research papers, scholars articulate a conceptual definition. Then, often later in the methods section, the operational definition is specified, meaning the specific questionnaire items used to measure the aggressive behaviors, or the particular behaviors coded as aggressive. Sometimes the conceptual and operational definitions are the same, and sometimes they are not. The following sections highlight both types of definitions and focus on questions posed and methods used by different teams of investigators. The findings of these important research projects are featured in the four chapters in Section II on the development of social aggression from infancy through adolescence.

INDIRECT AGGRESSION

Several researchers have proposed the term "indirect aggression" to describe more subtle, hurtful behaviors that girls might use more frequently than physical fighting. In 1961, A. H. Buss wrote,

> From the aggressor's vantage point, the best mode of aggression is one that avoids counterattack. Indirect aggression solves the problem by rendering it difficult to identify the aggressor. Indirect aggression may be verbal (spreading nasty gossip) or physical (a man sets fire to his neighbor's home). (p. 8)

However, Buss also argued against considering psychological harm as an acceptable criterion for defining aggression. As stated in the above quotation, Buss considered some forms of verbal aggression to be a subset of indirect aggression, and it is this type of indirectly aggressive behaviors that have been studied most by subsequent researchers. In discussing verbal aggression, Buss stated:

> Some psychologists have used the notion of injury to define not only physical aggression but also verbal aggression; they refer vaguely to "psychic injury." Injury in the usual biological sense is a clear term. Since adding the adjective *psychic* to it renders the term fuzzy and imprecise, it is preferable to avoid the notion of a bruised or wounded ego. (p. 6)

In making this statement, Buss seems doubtful that "psychic harm" can be defined and measured, which casts uncertainty on the viability of indirect aggression as a subject of scientific inquiry. Perhaps one reason that indirect aggression received so little research attention for so long is precisely these definitional problems.

In considering the history of research on indirect/relational/

social aggression, it is fascinating to note that the first published empirical investigations were conducted more than 30 years ago. Then, approximately 20 years after the first pioneering efforts, several different researchers began investigating these same phenomena, but used different terms and approaches.

Feshbach (1969; Feshbach & Sones, 1971) conducted early empirical investigations of indirect aggression in studies where she observed children interacting with a newcomer. Implicit in her choice of method is the assumption that indirect aggression corresponds to social exclusion and so the way to observe these behaviors is to create a situation in which two children might exclude a newcomer. In describing her construct of indirect aggression, she wrote, "Social exclusion and rejection, though indirect means of inflicting injury, are painful events, which like more direct methods such as physical attack can be used to satisfy hostile, aggressive motives" (Feshbach, 1969, p. 249). Feshbach continued, "The purpose of this investigation is to provide a situation in which the incidence of this kind of 'mean' behavior as well as the frequency of direct aggressive responses can be observed" (p. 250). She examined gender differences as well as the effect of the gender of the newcomer. Feshbach hypothesized that whereas boys would show more direct aggression toward the newcomer, girls would engage in more indirect aggression.

In a study with 6- to 7-year-old children, Feshbach (1969) paired children of the same gender and, in the first session of the experiment, encouraged them to think of themselves as a club, with a special name and badges; in the second experimental session, the pairs were observed as they interacted with a newcomer of either the same or the other gender. Several behaviors were included in the operational definition of indirect aggression: ignoring, avoiding (both of which could be nonverbal), refusals, and excluding.

In a similar study with adolescents, pairs of same-gender close friends interacted with a same-gender newcomer as they discussed problem situations (Feshbach & Sones, 1971). Indirect aggression was operationally defined here as rating the newcomer negatively on a questionnaire, verbally rejecting the newcomer, and failing to incorporate the newcomer's suggestions into the problem-solving discussion. Although Feshbach's laboratory methods were creative, it is less clear how well rating someone less positively and adopting their ideas less often map onto the construct of indirect aggression. As Feshbach and Sones (1971) acknowledged, "The issue is whether these sex differences are a reflection of differences in hostility" (p. 385); they went on to argue, however, that social exclusion does constitute a hurtful form of indirect aggression:

Nevertheless, insofar as aggression is conceived of as a motivated sequence of behaviors resulting in the infliction of pain, then a deliberate snub and social exclusion may be functionally equivalent to a verbal insult or even to a physical blow. (p. 383)

Note that Feshbach's conceptualization of indirect aggression included nonverbal behaviors (ignoring, snubs). Feshbach urged scholars to conduct empirical research to determine which behaviors included in indirect aggression are functionally equivalent and motivated by hostility. Surprisingly, researchers were slow to follow Feshbach's lead.

Nearly 20 years later, in 1988, a team of Finnish researchers led by Lagerspetz, Bjorkqvist, and Peltonen studied direct and indirect aggression in preadolescents, citing A. H. Buss's (1961) definition of indirect aggression. They also stated, "One feature of indirect aggression is that the aggressor may remain unidentified, thereby avoiding both counterattack from the target and disapproval by others" (p. 404). In a later paper, members of this same research group clarified their conception of indirect aggression as "a noxious behavior in which the target person is attacked not physically or directly through verbal intimidation but in a circuitous way, through social manipulation" (Kaukiainen et al., 1999, p.83).

Lagerspetz and colleagues (1988) sought "to study the prevalence of indirect aggression among 11- to 12-year-old boys and girls" (p. 405). They asked children to rate what they and specific classmates do when they are angry and then factor analyzed the children's responses to see which behaviors clustered together and which best differentiated between girls and boys. The factor analysis showed that indirect means of aggression included the following: "tells untruth behind [someone's] back"; "starts being somebody else's friend in revenge"; "abuses" (although this item also loaded on the direct aggression factor); "says to others, 'let's not be with [him/her]' "; "argues"; "sulks"; "takes revenge in play" (although this item loaded equally strongly on the direct aggression factor); "tries to put others to [his/her] side"; and "acts as if [he or she] didn't know" (p. 409).

Here note that many of the behaviors included in the operational definition of indirect aggression do not meet the researchers' criteria, namely, that the attacker cannot be identified. Items such as "argues," "abuses," and "says to others 'let's not be with [him/her]' " describe behaviors that might actually be quite direct and overt. In a subsequent study using a refined measure of indirect aggression with adolescents (Bjorkqvist, Lagerspetz, & Kaukiainen, 1992), items that loaded on the factor for indirect aggression were "gossiping, suggesting shunning of the other, spreading vicious rumors as revenge, breaking contact with the person in question, and becoming friends with someone else in revenge" (p. 125).

These studies of indirect aggression conducted by the Finnish research team led by Bjorkqvist and Lagerspetz have generated a fascinating developmental theory for why girls and boys may engage in different types of aggression during particular developmental periods (Bjorkqvist, 1994; Bjorkqvist, Osterman, & Kaukiainen, 1992). This theory is discussed in detail in the developmental accounts provided in Chapters 4 through 7. In addition to studying gender and age differences in indirect aggression among children, this research group has done pioneering work in suggesting that indirect aggression may be related to particular types of social skill, such as social intelligence, but negatively related to empathy (Kaukiainen et al., 1999). This team has investigated cross-cultural differences in direct and indirect aggression (Osterman, Bjorkqvist, & Lagerspetz, 1997; Osterman et al., 1994), sex differences in indirect aggression among adults (Bjorkqvist, Osterman, & Hjelt-Back, 1994), and published an edited volume of their papers on indirect aggression (Bjorkqvist & Niemala, 1992b). Their groundbreaking work merits careful attention by other researchers working in this area.

SOCIAL AGGRESSION

Cairns and colleagues proposed another term to describe aggression among girls: "social aggression" (Cairns, Cairns, Neckerman, Ferguson, & Gariepy, 1989); they set out to investigate "(a) changes in the nature of aggressive expression, (b) continuities of aggressive behavior over time in girls and boys, and (c) convergence between self-concepts and social attributions of others in ontogeny" (p. 320). They were conducting a longitudinal study in North Carolina in which every year from grades 4 through 10 they asked participants to describe recent conflicts with peers. The results showed that girls mentioned very few conflicts involving physical aggression but from fourth through seventh grade recounted increasing numbers of disputes involving social manipulation. By the seventh grade, more than one-third of girls' conflicts with other girls involved friendship manipulation. Cairns, Cairns, Neckerman, and colleagues (1989) proposed the term "social aggression" to describe these behaviors; they defined it as "the manipulation of group acceptance through alienation, ostracism, or character defamation" (p. 323). In subsequent years, the Cairns group did not focus on social aggression, although recently former members of this team and their associates have begun to explore the phenomenon by conducting reanalyses of this same longitudinal data set (Xie, Cairns, & Cairns, 2002, in press; Xie, Swift, Cairns, & Cairns, 2002).

RELATIONAL AGGRESSION

In 1995, Crick and Grotpeter proposed another term for the forms of aggression that may be more common among girls than physical fighting, namely, "relational aggression." They defined relational aggression as "harming others through purposeful manipulation and damage of their peer relationships" (p. 711). They wrote, "it seems important to initiate research in this relevant, but unexplored domain" (Crick & Grotpeter, 1995, p. 711) and "relatively little information has been generated to date regarding the aggressive behavior of girls" (Crick, 1995, p. 313). The goals of Crick and Grotpeter's initial study were to develop a measure of relational aggression, investigate gender differences, determine whether relational aggression was distinct from overt aggression (defined as physical and verbal aggression), and explore whether relational aggression was related to psychological maladjustment.

Crick and Grotpeter (1995) developed a peer nomination measure to assess relational aggression, for which children in the third through sixth grades nominated three peers who were most likely to engage in particular behaviors. Items assessing relational aggression included the following: "When mad at a person, gets even by keeping the person from being in their group of friends"; "Tells friends they will stop liking them unless friends do what they say"; "When mad at a person, ignores them and stops talking to them"; and "Tries to keep certain people from being in [his or her] group during activity or play time" (p. 713).

As useful as this peer nomination measure has been for generating subsequent research, the measure seems to have at least two problems. First, it is important to note that the original peer nomination measure also included an item assessing gossip: "Tells mean lies or rumors about a person to make others not like the person." However, even though this type of behavior seems to be well within the conceptual definition of relational aggression, it was dropped from further analyses because factor analyses showed that the item also loaded strongly on the factor for overt aggression. If nasty gossip is not relational aggression, what is? A second problem with the correspondence between the measure and the terms "overt" versus "relational" is that at least some of the relational behaviors seem quite overt, for example, "Tells friends they will stop liking them unless friends do what they say." In subsequent research, the gossip item was added to the measure and the distinction was characterized as physical versus relational aggression (e.g., Crick, 1997).

In addition to developing a peer nomination tool for measuring relational aggression, Crick and Grotpeter (1995) were the first researchers to argue explicitly that relational aggression is related to psychological maladjustment and maybe even later negative outcomes, perhaps in a manner similar to physical aggression. This interesting idea has generated a great deal of important research (see Crick et al., 1999, for an overview). Research on relational aggression seems also to have contributed to the provocative suggestion that girls are just as aggressive as boys, although girls might use different behaviors to express their hostility (Crick et al., 1999; but see also Bjorkqvist, 1994).

SOCIAL AGGRESSION REVISITED

In 1997, Galen and Underwood examined the three constructs previously proposed to describe aggression in girls (indirect, social, and relational aggression) and chose to work with the construct of social aggression because it seemed to best describe the function of these behaviors, namely, to do social harm. Galen and Underwood (1997) expanded the definition proposed by Cairns, Cairns, Neckerman, and colleagues (1989) slightly, stating, "Social aggression is directed toward damaging another's self-esteem, social status, or both, and may take such direct forms as verbal rejection, negative facial expressions or body movements, or more indirect forms such as slanderous rumors or social exclusion" (p. 589).

Galen and Underwood (1997) conducted a three-part study to explore whether social aggression is perceived to be hurtful in a manner similar to how physical aggression is perceived, whether elements of social aggression could be observed in a laboratory setting, and whether children would perceive actual videotaped examples of such behavior as hurtful.

In the first study, children in fourth-, seventh-, and tenth-grade classrooms were asked to read hypothetical vignettes, some describing physical aggression and some portraying social aggression. These vignettes included some examples of nonverbal exclusionary behavior. Here is one: "Four girls in your grade are talking about a movie they have just seen when you walk up to the group. The group sees you, stops talking, and turns away from you with their noses turned upward." Children rated how hurt they would be by these behaviors and how frequently they occurred in their peer groups. Factor analyses showed that responses to vignettes depicting physical and social aggression loaded on separate factors and that nonverbal exclusionary behaviors (e.g., the snub described in the vignette above) clearly loaded on the social aggression factor. In addition, nonverbal socially aggressive behaviors (such as nonverbal social exclusion) were among those reported to occur most frequently and were rated as equally hurtful as more verbal forms of social aggression.

In the second study, we attempted to create a laboratory context in which we might be able to observe elements of social aggression. Because social aggression involves manipulating relationships, it seemed important to observe children who had close relationships. Therefore, we observed a small sample of pairs of seventh-grade girls who had nominated each other as close friends. To enhance the likelihood that exclusionary behaviors might occur, we elaborated on Feshbach's (1969, 1971) newcomer methods in the following way. We invited girls who were close friends to play Pictionary with a third girl, whom they thought was a participant but who was really an actor. We trained our actor to engage in several annoying behaviors as she played the game. She made boastful statements (e.g., "My hair looks so hot today—check out my bangs!"), criticized participants ("Don't you know how to draw? That doesn't look like anything at all."), played the game poorly (showed others the cards, tipped over the hourglass timer), and bossed the other girls around ("I'm sitting there and I'm going first!"). We expected that these behaviors might invite social exclusion because previous research had demonstrated that unpopular children are more likely than their well-liked peers to behave in a bossy, attention-seeking manner (Gelb & Jacobson, 1988). Also, acting self-centered and disrupting others' play is related to difficulty in entering groups (Borja-Alvarez, Zarbatany, & Pepper, 1991). As the close friends interacted with our provocative actor, we carefully coded the verbalizations, facial expressions, and gestures by the close friends toward her. We were able to code reliably even subtle gestures, such as sneers and eye rolls.

In the third study, we selected video excerpts of nonverbal expressions of social aggression from these play sessions and showed these clips to youths unfamiliar with the girls on the tape. Girls and boys from elementary, junior high, and high school age groups viewed the video examples, then rated how much they thought the person displaying the mean nonverbal behavior was angry and how they would feel if they were the target of such behavior.

When we proposed to revive Cairns and colleagues' (1989) term "social aggression," we did so not only because the term best described an important goal of these behaviors—to do social harm—but also because we interpreted the term to leave open the possibility of including nonverbal exclusionary behaviors. The construct of relational aggression specifically excludes any nonverbal behavior (Crick & Grotpeter, 1995). The term "indirect aggression" seemed problematic because some of the behaviors involved are quite direct (e.g., telling someone "I won't be your friend unless you do what I say." In including nonverbal behaviors as part of the construct of social aggression, we believed that we were following in the tradition of Feshbach (1969, 1971) and the Finnish research team (Bjorkqvist, Lagerspetz, & Kaukiainen, 1992; Lagerspetz et al., 1988) in acknowledging that gestures can also hurt and exclude.

However, in recent years, others have interpreted social aggression to have a somewhat different meaning. In analyzing narratives of peer conflicts, one group distinguishes between direct relational aggression (overtly manipulating relationships) and social aggression (causing interpersonal harm in covert, nonconfrontational ways by involving the social community; Xie et al., 2002). Although this distinction between overt and covert relationship manipulations is theoretically interesting, it will be important to explore further the empirical evidence for direct relational aggression and social aggression as distinct constructs. To date, several factor analytic studies suggest that all of these behaviors cluster together (Bjorkqvist, Lagerspetz, & Kaukianen, 1992; Crick & Grotpeter, 1995), but this may be because items were not included to assess fully direct relational and social aggression.

OVERLAPPING, COMPETING CONSTRUCTS: PERILS, PITFALLS, AND POSSIBLE SOLUTIONS

After decades of research on aggression ignoring more subtle but still hurtful behaviors, the fact that such diverse research groups are working on indirect, social, and relational aggression represents remarkable progress. That these diverse groups focused on similar phenomena, seemingly independently, and arrived at such similar conclusions suggest that indirect/social/relational aggression is a robust phenomenon indeed.

Each of these research approaches has made important and unique contributions to our current understanding of aggression among girls. Feshbach (1969; Feshbach & Sones, 1971) led the way in focusing our attention on indirect aggression, arguing that these behaviors hurt, that they can be observed in the lab and coded reliably, and that they may be more common among girls. The Finnish research team (Bjorkqvist, Lagerspetz, & Kaukianen, 1992; Lagerspetz et al., 1988) developed a peer-rating instrument to assess indirect aggression,

conducted the first factor analyses to show that indirect and direct aggression may be distinct, and provided further evidence that "girls manipulate and boys fight" (p. 117). Cairns, Neckerman, and colleagues
(1989) provided the clearest developmental evidence that girls use
these behaviors in their peer conflicts during the junior high school
years. In their study, social aggression emerged in response to simple,
open-ended questions about peer difficulties. By using peer nomination methods that by definition identify the children who are most extreme in particular behaviors, Crick and colleagues took a more clinical
approach and suggested that engaging in relational aggression may
contribute to psychopathology (Crick & Grotpeter, 1995; Crick et al.,
1999). Our research group investigated whether nonverbal exclusionary behaviors could also inflict social harm (Galen & Underwood, 1997;
Paquette & Underwood, 1999; Underwood et al., 2001b).

Still, in its current state, our field is left with three largely but not
perfectly overlapping constructs. Scholars disagree as to whether the
constructs of indirect, social, and relational aggression describe similar
phenomena (Bjorkqvist, 2001; Underwood, Galen, & Paquette, 2001a).

In some ways, it is easiest to compare indirect and relational
aggression because both are assessed by peer instruments: indirect aggression by peer ratings, and relational aggression by peer nominations. Here it seems important to note that the use of peer ratings, in
which every peer rates every other peer on a 1–5 scale, seem to be a
particularly sensitive method for assessing peer perceptions of different forms of aggression and measuring levels of this behavior in normal samples. The use of peer nominations, where children vote for
only three people who engage in particular behaviors, provides a less
sensitive index of each child's relational aggression, although this
method works well for identifying extreme groups.

Although slightly different rating techniques are used, the items
on these measures seem remarkably similar. Table 2.1 lists the peer assessment items used to assess indirect and relational aggression. The
logic underlying the constructs also seems remarkably similar: Lagerspetz and colleagues (1988) wrote, "Peers may be used as means or ve-
hicles for harming the victim" (p. 405); Crick (1997) stated, "relational
aggression includes behaviors in which relationships specifically serve
as the vehicle of harm" (p. 610).

The main distinction between social aggression and the other constructs is that we argued explicitly that it is important to include nonverbal behaviors in the construct (Galen & Underwood, 1997). However, whether this was really different than indirect aggression is
debatable, depending on whether you interpret some of the codes used
by Feshbach (1969; e.g., avoiding) and the peer-rating items of Lager-

TABLE 2.1. Peer Items Used to Assess Indirect and Relational Aggression

Indirect aggression (Lagerspetz et al., 1988)	Relational aggression (Crick & Grotpeter, 1995)
When angry . . .	
• Tells untruth behind back.	• Tells mean lies or rumors about a person to make other kids not like the person (omitted in analyses because also loaded on overt aggression factor).
• Starts being somebody else's friend in revenge.	
• Says to others, "Let's not be with [him/her]."	
• Tries to put the other to his/her side.	• Tells friends they will stop liking them unless friends do what they say.
• Acts as if didn't know.	• When mad at a person, gets even by keeping the person from being in their group of friends.
• Sulks.	
• Abuses.	• When mad at a person, ignores them or stops talking to them.
• Argues.	
• Takes revenge in play (omitted because also loaded on direct factor).	
• Calls name (omitted in analyses because also loaded on direct factor).	

spetz and colleagues (1988; e.g., sulks) as including nonverbal behaviors.

In a way, it may be unproductive to attempt to deduce the subtle distinctions between these three constructs on the basis of conceptual definitions articulated so far. First, these definitions seem to be revised slightly from paper to paper as investigators refine their instruments, so it is difficult to tell what the boundaries of the category are. Second, of course each research team is motivated to promote its own construct—for personal as well as scientific reasons.

Why is it a potential problem for us to continue to work with these three overlapping constructs, as we will almost certainly continue to do, or for even more proposed constructs to spring up, as they most likely will? One difficulty is that if each research team continues to create and promote its own subtype to capture aggression among girls, we may find ourselves in a situation faced by our colleagues in cognitive psychology a decade or so ago. In reviewing theory and research to date on memory, Watkins (1990) wrote that theories had become so numerous that "we have entered a stage of personalized theorizing" (p. 328) in which theories become akin to toothbrushes in that everyone must have one of his or her own. I fear that if we are not careful, researchers studying aggression among girls will soon enter the era of personalized subtypes of aggression.

Why would it be harmful for each research team to propose its own subtype to describe aggression among girls? First, this would make it difficult to discriminate among definitions and we could easily end up with a perplexing array of only slightly different theories. Second, it would be difficult for studies to build on each other, because it would become increasingly complicated to understand which categories differ from each other in particular ways. Third, we scholars would be tempted to expend energy and resources tending and defending our personal subtypes, rather than working in concert with other research groups to try to understand this complex, far-reaching, fascinating phenomenon. Pursuing personalized subtypes would likely waste resources and leave us with the shared sense that our field is not moving forward.

How might researchers make progress in meeting these vexing challenges? First, it seems important to acknowledge that none of the existing definitions or theories is perfect. The term "indirect aggression" seems problematic because this construct includes behaviors that seem quite direct and overt (e.g., "Calls names"; Lagerspetz et al., 1988). Similarly, contrasting relational to overt aggression seems inaccurate because some of the relational aggression items seem quite overt, for example, "Tells friends they will stop liking them unless friends do what they say" (Crick & Grotpeter, 1995, p. 713). The terms "relational aggression" and "social aggression" both share the difficulty that they seem overly broad because most aggression occurs in the context of relationships and social interactions. As this book reviews research on indirect/relational/social aggression, I will examine carefully the empirical evidence for the distinctiveness of each of these constructs.

Second, given that none of our current terms is perfect and that it is tempting to construct a new, better term, it seems important that researchers take great care in introducing new constructs. If new subtypes are to be introduced, then it seems important that their proponents should argue carefully for why the new term is needed and how exactly the new construct differs from competing, already existing terms (Underwood et al., 2001a). Deducing differences among constructs when scholars themselves do not explain them is difficult indeed.

Third, it will be important for researchers to continue to articulate the conceptual basis on which they make distinctions between subtypes of aggression. As I discuss research on social aggression in different developmental periods in Part II of this book (Chapters 4–7), these conceptual issues are highlighted to the extent that they are apparent in the articles reviewed. In Chapter 10, some new models are proposed for defining and measuring social aggression.

Given that the focus of this chapter is definitions, it seems worth noting here that thus far investigators seem to have attempted to explain distinctions between subtypes of aggression on the basis of the means of harm (Crick & Grotpeter, 1995; Lagerspetz et al., 1988) or the goal the behavior is intended to serve (Galen & Underwood, 1997). However, as we argued in an earlier paper, these arguments are undermined by the fact that any form of aggressive behavior usually hurts others in multiple ways and serves multiple goals: to harm someone physically, to obtain access to objects, to demonstrate dominance in a group, to inflict emotional or psychological pain, or to harm relationships (Underwood et al., 2001b). All forms of aggression likely fulfill more than one of these goals. For instance, punching a classmate may hurt the victim physically, but it likely also harms that child's social standing, friendships, and self-esteem. Likewise, spreading a nasty rumor about a peer may result in harm to that child's friendships, but it may also be executed to serve more instrumental goals such as gaining status in a particular group.

Because almost all aggressive behaviors may serve multiple goals, we may be on shaky ground when we try to discriminate between boys' and girls' aggression on the basis of the type of harm inflicted. Other conceptual approaches may be needed (Underwood et al., 2001b), and some of these are described more fully in Chapter 10.

One possibility may be to consider subtypes of aggression to be less distinct categories and more prototypes—sets of associated features in which some features are more central and present in all category members, and others are more peripheral and less commonly shared. It seems possible to imagine a sort of categorical hierarchy of aggressive behaviors where some specific actions will fit clearly in one set or another but others overlap one or more categories.

Figure 2.1 presents one possible way to construct categories for understanding forms of aggression. This typology represents current thinking that the type of harm may be the best superordinate principal, but (as just stated) it is easy to imagine forms of aggression that do not fit neatly into these sets. For example, a boy who goes to his high school locker to find the word "Fag" spray-painted on its front has suffered property damage, harm to his social standing, and a verbal insult. In the next section, I explain this hierarchical system in more detail and why I use the term "social aggression."

Another important possibility is that we consider subtypes of aggression to be social strategies that exist on a continuum from more to less overtly hurtful (Archer, 2001). Once we are open to a more dimen-

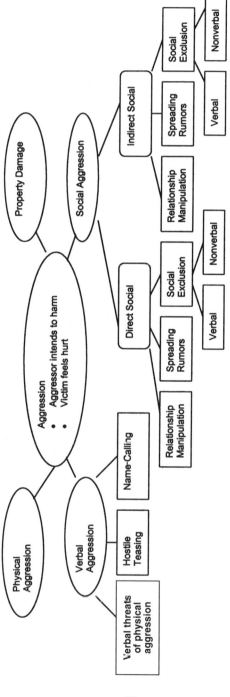

FIGURE 2.1. Forms of aggressive behavior.

sional model, it might also be interesting to consider whether some kind of multiaxial system of classifying aggression might be useful in which a particular aggressive act is evaluated on several important dimensions, such as physical–social, impulsive–deliberative, overt–covert, and reactive–proactive (Underwood et al., 2001b).

Considering aggressive behavior along several dimensions may help us to appreciate the richness and complexity of the phenomenon that is social aggression. It may also help us with the challenge that whatever category you prefer, indirect/relational/social aggression may be further divided into other subtypes that have been useful in understanding physical aggression. For example, to date, most researchers have focused on forms of social aggression that seem to be aimed at expressing anger and hurting others (Crick et al., 1996; Galen & Underwood, 1997). However, it seems just as likely that these behaviors might be used in the service of more instrumental or proactive goals, say, to improve one's standing in a group or for the sheer entertainment value of manipulating others. Likewise, some types of social aggression may seem more "hot" (angry, impulsive, dysregulated), whereas others may seem more "cool" (planful, deliberate, manipulative, and calmly executed with no seeming remorse).

Also, some forms of social aggression may actually be playful, similar to how rough-and-tumble play seems to be distinct from physical aggression in boys. For example, "playing the dozens" is a form of verbal banter common among African American boys (Lefever, 1981) in which insults are traded in a ritual, playful manner. Playing the dozens may well be an example of playful social aggression.

As tempting as it might be for the sake of precision and clarity, further dividing subtypes into smaller and smaller sub-subtypes seems like a hall of infinite regress. Given that some of the boundaries between these categories may be less than clear, some sort of multidimensional system may make more sense, especially if the dimensions are conceptualized as continua rather than categories with discrete boundaries.

Fourth, and most importantly, as important as conceptualization and theory are, our best hope for progress in clarifying which subtypes are most useful is likely to be empirical research (Underwood et al., 2001b). Investigators have already made good use of factor analyses to see which particular aggressive behaviors cluster together for peer ratings (Lagerspetz et al., 1988) and peer nominations (Crick & Grotpeter, 1995). However, for these factor analytic studies to be maximally useful, it is important that these measures include the items necessary to test competing constructs. It may also be enormously useful to conduct more qualitative research, to learn more about how children describe their experiences of perpetrating and being victimized by social aggression, and to see what features they perceive as most vivid and important. The deepest understanding of which subtypes are most helpful and useful will likely come from longitudinal research. Imagine a longitudinal study in which a large sample of children is followed from early childhood through adolescence and beyond, and assessed to determine which forms of aggressive behavior are stable, occur together, develop from similar causal factors, and most clearly predict important developmental outcomes. Clearly, such a study would be most productive if it included assessments of multiple types of hurtful behaviors.

WHY "SOCIAL AGGRESSION"?

Given the current state of the art and the fact that no construct is perfect, it seems necessary to explain why this book will use the term "social aggression." First, I prefer this term because, as stated earlier, to me it more clearly captures the defining goal of the behavior in question—to do social harm. Social aggression can certainly harm friendships, but these behaviors can also harm social standing and social self-concept. Second, this is the only category that explicitly includes nonverbal displays of social exclusion. Third, this construct seems to allow for both overt and covert forms of relationship manipulation.

As depicted in Figure 2.1, the core elements of social aggression are three behaviors that can be either direct and overt or indirect and covert ("behind the back): relationship manipulation, spreading rumors, and social exclusion (which can be verbal or nonverbal). The category of social aggression includes all behaviors that are intended to harm others by harming their social relationships, peer status, or friendships. In explaining how I conceive of these different categories, examples are provided (when possible, from the research literature to date). Direct socially aggressive behaviors include the following: relationship manipulation (saying, "Tells friends they will stop liking them unless they do what they say"; Crick & Grotpeter, 1995, p. 713); spreading rumors ("Tells mean lies or rumors about a person to make others not like the person"; Crick & Grotpeter, 1995, p. 713; the direct form of this behavior is openly maligning someone else to others with no pretense of benign intentions); verbal social exclusion ("During lunch, a group of girls are talking about the big party this Saturday. When you ask them if you're invited, they say, 'You?! I don't think so.' "; Galen & Underwood, 1997, p. 600); nonverbal social exclusion ("When mad at a person, ignores them or stops talking to them"; Crick & Grotpeter, 1995, p. 713; or "Four girls in your grade are talking about a movie they have just seen when you walk up to the group. The group sees you, stops talking, and turns away from you with their noses turned upward"; Galen & Underwood, 1997, p. 600). Indirect social aggression includes the same behavior types, but behaviors executed in a more covert, behind-the-back form: relationship manipulation (harming a person by secretly convincing someone else not to be his or her friend); spreading rumors (spreading hurtful information about someone discreetly, perhaps under the guise of helping that person or the group); verbal social exclusion (surreptitiously telling friends not to talk to a particular person just before he or she attempts to join the lunch table); and nonverbal social exclusion (exchanging glances with a friend behind someone else's back to communicate disdain and plans to exclude that person). Here, note that it is the more overt forms of social aggression that have been investigated thus far, rather than the truly indirect forms of this behavior.

As shown in Figure 2.1, social aggression does not include any type of aggression that inflicts only physical harm or property damage on others. Social aggression also does not include forms of teasing or name-calling that seem not to be explicitly intended to harm friendships or social standing.

Social aggression specifically does include nonverbal efforts at social exclusion. Our research group is not the first to claim that nonverbal behaviors can convey social exclusion. Olweus (1996) wrote, "negative actions can be carried out by physical contact, by words, or in other ways, such as making faces and nasty gestures or by intentional exclusion from a group" (p. 16).

We believe that the bulk of the empirical evidence suggests that specific types of nonverbal behaviors belong in any category proposed to describe aggression among girls. As stated earlier, we have found that vignette measures of social aggression including nonverbal social aggression show high internal consistency (Galen & Underwood, 1997), and seventh and eighth graders report that nonverbal forms of social aggression are experienced most frequently of all types of relationship manipulation (Paquette & Underwood, 1999). In a fascinating, more qualitative study in which groups of high school girls were asked to describe harmful peer behaviors, they described a number of nonverbal forms of social aggression (e.g., "they give you deaths," meaning threatening stares; Owens, Shute, & Slee, 2000a, p. 77). Finally, research suggests that experiencing peer victimization via disdainful facial expressions and gestures uniquely predicts depression and anxiety for adolescents, even above and beyond other forms of social aggression (Galen & Luthar, 2000). In this study, children provided self-reports of specific types of peer victimization, and being the victim of nasty glares and nonverbal social exclusion predicted variance in depression and anxiety, even beyond that predicted by verbal relational aggression behaviors (being the target of rumors or relationship manipulation).

Recent popular accounts based more on anecdotal evidence confirm that nonverbal social exclusion belongs in the category of social aggression. After interviewing hundreds of girls about "alternative aggressions," Simmons (2002) proposed that "mean looks and the silent treatment are the ultimate undercover aggression" (p. 47) and "there is no gesture more devastating than the back turning away" (p. 3). (Let me to take this opportunity to recommend Simmons's book *Odd Girl Out*, an extremely thoughtful account of social aggression among girls that suggests fascinating hypotheses for empirical research.) In another recent popular book by the author of a curriculum called empower to reduce aggression among youth, Wiseman (2002) repeatedly describes girls being crushed by friends suddenly falling silent, glaring, rolling eyes, or turning away. Thus, evidence from a wide variety of sources suggests that nonverbal forms of social aggression are important to examine.

As another point of clarification, although each of these terms has been proposed to describe forms of aggression that may be more common among girls than physical fighting, it is not at all clear that only girls engage in these behaviors, or even that girls engage in them more than boys do. As we discuss in Chapters 5–7 on social aggression in preschool, middle childhood, and adolescence, the evidence for gender differences is quite inconsistent (see Underwood et al., 2001b). Therefore, throughout this book, although our discussion will focus primarily on girls and on social aggression, we refrain from calling these behaviors "female aggression" or "girl aggression."

As important as definitions are, it seems that even if we had the perfect construct, the perfect definition of which behaviors do and do not belong in a subtype to describe aggression in girls, our task will have only begun. Even if we knew for sure that girls engage in social aggression much more than boys do, that would be only a partial clue to the much more interesting question of how and why these behaviors develop and where they lead. It is a well-worn maxim of science that careful description precedes explanation. Now that we have discussed the "what" of social aggression, how about the "why"? If it is true that girls engage in social aggression more than physical aggression and maybe even more than boys do, then why? Answers to this question may be intimately intertwined with both obvious and subtle qualities of girls' and boys' peer groups.

& Chapter 3

Gender and Peer Relations
Separate Worlds?

Who do you like to play with most at school?
　　Oh, girls. They like to play nice things, like Barbie Princesses and Mystical Unicorns. Boys play mean things, like Power Rangers and Bad Guys.
Are there ever times when you like to play with boys?
　　Yes. We play house. I like to play house with Chase.
　　　　　　　　—5-YEAR-OLD LOUISA, CONVERSING WITH HER PSYCHOLOGIST MOTHER

[W]hen boys and girls are engaged in social play, they congregate primarily with others of their own sex during the preschool and middle childhood years, and [those] different childhood "cultures" prevail in these gender-segregated playgroups.
　　　　　　　　　　　　　　　　—MACCOBY (1998, p. 1)

A more complex understanding of the dynamics of gender, of tensions and contradictions, and of the hopeful moments that lie within present arrangements, can broaden our sense of the possible.
　　　　　　　　　　　　　　　　—THORNE (1993, p. 173)

In beginning to unravel the possible reasons why girls may engage in social aggression, scholars have relied heavily on theories of gender differences in children's peer groups. These theories seem compelling as tools for understanding social aggression because this construct was proposed to capture more subtle forms of aggression that might be more characteristic of girls and a good proportion of the evidence so far suggests that girls may be more socially or relationally aggressive (see Crick et al., 1999, for a review).

　　Notice, however, that the argument "girls are more socially aggressive" has embedded within it at least two different claims, one much stronger than the other. The less controversial claim is that girls are

more socially aggressive than they are physically aggressive. This assertion is almost certainly true, because girls engage in low rates of physical aggression at most points during the lifespan (Coie & Dodge, 1998).
The second possible meaning of the statement "girls are more socially
aggressive" is that girls engage in social aggression more than boys do.
The evidence for this stronger claim is more mixed, as we will discuss
in Chapters 4–7.

Implicit in both claims about how girls may be more socially aggressive is the assumption that girls engage in social aggression because
they are girls, as a natural result of distinctive characteristics of girls'
peer groups. This assumption may be dangerous for several reasons.
First, blithely assuming that girls engage in social aggression because
they are girls is global and imprecise in the manner of most gender stereotypes about behavior and emotion (Brody, 1997), and this assumption does not challenge us to test specific questions about the interactions between individual differences and social contexts. Second,
accepting that girls engage in social aggression because they are girls
somehow tempts us to assume that these behaviors are natural and
right. Some are willing to argue that "boys will be boys," that physical
aggression among males is inevitable and not worth trying to prevent
or reduce. It would be a shame if concluding that "girls will be girls"
leads researchers, educators, and parents to minimize the importance
of social aggression in similar ways. Third and finally, when we assume
that girls engage in social aggression because they are girls, we blind
ourselves to the very real possibility that many boys also engage in and
are victimized by social aggression. For all of these reasons, it is critically important to examine carefully the evidence for gender differences in children's peer groups and how these may relate to social aggression among girls and boys.

Qualities of girls' and boys' peer groups have been studied from at
least two perspectives (see Underwood, in press, for a similar discussion). One group of scholars primarily interested in gender has used
both quantitative and qualitative methods to observe children in a variety of social settings, documented the robust phenomenon of gender
segregation, and identified differences in how girls' and boys' groups
behave. Some of these theorists have concluded that differences between girls' and boys' groups are so strong and significant that the genders grow up in separate peer cultures, at least from preschool through
middle childhood (for clear and compelling accounts of this perspective, referred to hereafter as "Two Cultures Theory," see Maccoby,
1990, 1998; Thorne, 1986; Thorne & Luria, 1986). The other group of
researchers interested primarily in children's peer relations has used
mostly quantitative methods to assess children's friendships, social net-

works, social status, and long-term negative outcomes associated with childhood peer problems. Peer relations researchers seek to understand the forms and functions of the peer group. Such researchers have less frequently focused on gender and seem to find more modest gender differences.

This chapter reviews Two Cultures Theory and its supporting evidence, then discusses what this provocative conceptual approach suggests for how and why girls engage in more social aggression than physical aggression, and possibly engage in more social aggression than boys do. Then, I contrast the claims of Two Cultures Theory with evidence from research on children's peer relationships. (Here it should be noted that to distinguish between these two approaches and groups of researchers is at least in part contrived, but—as I argue below—the aims and findings of these groups seem different enough to merit discussion.) I then consider why researchers using these approaches might sometimes reach different conclusions and how discrepant findings might be reconciled. Last, I propose how future research could even more carefully test the claims of Two Cultures Theory with respect to social aggression.

TWO CULTURES THEORY

Two Cultures Theory emerged in the 1980s on the basis of research on children's discourse (Maltz & Borker, 1982), ethnographies of children on elementary school playgrounds (e.g., Thorne, 1986; Thorne & Luria, 1986), and developmental psychologists' observations of children's playmate choices in the lab and at schools (Maccoby & Jacklin, 1987). The basic tenet of Two Cultures Theory is that "the distinctive play styles of the two sexes manifest themselves in distinctive cultures that develop within boys' and girls' groups as the children grow older" (Maccoby, 1998, p. 78). Space constraints here prevent a thorough, detailed exposition of such a comprehensive conceptual framework; this summary relies heavily on the clear and authoritative review provided by Maccoby (1998). In Chapters 5–7, I focus more precisely on how girls' peer groups function during preschool, middle childhood, and adolescence, and how social aggression may develop in these groups. The following few paragraphs will provide an overview of how Two Cultures theorists characterize the world of girls.

Two Cultures Theory logically begins with the striking phenomenon of gender segregation in children's peer groups. Both boys and girls strongly prefer to interact with same-gender partners beginning in the third year of life (Serbin, Moller, Gulko, Powlishta, & Colbourne,

1994) and continuing during the elementary school years through preadolescence (Gottman & Mettetal, 1986; Maccoby & Jacklin, 1987). Boys and girls may interact primarily in same-gender groups because same-gender peers are more compatible in their play styles (Serbin et al., 1994) and ways of regulating emotions (Fabes, 1994), because children are rewarded more by peers and teachers for same-gender interaction (Fagot, 1994), and because children prefer other peers "like me" (C. L. Martin, 1994). Gender segregation appears across cultures (Whiting & Edwards, 1988). The fact that gender segregation is such a widely observed, long-lasting phenomenon allows for the possibility that girls' and boys' groups not only operate separately, they somehow function differently.

According to Two Cultures Theory, girls' and boys' peer groups differ on several important dimensions: play styles and activity preferences; discourse; friendships; and group size, strength, and power (Maccoby, 1998). Because girls are the focus here, this summary highlights that which is proposed to be distinctive about girls' peer culture.

Two Cultures Theory posits that girls' social encounters emphasize relationships rather than structured games or activities. One observational study of children during free play showed that girls are more likely than boys to do cooperative activities that involve more turn taking and reciprocity; 21% of girls' games involve turn taking as compared to less than 1% of boys' games (Crombie & Desjardins, 1993). Girls less frequently play organized sports (Lever, 1976) and are much less likely to engage in direct competition when playing games than are boys (less than 1% of the time as compared to 50% of the time for boys; Crombie & Desjardins, 1993). Girls' interactions involve less rough-and-tumble play than those of boys do (Coie & Dodge, 1998; Smith & Boulton, 1990). For girls, social dominance hierarchies are less clearly defined than for boys' groups (Charlesworth & Dzur, 1987). Although most girls typically refrain from particular activities that are stereotypically male (competitive games, rough-and-tumble play), girls are more likely to engage in activities that are stereotypically masculine than boys are to engage in stereotypically feminine pursuits (Bussey & Bandura, 1992).

In social conversations with peers, boys' and girls' language and manner of speaking appear to be similar in many ways, although there are some intriguing differences (Maccoby, 1998). Girls are more likely to take turns and to refer to what another has said than are boys (see Maltz & Borker, 1982, for a review). Girls are more likely than boys to try to avoid conflicts by cooperating with others' wishes; when conflicts do occur, girls are more likely than boys to express anger covertly, compromise, and try to clarify the other person's desires (P. M. Miller,

Danaher, & Forbes, 1986). Girls generally say they prefer not to yell but to assert their goals more politely (Crick & Ladd, 1990). Whereas boys often take great glee in encouraging each other to take risks and engaging in risqué talk about sex, girls are more likely to enjoy discussing close relationships and themes of great romance (Thorne & Luria, 1986).

Two Cultures Theory posits that girls' friendships are more intense and intimate than are those of boys (Maccoby, 1998). Girls are characterized as self-disclosing more, touching each other more, and being more concerned about who is best friends with whom. Girls' friendships are described as more closed and exclusive than boys' friendships are (for reviews, see Daniels-Bierness, 1989; Hallinan, 1980).

Two Cultures Theory posits that perhaps because girls are so focused on dyadic relationships, they tend to play in smaller groups and have smaller social networks than do boys. One study with 4- and 6-year-olds observed children in laboratory play groups in which six children of the same gender had the opportunity to play in a confined area with dolls and balls (Benenson, Apostoleris, & Parnass, 1997). The results showed that boys and girls engaged in equal amounts of dyadic play, but girls' episodes were longer and boys engaged in shorter, more frequent episodes of dyadic engagement. Six-year-old boys engaged in more group play then did 6-year-old girls. In another study, 4- and 6-year-old children were given a sociometric measure in which they were asked to rate each classmate for whether he or she liked to play with the person "(1) a little bit, (2) a medium amount, or (3) a lot" (Benenson, 1994, p. 480). Children rated highly were considered to belong to a particular child's social network. The results of the study showed that girls' social networks decreased in size from age 4 to age 6, whereas boys' networks remained the same size. Ethnographic research with older elementary school children also suggests that boys generally tend to interact in larger social groups than girls do (Thorne & Luria, 1986).

Girls' peer groups may be more subject to outside influence than boys' groups, both by members and activities of the other gender and by adults' instructions. Even though girls and boys express similarly strong preferences for same-gender peers (Serbin, Powlishta, & Gulko, 1993), girls' groups are less likely to exclude boys than vice versa. Girls are less inclined to chastise each other for engaging in masculine activities, whereas boys mercilessly tease other boys who do anything bordering on feminine (Feiring & Lewis, 1987).

Girls' groups are more open to the input of adults than are boys' groups (Maccoby, 1998). Girls play closer to teachers than do boys, and are more responsive to teachers' directives. Girls' groups engage in less furtive rule-breaking than boys' groups do (Thorne & Luria, 1986).

In light of the foregoing outline of the Two Cultures view on girls' peer groups, it is easy to see why this theory has been attractive as an explanation for why girls might engage in social aggression. Two Cultures Theory certainly fits with the hypothesis that girls engage in social aggression more often than physical aggression. If girls' groups are characterized by more mitigation of conflicts and less rough-and-tumble play, then it seems sensible that physical aggression would be all the more unwelcome and girls might instead express anger in more subtle ways. Furthermore, if girls are playing in groups closer to adult supervision and are more sensitive to adult reactions to their behavior, it only stands to reason that they might resort to less obvious means of harming one another, behaviors less likely to be punished than physical aggression.

Two Cultures Theory also offers other intuitively appealing explanations for why girls may engage in social aggression more than boys do. Given that girls are portrayed as valuing close relationships more than status and dominance, it seems logical that a powerful way for girls to hurt one another may be to harm each other's friendships. If girls' social encounters indeed focus more on relationships than on sports and activities, then no wonder girls care so deeply about having friends as a way of fitting in—just joining in an organized game may well not be an option. If girls' dominance hierarchies are less well defined than those of boys (Charlesworth & Dzur, 1987), it follows that girls may need to jockey for social position more frequently, to engage in relationship manipulation as a way of securing their own status. If girls' friendships are more intimate and involve more self-disclosure than boys' friendships, it is easy to imagine why girls might be more vulnerable to gossip and to relationship manipulation. If girls are interacting in smaller groups and if dyads are interlocking and best friendships shifting often, then girls may be well justified in worrying about fitting in and may even be tempted to exclude others as a way of confirming their own status.

Indeed, researchers studying the various subtypes proposed to describe aggression among girls have been quick to invoke elements of Two Cultures Theory as possible explanations for why girls engage in indirect/relational/social aggression. As early as 1969, Feshbach (p. 256) interpreted her results showing that pairs of first-grade girls were initially more unkind to a newcomer than were boys by writing, "The finding that girls displayed more of these behaviors is consistent with the general empirical finding that girls are more socially oriented than boys (Maccoby, 1966)." In arguing for why girls might engage in more relational aggression than do boys, Crick and Grotpeter (1995, p. 710) stated, "In contrast to boys, girls are more likely to focus on relational issues during social interaction (e.g., establishing close, intimate connections with others) (see Block, 1983, for a review)."

These broad, sweeping claims about girls' peer relationships demand careful consideration of evidence from research conducted by investigators primarily interested in peer relationships. Two Cultures theorists consistently emphasize the importance of children's peer groups for the development of gender differences in social interaction. Maccoby (1990) writes, "I would place most of the emphasis on the peer group as the setting in which children first discover the compatibility of same-sex others, in which boys first discover the requirements of maintaining status in the male hierarchy, and in which the gender of one's partners becomes supremely important" (p. 519). If peer groups really are the context in which gender differences emerge and are most salient, then it stands to reason that the results from studies of children's peer relations would converge with some of the most important claims of Two Cultures Theory. To what extent has this been true?

TWO CULTURES THEORY AND RESEARCH ON PEER RELATIONS

Whereas gender scholars and Two Cultures theorists set out to test questions related to gender, peer relations researchers have often begun with different goals and seem to have been disinclined to focus on gender, at least initially (see Underwood, in press). Many of the early, groundbreaking studies of children's peer relations examined the behavior correlates of peer acceptance and were conducted with samples of boys only (e.g., Coie & Kupersmidt, 1983; Dodge, 1983; Putallaz, 1983). Other even earlier studies included girls but either did not examine gender differences (Gottman, Gonso, & Rasmussen, 1975; Hartup, Glazer, & Charlesworth, 1967) or examined but did not find gender differences (Putallaz & Gottman, 1981).

Although reasons for studying boys only or not examining gender differences were often left unstated, several explanations seem likely. First, the explosion of interest in children's peer relations during the 1970s and 1980s was at least in part fueled by evidence that peer problems in childhood predict later negative outcomes, particularly delinquency and antisocial behavior (Kohlberg, LaCrosse, & Ricks, 1972). These antisocial outcomes initially linked to peer problems were those that had higher base rates in males (Coie & Dodge, 1998), so perhaps understanding boys' childhood peer relations seemed more urgent. Second, this focus on peer rejection naturally led to interest in one of its strongest correlates, physical aggression (Coie & Kupersmidt, 1983), a behavior more frequent among boys. Another more pragmatic reason for the early focus on boys may have been limited resources; the pioneering studies in this field involved observational methods and fine-grained coding, and doubling the size of the sample by including girls may have not been possible. Conceptual frameworks for peer relations quickly become so complex that sophisticated designs are required to answer pressing questions for one gender, and sometimes to study both is not a practical option (Coie et al., 1999). Last, it may also be the case that the tendency of peer relations researchers to study boys only or at least boys first was part of a larger trend among developmental psychologists to dismiss the importance of gender or to consider girls' relationships "hard to trace, a territory where violence is rare and relationships remain safe" (Gilligan, 1982, p. 62).

Historical precedents aside, what continues to be striking is the current reluctance of many peer relations researchers to consider gender seriously. Progress is apparent in that most investigators have begun to include girls in their samples, but evidence for gender differences seems mixed and theories of gender development, including Two Cultures Theory, rarely guide the design of research on children's peer groups. On the basis of almost three decades of large-scale systematic studies of children's peer relations, recent literature reviews still assert that the role of gender is unclear and that future research is needed (e.g., Newcomb & Bagwell, 1995; Newcomb, Bukowski, & Patee, 1993). In a recent *Handbook of Child Psychology* chapter on peer relations, gender is discussed in a single paragraph near the end of the large-scale review, which notes that, "not much is known about the possibility that the peer culture can play different functions for boys and girls" (Rubin, Bukowski, & Parker, 1998, p. 682).

Clearly, this conclusion stands in stark contrast to the claims of Two Cultures theorists about gender differences in boys' and girls' peer groups. To more closely examine how the claims of Two Cultures Theory fit with recent research on children's peer relations, the following discussion will consider the evidence for gender differences in friendships and social networks.

Peer Relations Evidence for Gender Differences in Children's Friendships

In contrast to the Two Cultures assertion that girls are more concerned with close relationships than boys are and that girls' friendships are more intimate and exclusive than are those of boys, peer relations research suggests that gender differences may be more subtle and complicated. Gender differences in activity preferences may be more apparent for younger children than for older ones. A time-sampling study of 2- and 4-year-olds found that girls spent more time socializing and boys spent more time playing video games (Huston, Wright, Marquis, & Green, 1999). Another time-sampling study with older children, fifth through eighth graders, found that girls and boys did not differ in the time reported interacting with same-gender peers but girls reported thinking more about same-gender companions than did boys (Richards, Crowe, Larson, & Swarr, 1998). Whereas Two Cultures Theory implies that girls participate mostly in communal, relationship-focused activities and boys participate more in structured, agentic activities, a recent study of fifth and sixth graders showed considerable overlap between activities reported by boys and girls (Zarbatany, McDougall, & Hymel, 2000).

Peer relations researchers have been more reluctant than Two Cultures theorists to claim that girls' and boys' friendships differ in dramatic ways (Berndt, 1982), and recent evidence suggests that this caution may be warranted. Peer relations research does not support the Two Cultures claim that girls have fewer friends than boys do. When children are asked to name classmates as friends, there are typically no gender differences in the number of friends named (Berndt, 1982; A. J. Rose & Asher, 1999).

Whether gender differences in friendships are apparent seems to depend in part on the research method used. When children respond to questionnaires, interviews, or vignettes about hypothetical friends or ideas about friendships in general, gender differences are larger than when children are asked to describe particular friendships. When asked to describe friends in the abstract, girls are more likely than boys to focus on intimate interactions, self-disclosure, and mutual support (Blyth & Foster-Clark, 1987; see Buhrmester & Prager, 1995, for a review). Girls report worrying more about friends' loyalty and betrayal than boys do (Berndt, 1981). In response to hypothetical vignettes about friendship conflicts, girls more strongly advocate relationship-preserving goals than do boys, and boys more strongly endorse instrumental and revenge goals than do girls (A. J. Rose & Asher, 1999).

However, in studies where preadolescents are asked to describe intimate self-disclosure and close knowledge of a particular best friend, gender differences are less consistent. Some studies find no gender differences (e.g., Sharabany, Gershoni, & Hofman, 1981); Zarbatany and colleagues (2000) found gender differences for friendship intimacy for sixth but not for fifth graders. However, another investigation with a large sample of third through sixth graders found that girls reported more intimate exchange in their best friendships than did boys (Parker & Asher, 1993).

Another explanation for seemingly inconsistent findings for gender differences in intimacy may be that these are confounded with social context. Rather than girls' friendships being consistently more intimate, maybe girls spend more time engaged in activities in which intimacy is more likely, for example, conversing in small groups. Therefore, questionnaire measures of overall intimacy across contexts yield gender differences more often than do observational studies of girls and boys in the same social setting.

When girls and boys are observed in the same social contexts, many of the gender differences in children's discourse are less dramatic and girls' and boys' conversations appear more similar than different (Leaper, 1994; Leaper, Tenenbaum, & Schaffer, 1999). In an observational study of triads of third, fourth, and fifth graders interacting, girls' triads engaged in more intimacy and information exchange than did boys' triads (Lansford & Parker, 1999). However, there were not gender differences for many other variables related to the claims of Two Cultures Theory: individual versus collective orientation, exuberance, hierarchical structures and leadership imbalance, responsiveness, and contention and conflict. In one of the few peer relations studies specifically designed to test Two Cultures Theory, the intimacy of both boys' and girls' friendships was related to participating more in communal activities, such as telling secrets and going to restaurants with friends (Zarbatany et al., 2000). These findings suggest that gender differences in friendships may be closely tied to activity preferences and time spent in particular social contexts.

Whereas Two Cultures theorists have proposed that girls' friendships are more exclusive than are those of boys (see Daniels-Bierness, 1989, and Maccoby, 1998, for reviews of the evidence for this position), recent peer relations research casts doubt on this assertion. Girls do not prefer dyadic to triadic interaction more than boys do (Lansford & Parker, 1999). Although some of the earliest studies of gender differences in indirect aggression found that girls were less welcoming to newcomers than were boys (Feshbach, 1969; Feshbach & Sones, 1971), recent studies have not replicated these findings. In a laboratory study of triads of 7- to 9-year-olds in which a "guest" participant attempted to join two "hosts" of either the same or the other gender, host girls were actually more welcoming to guests than were host boys, and girls' dyads were easier to join than were boys' dyads (Borja-Alvarez et al., 1991). In another study with 10- to 12-year-olds, dyads of host friends were asked to choose between including a third child or winning a larger prize (Zarbatany, Van Brunschot, Meadows,

& Pepper, 1996); girls were more likely to choose to admit the guest than were boys.

Although this brief discussion of gender differences in friendships is by no means a comprehensive review, it seems that peer relations research does not unequivocally support the Two Cultures assertion that girls' friendships are more intimate and exclusive than boys' friendships are. Overall, gender differences in friendship variables are more dramatic for questionnaire studies that assess overall intimacy across settings, and they are less apparent in observational investigations of girls and boys in the same social contexts. The questionnaire studies may find that girls report more overall intimacy with close friends than boys do because girls are more likely to seek out social situations that foster intimate exchange, such as small-group interactions. However, studies of girls and boys interacting with friends in the same social context suggest that boys may also have the capacity for intimate exchange and exclusiveness when they find themselves in settings that elicit these behaviors.

Peer Relations Evidence for Gender Differences in Children's Social Networks

Two Cultures Theory proposes that girls' and boys' social networks differ in size, structure, and strength of influence (see Maccoby, 1998, for a summary of this perspective). Once again, peer relations research does not provide strong support for these claims.

Two Cultures Theory describes girls' social networks as smaller and more horizontal in structure, whereas boys' networks are described as larger and more hierarchical (Daniels-Bierness, 1989; Maccoby, 1998). Here again, at least for children beyond the preschool years, contemporary peer relations research does not confirm these predictions. Cairns and Cairns (1994) refined elegant social cognitive mapping procedures to measure social networks in which many members of the peer group report who hangs around together, and the strength of the associations is mapped to assess children's social networks. These procedures take advantage of multiple informants and avoid many of the biases of self-reports. Having used these procedures now for years with large samples of school-aged children and adolescents, Cairns and Cairns repeatedly found that boys' and girls' social networks do not differ in size. In another study using similar methods to identify peer cliques for a large sample of preadolescents, there were no gender differences in the size of social networks, and girls and boys were equally likely to be central members of their respective groups (Bagwell, Coie, Terry, & Lochman, 2000).

Whereas Two Cultures Theory proposes that boys' social networks are more influential than girls' groups in encouraging members to take risks and engage in deviant behaviors (Thorne & Luria, 1986), contemporary studies of peer group influence do not yield strong gender differences in the strength of peer group socialization. In several studies, gender accounted for little to none of the variance in peer group influence on several important outcomes: adjustment to junior high school (Berndt, Hawkins, & Jiao, 1999), school engagement (Sage & Kindermann, 1999), cigarette smoking (J. S. Rose, Chassin, Presson, & Sherman, 1999), and alcohol consumption (Pilgrim, Luo, & Urberg, 1999; Schulenberg et al., 1999). However, it is probably premature to conclude that gender is unrelated to peer group influence, because so few studies have considered both the gender of the child being socialized and the gender of the person or group doing the socialization (Hartup, 1999). At present, evidence does not warrant concluding that boys' peer groups exert more influence on their members to engage in deviant behaviors than do girls' groups.

Overall, peer relations research to date does not offer resounding support for the claims of Two Cultures Theory, at least not for those tenets related to friendships and social networks. Whereas some describe the differences between girls' and boys' friendships as to be "so sweeping as to be almost irreconcilable" (as noted by Lansford & Parker, 1999, p. 90), peer relations evidence suggests that gender differences are, at the very least, more modest.

RECONCILING DISCREPANT FINDINGS

If our goal is to understand how and why girls engage in social aggression, we must try somehow to make sense of the discrepant findings of gender scholars and peer relations researchers. These sets of findings have different implications for the development of social aggression in girls. Two Cultures Theory suggests compelling arguments for why girls may engage in social aggression much more than boys do, and implies that social aggression may only be frequent and hurtful among girls. However, peer relations research suggests a different possibility: Peer cultures are not so different after all, and both boys and girls may engage in and be victimized by social aggression. How it is possible that research from these two different perspectives points to at least somewhat different conclusions, and how can these conflicting bodies of evidence best guide our efforts to understand social aggression?

One likely reason that gender scholars and peer relations researchers reach somewhat different conclusions is that they have preferred to use different methods, particularly when studying older children. The claims of Two Cultures Theory for middle childhood and beyond, perhaps the age range most relevant for understanding social aggression, are based in large part on ethnographies (e.g., Thorne & Luria, 1986). Ethnographies provide rich descriptions and generate fascinating hypotheses, but they are less helpful for investigating specific claims about the size, composition, and developmental functions of children's groups. Ethnographies also naturally lead investigators to observe the highest-profile, most visible children, who may not be representative of the larger group (Thorne, 1993).

Even though Two Cultures scholars and peer relations researchers have both used observational methods to good effect, they may find different results because they tend to observe in different contexts. Ethnographers generally prefer to observe children in naturalistic settings, often during free play when children are far from adult supervision and have more choice of activities (Thorne & Luria, 1986). Peer relations researchers are more likely than ethnographers to observe children's social interactions in controlled laboratory settings (Coie & Kupersmidt, 1983), or in classrooms where adults are present (Gottman et al., 1975). Thorne (1986) has cogently suggested that other-gender interactions among children are more frequent and comfortable when they are involved in a fascinating activity, when they need not choose who is involved in the group, when the group has been formed on the basis of something other than gender, and when the setting is more private. Laboratory playrooms, classrooms, and playgrounds differ enormously on most of these dimensions, and it seems likely that these contextual factors influence social interactions within and across children's gender groups.

Another likely explanation for why gender and peer relations researchers may come to somewhat different conclusions is that, although they sometimes make use of similar methods and sometimes not, their choices of methods may be confounded with the age groups they study. In marshalling the evidence for Two Cultures Theory, scholars most often cite laboratory studies with preschool and early school-age children (see Maccoby, 1998, for examples) and ethnographic studies of children in the later elementary (Thorne & Luria, 1986) and middle school years (Eder, Evans, & Parker, 1995). Many peer relations researchers prefer sociometric and questionnaire methods, especially with older children. When they do observational studies, these typically involve quantitative, microanalytic coding systems with larger samples of children and are conducted in controlled laboratory settings (e.g., Coie, Dodge, Terry, & Wright, 1991; Coie & Kupersmidt, 1983), or in classrooms with younger samples (e.g., Vaughn, Colvin, Azria, Caya, &

Krzysik, 2001). Given that gender and peer relations scholars sometimes use different methods with different age groups, it is hardly surprising that their findings do not always converge.

Perhaps the most important reason why gender and peer relations
researchers might find different results is that their research has sought
to answer different questions. Gender scholars design their research
with gender as a central focus, and their hypotheses and research designs are driven by theories about the development of gender. This often leads them to make methodological choices so that the effects of
gender are most likely to be detected, for example, making sure to observe children in contexts that are meaningful for both boys and girls
(see Thorne & Luria, 1986, for an interesting discussion of the
pragmatics of gaining access to girls' groups and to boys' groups). For
example, ethnographers tend to observe closely conversations among
small groups (e.g., Thorne & Luria, 1986), a setting in which intimate
exchange is likely (Zarbatany et al., 2000), particularly for girls. Ethnographers also tend to watch children on playgrounds, which allows them
to observe the larger, game-focused interactions of boys. On the other
hand, peer relations researchers tend to use more microanalytic systems to code overt behavior, either from afar or from videotape, therefore making it less likely that they could detect gender differences in intimate exchanges in small groups. Two Cultures Theory suggests that
specific settings may be important for each gender, perhaps dyadic
conversations for girls and group games for boys, and peer relations researchers might make an effort to observe both genders in both types
of settings to sort out the effects of gender and social context. However, methodological choices driven too strongly by Two Cultures Theory may make it less likely that the theory will fail to be supported: "the
wheels of description and analysis slide into the contrastive themes and
move right along" (Thorne, 1993, p. 96).

Peer relations researchers focus primarily on carefully measuring
and understanding children's social behavior, friendships, social networks, and social status. Peer relations researchers quite naturally prefer questionnaires that can be administered easily to larger numbers, or
observation in more controlled settings such as laboratories or classrooms. Their hypotheses are rarely guided by theories about gender;
these theories are usually invoked only briefly in discussion sections,
and only if gender differences reveal themselves. As a result, peer relations research is not always designed to test fairly the effects of gender,
and gender differences that appear are not integrated into the major
conceptual frameworks that drive this research area. Fair tests of the
role of gender and gender differences might involve hypotheses guided
by Two World Theory or other gender theories, methods that assess

children's social behaviors in contexts that are meaningful for girls and boys, analyses that carefully examine not only gender differences in mean scores but also gender differences in the relations among variables, and interpretations of findings with reference to gender theories.

DANGERS OF ACCEPTING TWO
CULTURES THEORY WHOLESALE

Although it is easy to understand possible reasons why gender and peer relations researchers arrive at sometimes different conclusions, we are still left with discrepant claims that can be difficult to integrate. On the one hand, Two Cultures Theory offers intuitively clear and compelling explanations for why girls engage in social aggression, explanations that match our cultural stereotypes about boys and girls and logically lead to clear and direct hypotheses. On the other hand, we have a body of empirical evidence from peer relations research that is less clear about gender differences overall, rather confusing in its array of nonreplicated findings, yet suggesting that gender differences in social aggression may be less dramatic.

To make matters even more complicated it is possible that, even in the peer relations literature, gender differences may have been exaggerated due to the possibility of Type I error. Type I error occurs when the null hypothesis, in this case not finding gender differences, is erroneously rejected on the basis of chance findings (which, following the logic of statistics, will occur approximately 5% of the time). The likelihood of Type I error may be increasing in recent times as more investigators study boys and girls and routinely test for gender differences. If only those differences that achieve significance make it to publication and many more null findings remain in file drawers, what we will end up with is a distorted, exaggerated picture of gender differences.

Of these two sets of findings, the Two Cultures perspective offers the more easily understandable, exciting story. Given that our focus here is girls and that this theory highlights what is distinctive about a group that has long been ignored in research on aggression, it is sorely tempting to embrace Two Cultures Theory wholeheartedly. Two Cultures Theory fits many women's experiences of their own childhoods and confirms deeply held cultural beliefs about the nature of girls and boys. Some of these schemas about gender become lenses through which we view the world (Bem, 1993), and researchers seeking to understand children's peer groups are not exempt from "stereotypes and ideologies that should be queried rather than built upon and perpetu-

ated as social fact" (Thorne, 1993, p. 91). Indeed, recent theory and research suggest that prematurely adopting a strong Two Cultures view
may be dangerous.

Interestingly, some of the most thoughtful criticism of Two Cultures Theory has come from one of its earliest advocates. On the basis
of her more recent ethnographic research and her readings of the evidence from peer relations studies, Thorne (1993) has questioned some
of the central principles of Two Cultures Theory. First, Two Cultures
Theory fails to consider that the importance of gender fluctuates in
children's ongoing social interactions; some other-gender interactions
are relaxed and comfortable, and some children seem to defy the
norms of their gender cultures with impunity. Second, Two Cultures
Theory does not account for the variation within gender groups and instead highlights group differences "in static and exaggerated dualities"
(p. 91). Third, Two Cultures Theory characterizes the two genders as
separate and different, rather than focusing on the effects of gender in
particular social contexts. Fourth, perhaps because Two Cultures Theory has relied heavily on ethnographies especially with older children,
the theory has been based on more observations of dominant, high-
profile children and less on those who are quieter and marginalized.
Thorne refers to this as "Big Man Bias" (p. 98), similar to the bias in an-
thropological research that assumes that characteristics of the strongest, most powerful men represent qualities of men as a group. As a result, Two Cultures Theory has rarely acknowledged that children can
be masculine and feminine in a variety of ways. Last, Thorne accurately
points out that Two Cultures Theory has been developed on the basis
of research done almost entirely with middle- to upper-class white children. We know little about whether separate gender cultures exist in
other socioeconomic or ethnic groups.

Adopting Two Cultures Theory wholesale for understanding social
aggression could be dangerous in similar ways. Researchers might be
tempted to believe that social aggression is characteristic of only girls
and to expect dramatic, consistent gender differences instead of variation within gender groups. Investigators might be tempted to view social aggression as more of a trait, a personal quality that is invariant
across settings, rather than behaviors that are more or less likely in particular social contexts. Researchers might be enticed to use methods
that best assess only the most visible or high-profile children, leading to
a "Big Girl Bias" in research on social aggression. If we enter our research efforts believing that girls engage in social aggression because
they are girls, we may not be as energetic in studying this phenomenon
in different ethnic or socioeconomic groups.

Thorne's (1993) interpretation of more recent evidence has led her to extreme disenchantment with Two Cultures Theory, which she refers to as "a conceptual dead end" (p. 91). She suggests that the theory has outlived its helpfulness and that it is time "to move our research wagons out of the dualistic rut" (p. 109) by focusing on understanding how gender interacts with individual differences in particular social contexts.

However, to dismiss Two Cultures Theory and all of its compelling ideas and evidence seems to me premature. Many of its fascinating claims have yet to be put to the most rigorous empirical tests, and many peer relations researchers have been slow to join the effort to understand gender and its effects on the peer culture. Also, although gender differences in observable behavior or quantifiable dimensions of the peer group may not always be dramatic, even small or subtle differences may matter a great deal. Some of these subtle differences may bear less on behavior and more on children's self-conceptions. Cross and Madson (1997) have argued convincingly that males' self-construals are more independent in that they are based on individual qualities and distinguishing the self from others, whereas women's' self-construals are more interdependent, more tied to relationships and to preserving harmony. Even if these gendered self-construals do not manifest themselves in massive behavioral differences in all domains, they may well affect how girls and boys evaluate and experience social aggression.

SOCIAL AGGRESSION AND TWO CULTURES THEORY: TESTABLE QUESTIONS

Rather than abandon Two Cultures Theory altogether, I hope that gender scholars and peer relations researchers will begin to collaborate to test some of its compelling claims, using varied and sophisticated empirical methods. Very few studies to date have benefited from both the guidance of Two Cultures Theory and methods refined by peer relations researchers, but the notable exceptions seem extremely promising.

One recent study examined the claim of Two Cultures Theory that gender differences in friendship intimacy are related to participation in girls' and boys' peer subcultures (Zarbatany et al., 2000). The research assessed two dimensions of peer culture: the gender composition of children's peer networks, and preferences for activities characterized as agentic and communal. Agentic activities were primarily team sports, and communal activities were various types of socializing. If Two Cultures Theory is correct, then girls should rate their friendships as more intimate and intimacy of friendships should be related to engaging in communal activities more than agentic activities.

The results supported some claims of Two Cultures Theory but not others. As noted earlier, although sixth-grade girls described their friendships as more intimate than did sixth-grade boys, the expected gender difference was not found for fifth graders. Also, there was ample overlap in girls' and boys' preferences for agentic and communal activities, more than would be predicted by Two Cultures Theory. As hypothesized, engaging more in communal activities was related to greater friendship intimacy for both girls and boys, but somewhat surprisingly children reported intimacy with friends outside of the expected communal activities. Some agentic contexts seemed to advance both types of goals, especially boys engaging in team sports. Also, the relationships between the peer culture variables and friendship intimacy were stronger for girls than for boys, suggesting that other dimensions may be important for explaining intimacy among young males.

This well-conducted, theoretically driven investigation highlights how Two Cultures Theory and peer relations research might profitably enhance one another. The research was designed to test specific claims of a powerful and compelling theory, and sophisticated quantitative methods were used to measure important variables such as peer networks, activity preferences, and friendship qualities. The questionnaire methods allowed assessment of a large sample, including more- and less-visible children, perhaps avoiding the danger of "Big Girl Bias." The analyses examined not only gender differences in mean scores for variables but also gender differences in the relations among intimacy and activity preferences. Last, Zarbatany and colleagues (2000) interpreted these results with reference to both Two Cultures Theory and peer relations research, providing a model for how integrating these approaches is not only possible but also highly beneficial.

How might researchers investigate the claims of Two Cultures Theory as they relate to the development of social aggression? This effort has already begun in one fairly straightforward way, examining whether there are gender differences. If the claims of Two Cultures Theory hold true, then we expect girls to be more socially or relationally aggressive than boys. As we discuss next in Chapters 4–7, gender differences are neither large nor consistent, and whether they appear depends on the method used and the developmental period studied.

Two Cultures Theory suggests many other testable questions related to social aggression. Do children actually perceive that social aggression primarily harms relationships, and do girls hold this view more strongly than do boys? Is perpetrating social aggression related to children's perceptions that relationships are paramount? Do children more strongly identified with the girls' same-gender group more often engage in and experience social aggression? Does social aggression occur in boys' groups, and is it particularly effective? Do girls' and boys' peer groups sanction and condone socially aggressive behaviors in similar or different ways? Is engaging in social aggression more likely in the context of particular types of communal activity? Do girls feel more hurt by social aggression because it harms that which they are reputed to most value?

Because Two Cultures Theory is such a broad, sweeping conceptual approach, already existing evidence can be consulted to test its claims—that produced by research on peer relations in particular developmental periods. In Chapters 4 through 7, I discuss what research on peer relations, emotion regulation, aggression, and gender suggests for the forms and developmental functions of social aggression during infancy, the preschool years, middle childhood, and adolescence. In reviewing the evidence, it seems important to remain cognizant of our own gendered lenses (Bem, 1993), to at least try to consider carefully the role of gender with fresh eyes.

PART II

DEVELOPMENT

Chapter 4

Girls' Anger in Infancy
Early Lessons That Anger Is Unwelcome

[The results indicate that] socialization of affect expression is occurring during early infancy and that the infants' expressiveness is becoming appropriate according to cultural, gender, and familial demands far before the first birthday.
—MALATESTA AND HAVILAND (1982, p. 991)

Nothing that human infants do during the first year can properly be considered aggressive if we use the term to mean actions directed toward a specific other person that are intended to hurt or frighten.
—MACCOBY (1980, p. 116)

Mothers' reports on the frequency of physical aggression of their 17-month-old children and the age of onset of these behaviors provide evidence that physical aggression by humans can appear before the end of the first year after birth, and that the rate of cumulative onset increases substantially from 12 to 17 months.
—TREMBLAY ET AL. (1999, p. 19)

For the most complete understanding of anger and aggression in girls, it is critically important that we understand the early developmental origins of behaviors such as social aggression. This chapter will explore how girls' expressions of anger and contempt may be shaped by lessons they are taught about how to regulate negative emotions, lessons that start as early as infancy.

HOW EARLY DO CHILDREN SHOW ANGER?

Experts have long disagreed as to when infants begin to express the specific emotion of anger, although most concur that expressions resembling anger can be detected in the first year of life (see Lemerise &

Dodge, 2000; Stenberg & Campos, 1990). How can we know when an infant is angry? Some investigators have observed infants interacting with mothers in seminaturalistic contexts and have carefully examined infants' facial expressions resembling anger, using well-validated coding systems for emotions such as Izard's (1970) MAX (Maximally Discriminative Facial Movement Coding System; see Malatesta, Culver, Tesman, & Shepard, 1989, for an example). Other investigators have similarly coded infants' emotional responses, but in naturalistic settings in which pain and rage might be likely, such as when infants are given inoculations in pediatric offices (Izard, Hembree, & Huebner, 1987).

Other investigators have devised clever laboratory tasks to elicit anger in very young children. Stenberg, Campos, and Emde (1983) provoked 7-month-olds to anger by seating them in high chairs, with either the child's mother or an experimenter sitting 4 feet away. The adult gave the infant a teething biscuit and let the child suck it for 3 seconds. Then, the adult slowly and deliberately grabbed the teething biscuit and took it out of the baby's mouth. This procedure was repeated 10 times with the stranger and 10 times with the familiar adult (unless the child engaged in wrathful wailing, at which time the experiment was stopped). Not surprisingly, the results showed that most 7-month-olds in this situation appeared to be furious; their facial expressions could be coded reliably by adults and did not show features of sadness or of other negative emotions. In a similar study, an arm restraint procedure provoked infants to see whether anger could be reliably coded in 1-, 4-, and 7-month-olds (Stenberg & Campos, 1990). The results showed that it was difficult to detect anger in 1-month-olds, that 4-month-olds' anger could be coded reliably but seemed less socially motivated, and that 7-month-olds' anger was more often directed at social targets. Other clever methods for eliciting anger in young infants have included presenting an attractive toy behind a clear plastic barrier (K. A. Buss & Goldsmith, 1998), and buckling the infant into a tight car seat and taking away an attractive toy (Kochanska, Coy, Tjebkes, & Husarek, 1998).

BEGINNING AUTONOMY AND ANGER

Although we still have much to learn about the development of anger over the first year of life, infants may begin to show more anger around 7–9 months of age due to their increasing abilities to assert their own desires. In the Izard and colleagues (1987) study of infants' responses to shots, pain expressions decreased from 2 to 18 months, but the frequency and intensity of anger increased, especially between 7 and 19 months. Izard et al. suggested that the increase in anger is related to older infants' advanced cognitive abilities allowing them to identify the person who is interfering with them in some way, and to neurological maturation that might allow them to terminate the more automatic pain response and instead express rage.

Another developmental accomplishment may contribute to the increase in infants' anger expression during the first year of life—the onset of independent movement by crawling or walking (Campos, Kermoian, & Zumbahlen, 1992). Babies who can move on their own likely elicit and observe more anger from adults. The onset of locomotion may intensify expressions of anger because as children move they likely incite more anger in their parents because the child appears autonomous. Independent movement prompts infants to have higher aspirations and therefore more chances to feel really frustrated; moreover, infants' movements at times elicit vigorous emotional responses in their parents that infants might model, and movement alters the quality of the attachment relationship (Campos et al., 1992). As compared to parents of children who are not yet moving independently, parents of infants who can crawl describe both themselves and their infants as more angry. Because boys as a group have higher activity levels than do girls (Eaton & Ennis, 1986), perhaps they experience parents' anger more frequently.

GENDER DIFFERENCES IN INFANTS' ANGER EXPRESSIONS

Are there gender differences in infants' expression of anger, and what would it mean if there were? When studying young infants, it is tempting to believe either that gender differences are unlikely or that any gender differences that appear must be biological in origin because the children are too young to have been affected much by socialization. As we shall see, however, parental socialization may begin very early, and it may differ for girls and for boys. To make matters more complicated, even when parents treat girls and boys similarly, girls and boys may respond differently (Brody, 2000).

Overall, the evidence for gender differences in infants' expressions of anger is mixed. Some investigators do not report testing for gender differences (e.g., K. A. Buss & Goldsmith, 1998; Campos et al., 1992), and others do not find them when they do (Kochanska et al., 1998). When gender differences appear, they are slight and sometimes inconsistent across age ranges and social contexts. For example, in their arm restraint study, 4-month-old girls tended to show more facial components of anger than did boys whereas 7-month-old boys appeared angrier than did 7-month-old girls (Stenberg & Campos, 1990). In the study of infants who were receiving painful inoculations, no gender differences were evident in emotions at any of the ages studied, except that 4-month-old girls exhibited more anger than did boys (but boys showed more pain; Izard et al., 1987). In an observational study of mothers interacting with 3- and 6-month old infants, the only gender difference in facial expressions was that girls showed more frequent expressions of interest (Malatesta & Haviland, 1982). So, it seems that at least around 4 months of age, girls show more facial expressions of anger when their arms are held down or when they get a shot, but not in ongoing social interactions with their mothers. Although there are not clear and consistent gender differences for negative emotions such as sadness or anger, the gender difference in expressions of interest may be particularly important because it was quite large and because it may contribute to parents' impressions that their infant daughters are more sociable than their infant sons.

CHILD GENDER AND PARENTAL SOCIALIZATION

Although gender differences in infants' anger expressions are often not large or consistent, gender differences are more apparent when investigators examine the effect of the child's gender on how parents respond to the infants' emotional expressions. A growing body of research suggests that there are differences in how parents socialize emotions in boys and girls (see Brody, 2000, for a review). Most of these studies are investigations with children beyond infancy, but one intriguing investigation suggests that mothers may respond differently to boys' and girls' emotional expressions as early as 3 months of age (Malatesta & Haviland, 1982). Mothers of 3- and 6-month-old infants were observed interacting with their babies during play and during a reunion after a short separation. Infants' emotions and mothers' responses to these were coded. The results showed that mothers of both boys and girls were highly unlikely to acknowledge the infant's anger as well as other negative emotions, but that for all emotions in general mothers were more likely to respond to boys' emotional displays than to those of girls.

Some of these differences may be responses to real differences in boys' and girls' behaviors (Brody, 1993), such as girls' more frequent expressions of interest noted in the previous study (Malatesta & Haviland, 1982). Although a comprehensive review of early gender differences in social behavior is beyond the scope of this chapter, Brody (1999, 2000) has summarized evidence that suggests that early differences in temperament and language ability may lay the groundwork for boys and girls to be socialized to express emotions in different ways. For example, newborn girls prefer to look at a female human face, whereas newborn boys prefer to gaze at a mechanical object (composed of parts of the same woman's face; Connellan, Baron-Cohen, Wheelwright, Batki, & Ahluwalia, 2000). Infant girls have lower activity levels than do boys (Eaton & Ennis, 1986). Girls initiate more social interactions than boys do at 6-, 9-, and 12-months of age (Gunnar & Donahue, 1980). Six-month-old girls fuss less than do boys when their parents refuse to smile at them in "still-face" studies (Weinberg, Tronick, Cohn, & Olson, 1999). Girls learn language earlier than do boys (Schacter, Shore, Hodapp, Chaflin, & Bundy, 1978). At the age of 1 year, girls show more empathy and distress than boys do when they observe adults pretending to be hurt (Zahn-Waxler, Radke-Yarrow, Wagner, & Chapman, 1992). In a study of social referencing, 1-year-old girls were more responsive to their mothers' appraisals of novel objects, despite the fact that mothers displayed stronger fear signals to their infant sons (Rosen, Adamson, & Bakeman, 1992). Brody (2000) argues that because girls are more verbal, responsive, and socially outgoing, parents might emphasize more positive emotions in their interactions with girls than with boys, and might tend to use more emotion words. With infant boys, parents might try to help them minimize their emotions due to their greater arousability and might talk with them less because of their less sophisticated language abilities. As I discuss in the next section, much of the research on parental socialization of preschooler's anger fits with this theory. Still, there may be another explanation.

Some of the differences in how parents socialize emotions in young girls and boys may also be due to parental stereotypes about gender (Brody, 2000). Simply being told that a particular infant is male or female changes how adults interpret infants' facial expressions (Haviland, Malatesta, & Levlivica, 1984). When undergraduate raters view brief video segments of a boy and a girl exhibiting carefully matched emotional expressions, they more often describe girls' faces as surprised or joyful and boys' faces as angry, distressed, or scared. Interestingly, undergraduates' ratings follow these same patterns when they are misinformed of the infant's gender, suggesting that differences in such ratings of boys and girls are determined less by featural or behavioral differences and more by adults' conceptions of which emotions are likely or appropriate for girl and boys. Haviland and colleagues (1984) found similar results for a study with elementary-school-age raters. This suggests that stereotypes about gender and emotion may be well learned by middle childhood, and that these stereotypes might influence how children perceive and respond to the emotional expressions of their peers. How might gender differences in young children's behaviors and parents' and peers' differential responses set the stage for gender differences in anger regulation during the preschool years?

WHAT IS THE AGE OF ONSET FOR PHYSICAL AGGRESSION?

As indicated by the quotation at the beginning of this chapter, experts disagree somewhat as to the age of onset for physical aggression. Maccoby (1980) argued that nothing that young infants do meets the criteria for intention to harm. Similarly, Fagot and Hagan (1985) noted that psychologists typically consider the hitting and grabbing behaviors of toddlers to be assertive rather than aggressive. Early approaches to studying toddlers' disputes assumed that conflict in this age group is not particularly social, but instead "best viewed as a serendipitous encounter occurring when two children accidentally seek access to the same toy at the same time" (Caplan, Vespo, Pederson, & Hay, 1991, p. 1513).

However, recent empirical evidence suggests that some mild forms of aggression appear at least as early as about 1 year of age, may be quite common by 18 months, and may be motivated by social as well as instrumental goals. In an observational study with triads, 1-year-olds were engaged in conflict during 16% of the time spent interacting in play sessions and 2-year-olds for 26% of the time (Caplan et al., 1991); 39% of conflicts featured instrumental force (grabbing toys), and 9% included personal force (hitting a peer). Contrary to hypotheses, triads dominated by girls (two girls and one boy) were higher on use of force and lower on prosocial behavior in resolving conflicts than triads dominated by boys. This finding was surprising in light of studies with preschoolers showing that physical aggression is higher among boys' groups (e.g., Smith & Green, 1975). Furthermore, boys in the Caplan and colleagues (1991) study were more likely to resolve disputes using prosocial behavior than were girls, especially if duplicate toys were available. Although these results await replication, they suggest that at least in the context of triads, very young girls are capable of being assertive and hanging on to what they consider to be theirs.

Other results from this same study suggested that 1- and 2-year-old's conflicts were quite social in nature: conflicts occurred in the context of positive social interactions and conflicts were more frequent when toys were abundant than when they were scare. In fact, in 25% of the conflicts over toys in a condition where duplicate toys were available, one of the children held the matching toy in their laps as they tried to take its twin from a peer.

Other evidence that some forms of aggression may begin quite early in life comes from large-scale survey in Canada. According to maternal reports, 80% of children have initiated physical aggression by the time they are 17 months old (Tremblay et al., 1999). Aggressive behaviors included in the survey were "Takes things from others" (74% of mothers reported that their 17-month-olds engaged in this behavior "sometimes" or "often"), "Pushes to get what [he/she] wants" (46%), "Bites" (27%), "Kicks" (24%), "Fights" (23%), "Threatens to hit" (22.5%), "Physically attacks" (20.6%), "Hits" (15%), "Starts fights" (12%), "Bullies" (8%), and "Cruel" (3.9%) (Tremblay et al., 1999, p. 15). Whether more boys or girls engage in physical aggression by this age depends on the family context—whether the child has siblings or not. For girls and boys who had siblings, there were no gender differences in maternal reports of physical aggression. For only children, more mothers of boys reported that their sons were physically aggressive than did mothers of girls (Tremblay et al., 1999).

Gender differences aside, these results suggest that aggression is well underway for many children by 18 months or so. In fact, the majority of children who refrain from physical aggression in the early elementary grades may in fact be early desisters from higher levels of aggression when they were younger (Tremblay et al., 1999). Why do some young children apparently become less aggressive after 18 months of age and some not? One longitudinal study of children from ages 1–3 years suggests that early precursors of aggressive disruptive behavior may differ for girls and for boys (Shaw, Keenan, & Vondry, 1994). For boys, aggressive behavior at age 3 was predicted by earlier maternal unresponsiveness, attention seeking in infancy, aggression, and noncompliance in toddlerhood. For 3-year-old girls, aggressive behavior was predicted only by toddler noncompliance. Additional research with younger samples is needed to clarify the early developmental course of aggression and whether causal factors differ for girls and boys.

SUMMARY AND CONCLUSIONS

Although it is clear that young infants are likely not extremely aggressive in the strictest sense of the word (Maccoby, 1980), contemporary research has been helpful in illuminating some important elements of aggressive behavior that may be evident by the end of the first year of life. Research with infants demonstrates that anger is apparent as early as 3–4 months of age, then begins to intensify around age 7 months as children develop the motor abilities to move independently and to assert their desires, as well as the cognitive skills to recognize when others are interfering with what they want. There seem not to be dramatic, consistent gender differences in anger or aggression during infancy, but parents may respond differently to girls' and boys' anger, due either to subtle gender differences in infants' behaviors or to parental gender stereotypes. Parents might ignore girls' anger more and instead focus on positive emotions, and they might expend greater effort in helping young boys to control their arousal and negative emotions. Still, at least some evidence suggests that many infant girls are capable of asserting themselves quite forcefully in particular social contexts such as with their siblings and in triads composed of two girls and one boy. Why do some children desist from early physical fighting and some persist, and how might this be related to how girls may begin to express anger and contempt in more subtle ways?

Chapter 5

Girls' Anger and Aggression in Preschool

"If You Don't Do What I Say, I Won't Be Your Friend"

How was your day at school?
> Great. Nicole told the whole class that she made a list of who could come to her birthday party, and that she crossed off all of the girls but me.

How did that make you feel?
> Good. But, then she told me that I would not get a goody bag at the party unless I play what she wants every single day.
> —5-YEAR-OLD LOUISA, TALKING WITH HER MOTHER

Preschool children as young as age 3 engage in social aggression (Crick, Casas, & Mosher, 1997; McNeilly-Choque, Hart, Robinson, Nelson, & Olsen, 1996). Consider how fascinating it is that such young children seem to understand the power of social exclusion to hurt, manipulate, and perhaps even achieve instrumental goals. Around this same developmental period, gender differences emerge for physical aggression, with girls becoming less aggressive than boys (Loeber & Hay, 1997). How can we understand and explain these amazing developments?

This chapter examines how preschool aged girls (approximately 2–5 years old) express anger and behave aggressively, with special attention to social aggression, and how and why it develops. The first section describes, in several subsections, what we know about the nature of girls' anger and aggression from ages 2–5: expressions of anger, peer conflicts, verbal aggression, rough-and-tumble play, physical aggression, and social aggression. To examine what is and is not distinctive about girls' anger and aggression, these subsections examine a great deal of research with both genders. The next section considers possible reasons why social aggression might become more prominent in girls' behavioral repertoires than physical aggression: temperament, socialization by parents and teachers, gender stereotypes and peer responses to particular types of angry, aggressive behavior. Because little research to date has directly examined developmental origins of social aggression, this section is in part speculative in linking other bodies of evidence to early social aggression. The chapter concludes by summarizing what we do and do not know about girls' anger and aggression in the preschool age range, and by outlining questions for future research.

FORMS OF ANGRY, AGGRESSIVE
BEHAVIOR AMONG PRESCHOOL GIRLS

Anger

Most experts agree that preschool aged children struggle to regulate angry feelings, perhaps especially with peers. A classic diary study found that mothers reported increases in children's angry tantrums from 12 to 30 months (Goodenough, 1931). In one of the few attempts at a comprehensive theory of emotional development, Gottman and Mettetal (1986) described early childhood as a time when children expend considerable effort to contain negative emotions so that they can begin to engage in coordinated play. Ethnographic research with children from working class families in Baltimore suggests that, by age 2½, children understand that feeling and behaving angrily requires justification (P. M. Miller & Sperry, 1987). By age 4, children seem to understand the importance of masking anger in interactions with friends, reporting that they expect peers to respond more negatively to displays of negative emotions than do parents (Zeman & Penza, 1997).

One of the few observational studies that focused specifically on preschooler's anger in peer interactions examined the relation between peer status and coping with anger (Fabes & Eisenberg, 1992). Children often coped with anger by active resistance (protecting one's property or position through verbal or nonaggressive physical means—e.g., trying to take back a toy that someone else had swiped) and by venting (displaying emotions without taking any direct steps to rectify the situation—for example, crying or having a tantrum). Young children were about equally likely to seek adult help for physical and verbal aggression (12% and 10% of episodes, respectively), but less likely to seek adult assistance for social rejection (4% of the time). Although there were no gender differences for the overall frequency of showing anger or for the causes of disputes, girls and boys differed in more subtle ways. Compared to boys, girls were more likely to manage anger by active resistance and less likely to vent. For girls, age was positively correlated with the likelihood of responding angrily to interpersonal rejection, defined as being ignored or not allowed to play with peers. Interestingly, for girls, being liked by peers was negatively related to venting and to being angered by social rejection.

Although these subtle gender differences are interesting, it is important to remember that girls and boys respond similarly in many ways and some of the differences are not found consistently for different samples. For example, a study using a coding system similar to that of Fabes and Eisenberg (1992) with a lower-income, mostly African American sample found no gender differences in observed anger and sadness (Garner & Spears, 2000).

In another study using similar methods, preschool children were observed in classrooms to compare how they responded to provocation by children they liked well and those they did not like (Fabes, Eisenberg, Smith, & Murphy, 1996). Each child's liking of each other child was assessed using the interview procedures developed by Asher, Singleton, Tinsley, and Hymel (1979), in which children designate each peer as someone they "really like to play with," "like to play with some," and "like to play with only a little." Although the degree of liking was unrelated to the intensity of the provocation, when responding to challenges by peers whom they liked, children were more controlled and regulated. Boys' responses to provocation were more strongly associated with whether the individual child liked the provocateur than were girls' reactions. Interestingly, girls were more likely to socially reject provocateurs than were boys.

Other research shows that there are individual differences in the extent to which children perceive and evaluate interpersonal provocation. The *Hostile Attribution Bias* is a tendency to perceive ambiguous social cues as hostile, especially when those cues are relevant to the self (Dodge & Somberg, 1987; the same phenomenon was referred to as the *Anger Attribution Bias* by Schultz, Izard, & Ackerman, 2000). Some children are more vulnerable to becoming angry because they are more likely than other children to perceive that they have been slighted, maligned, attacked, or wronged, in the face of events or feedback that others might perceive as ambiguous or even benign. Although most studies of the Hostile Attribution Bias have focused on middle-childhood samples, recent research suggests that this bias can be assessed as early as 4 years of age. In one study using a vignette measure of the Anger

Attribution Bias for preschoolers, girls scored lower than boys did (Schultz et al., 2000). Interestingly, whereas physically aggressive boys in the sample were higher on the Anger Attribution Bias than were nonaggressive peers, there was no difference between aggressive and nonaggressive girls. Schultz and colleagues (2000) acknowledge that this may be due to the fact that their measure of aggression emphasized physical fighting. Some girls may indeed overattribute hostility but may still choose not to respond or even to retaliate more indirectly.

Although few longitudinal studies have addressed the long-term consequences of particular forms of anger expression in preschool, one investigation suggests that ways of coping with anger at age 4–6 years of age are related to social functioning 2 and 4 years later (Eisenberg, Fabes, Murphy et al., 1999). Responding to anger with non-abusive verbal assertions during preschool/kindergarten predicted being rated by teachers as socially skilled 2 and 4 years later, and predicted being low on problem behaviors according to parent reports. Responding to anger with physical retaliation predicted later social problems. Some of the findings were gender specific; girls who vented when angry during preschool were rated as less socially appropriate by teachers 2 and 4 years later.

Overall, these studies suggest a very interesting portrait of preschool girls' anger. Girls are perfectly capable of asserting themselves by active resistance, but they are less likely to vent and are lower on the Hostile Attribution Bias. Older preschool girls are more likely to be angered by social exclusion than are younger girls. For girls only, venting and expressing anger following interpersonal rejection are related to being disliked by peers, and venting predicts later social problems. Girls are more likely than boys to socially reject a child who has recently provoked them.

Conflicts with Peers

Whereas research on children's anger focuses on encounters in which one of the participants exhibits angry emotion that is overt enough to be detected by observers, research on conflict examines disputes, whether or not the children involved become angry. Researchers differ in exactly how they define conflict: some code conflicts as any interaction featuring overt or covert disagreements (e.g., P. M. Miller et al., 1986); other investigators use a more strict definition requiring a specific sequence of opposition ("any interaction in which Child A attempted to influence Child B, B resisted the influence, and A persisted in his or her influence attempts"; D. W. Shantz, 1986, p. 1324). Regardless of exactly how conflict is defined, investigating conflicts is important because children manage disputes in a range of positive and negative ways that would not be observed in studies focusing only on anger or aggression.

Observational studies indicate that many peer conflicts among preschool children are quite brief and do not involve anger or aggression (Laursen & Hartup, 1989; Vespo, Pedersen, & Hay, 1995). In one naturalistic study with 4- and 5-year-olds observed during free play at a summer day camp, all disputes were less than 1 minute long and anger was not strongly linked to conflict behavior (Arsenio & Lover, 1997). Even in the family context where emotions might run hot and open displays of anger might be more likely, only 5–10% of children's disputes with their mothers and their siblings featured anger (Dunn & Munn, 1987).

Observational research shows that young children are capable of resolving conflicts in fairly sophisticated ways. In preschool classrooms, children most frequently resolve peer conflicts by insistence, negotiation, or disengagement (Laursen & Hartup, 1989). In an observational study with 5- and 7-year-old children in experimental playgroups, the most common strategy for resolving disputes was moderate persuasion (including behaviors such as justification, explanations, and entreaties; P. M. Miller et al., 1986). The extent to which conflict episodes among preschoolers involve social aggression remains largely unknown. However, one observational study of 4- and 5-year-olds playing with table toys in triads showed that 8% of children's conflicts featured psychological harm or social exclusion (Arsenio & Killen, 1996).

Many observational studies of younger preschool children do not find gender differences in children's responses to peer conflicts (e.g., see Laursen & Hartup, 1989, for a study with 3- to 5-year-olds, and Vespo, Pedersen, & Hay, 1995, for a study with 3- and 4-year-olds). However, studies with slightly older children suggest that gender differences may emerge just a bit later. One study observed rates of agonistic behavior (conflicts over toys and space) among children ages 2, 3, and 5 in a day-care setting (Legault & Strayer, 1990). For 2-year-olds, there were no gender differences. For 3- and 4-year-olds, girls' frequency of agonistic behavior decreased and boys' rates increased slightly such that boys' rates of agonistic behavior were twice as high as girls' rates. In a study of experimental playgroups of 5- and 7-year-olds, boys were more likely to be involved in conflicts than were girls (P. M. Miller et al., 1986). Although both boys and girls were likely to resolve disputes with moderate persuasion, boys were more likely to use threats and physical force, whereas girls were more likely to try to mitigate conflicts, especially the older girls in the sample. Interestingly, how girls resolved conflicts depended on the gender of their interaction partners. Girls were more forceful and less mitigating in their conflict strategies when interacting with boys than when interacting with other girls. Boys used more forceful conflict strategies regardless of whether they were interacting with girls or boys. (For a thorough discussion of gender-of-partner effects across domains and age groups, see Maccoby [1998].)

Taken together, these fascinating findings suggest that by the end of the preschool period girls may be more likely to try to smooth over disputes, and less likely to resolve disputes in ways that might threaten relationships. Girls' tendency to try to mitigate conflicts may be more pronounced in their interactions with other girls than in their encounters with boys. However, it is important to remember that gender differences in conflict behavior may depend on the social context. Two longitudinal studies in the United States and the United Kingdom did not find gender differences in preschool children's conflict behaviors with close friends, siblings, and mothers (Dunn, 2001). Girls and boys may not differ in how they handle conflicts in close relationships, although girls may be more mitigating with classmates in play group studies.

Rough-and-Tumble Play

That girls may be involved in fewer, less physical conflicts than boys may also be related to the fact that they are less likely to be involved in rough-and-tumble play (Coie & Dodge, 1998; DiPietro, 1981; Smith & Boulton, 1990). Rough-and-tumble play is physical, often involving play fighting or chasing, but occurs between friends and features benign intent, positive affect, restraint, and role reversals (Smith & Boulton, 1990). In an observational study of triads of 4-year-old girls and boys, boys' play featured more "playful physical assault," defined as:

> Discrete action consisting of hitting other child with body part or object; grabbing clothing or appendage; pushing; tripping. Facial features of both actor and recipient must convey excitement or positive affect. Accompanying vocalizations of actor must be non-threatening and verbal response of recipient, non-prohibitive. Outcome must not be accidentally injurious or distressing. (DiPietro, 1981, p. 53)

Researchers argue that rough-and-tumble play requires and perhaps even teaches social skills because it entails a willing partner, correctly inferring playful intent, changing roles, and both members of the dyad expressing but containing exuberance well enough that the interaction does not get out of hand (DiPietro, 1981; Smith & Boulton, 1990). Experts also acknowledge that rough-and-tumble play can often become conflictual or even aggressive when one or both participants loses control or suddenly feels mistreated and angry rather than playful and excited (Coie & Dodge, 1998). One partner may mistakenly infer hostile intent, or a child might send deliberately ambiguous signals as a form of social manipulation to increase status or do social harm, by making it difficult for the partner to know how to respond (Smith & Boulton, 1990). That girls engage in less rough-and-tumble play than do boys suggests that they might have fewer opportunities for both practicing and losing emotional control in peer encounters, perhaps making them more prone to masking anger and inhibiting physical aggression.

Physical Aggression

Although gender differences in physical aggression are well documented for older children (Coie & Dodge, 1998; Maccoby, 1998), they are much less clear for young preschoolers. In comprehensive reviews of developmental trajectories of aggression for girls and for boys, Loeber and Hay (1997) concluded that there are few gender differences in physical aggression in toddlerhood, and Keenan and Shaw (1997) surmised that gender differences in problem behaviors are not evident until age 4. Observational studies to date have yielded conflicting findings for gender differences in the early preschool years. One study of children from low-income families in which children were observed at 18 and 24 months old found no gender differences for physical aggression (Keenan & Shaw, 1994). Similarly, a longitudinal study in which children were observed interacting with a best friend at ages 2 and 5 found no gender differences in the frequency or type of physical aggression (Cummings, Iannotti, & Zahn-Waxler, 1989). However, in one study with 2-year-olds, boys were observed to be more aggressive than girls in a 35-minute session of same-gender play (Rubin, Hastings, Chen, Stewart, & McNichol, 1998). Additional observational research in different social contexts might be helpful in reconciling these discrepant findings and in determining when and in what settings gender differences in physical aggression may begin to emerge.

Whether teachers rate preschool girls as less physically aggressive than preschool boys depends on the sample and the specific behaviors assessed. In one investigation with 3- to 5-year-olds at a university preschool in the midwestern United States, teachers rated girls as lower on overt aggression than boys, although peer nominations indicated no gender differences (Crick, Casas, & Mosher, 1997). Another study using this same teacher measure found no gender differences for teacher ratings of overt aggression for a sample of nursery school children in Russia (Hart, Nelson, Robinson, Olsen, & McNeilly-Choque, 1998). For a large, diverse sample or preschool children in the southeastern United States, gender differences were not apparent for teacher ratings of overt antisocial behavior (including physical and verbal aggression; Willoughby, Kupersmidt, & Bryant, 2001).

However, other studies suggest that between ages 3 and 5, gender differences in aggression may become more prominent. Coie and Dodge (1998) reviewed many classic studies of early gender differences in aggression; they concluded that, across settings, methods, and even cultures, girls become less aggressive than boys during this developmental period. For example, in a longitudinal study of children of depressed and well mothers, 2-year-old girls and boys were similar on interpersonal physical aggression and object-oriented aggression in peer interactions (although boys were higher on out-of-control aggression; Zahn-Waxler, Iannotti, Cummings, & Denham, 1990). When this same sample was 5 years old, mothers completed the Child Behavior Checklist and boys were rated by their mothers as higher on externalizing problems than were girls. Coie and Dodge (1998) surmised that girls might become less aggressive than boys during the later preschool years because girls are less impulsive, more deliberate in resolving conflicts, and more likely to use verbal strategies such as negotiation than are boys. Other research suggests that gender differences emerge between 21 and 40 months because girls' becoming less aggressive is related to their learning to label gender. In one study, girls who could accurately label gender behaved less aggressively than boys and than nonlabeling girls in laboratory play groups (Fagot, Leinbach, & Hagan, 1986).

Research indicates that stable aggressive behavior can be identified in children as young as 2 and 3 years of age, although some of these studies define aggression more broadly than as just physical fighting. For example, Kingston and Prior (1995) identified a stable aggressive subgroup ($n = 53$) from a large sample included in the Australian Temperament Project ($N = 1,721$) on the basis of maternal reports indicating that the child was 1 standard deviation above the mean on aggression at annual assessments from ages 3 to 8 years. Their definition of aggression included both physical and verbal aggression. Still, most members of the highly aggressive subgroup were boys (41 of 53).

Interestingly, although observational studies of younger preschoolers often do not find gender differences in preschoolers' physical aggression, some of these same studies do find gender differences in the stability of physical aggression. One study observed children ages 18–27 months in ongoing yearly playgroups, examining stability across 1 and 2 years (Fagot, 1984). For boys, conduct problems with aggression were quite stable over 1 year ($r = .78$) and 2 years ($r = .68$). For girls, aggression was less stable across 1 year ($r = .23$) and 2 years ($r = .15$). Similarly, another longitudinal study found higher stability for boys' aggression from age 2 to age 5 ($r = .59$) than for girls' aggression ($r = .36$) (Cummings et al., 1989).

Taken together, many of these studies suggest that gender differences emerge during the later preschool years because girls become less physically aggressive. Perhaps one reason for this is that preschool girls may prefer to aggress using their developing verbal skills (Bjorkqvist, 1994).

Verbal Aggression

One challenge in determining the onset of aggression and the emergence of gender differences has been that studies confound different types of aggression: physical versus verbal; direct versus indirect (Bjorkqvist, 1994; Tremblay et al., 1999). Some experts have argued that gender differences will become more clear if we focus on certain forms of aggression—in particular, verbal aggression.

However, verbal aggression has been extremely difficult to define because human speech is so widely varied, tone of voice can be difficult to classify, and determining a speaker's desire to harm is hard to do objectively (McCabe & Lipscomb, 1988). For example, it can be difficult to separate verbal aggression from teasing. Perhaps because of a lack of consensus about how to define verbal aggression, previous research has yielded conflicting findings for gender differences. Some investigators conclude that there are no gender differences in verbal aggression (e.g., Bandura, Ross, & Ross, 1961; Blurton-Jones & Konner, 1973; Dawe, 1934; Madsen, 1968; Roff & Roff, 1940; Whiting & Edwards, 1973; T. M. Williams, Joy, Kimball, & Zabrack, 1983—as cited in McCabe & Lipscomb, 1988). Other experts assert that boys are more verbally aggressive than are girls (Maccoby & Jacklin, 1974; Parke & Slaby, 1983; J. H. Williams, 1977—as cited in McCabe & Lipscomb, 1988).

McCabe and Lipscomb (1988) attempted to solve the definitional problems by using formal linguistic criteria to define verbal aggression as "any sentence or phrase standing alone and judged to be a reprimand, harsh command, tattle, tease, insult, rejection, hostile assertion of ownership or priority, callous factual statement, accusation, criticism, obscenity, or other expletives" (p. 393). According to this definition, they observed verbal aggression in 4-year-olds in preschool classrooms and found no gender differences.

Although this definition of verbal aggression was formulated to distinguish it from physical aggression, note that it seems to confound verbal and social aggression. Included in this construct are behaviors that sound like venting or like the more forceful overt conflict resolution strategies preferred by boys (Fabes & Eisenberg, 1992; P. M. Miller et al., 1986) but also behaviors that sound a lot like social aggression, such as rejection, which some argue is more characteristic of girls (Crick & Grotpeter, 1995). Therefore, the lack of gender differences observed here might once again be due to the breadth of the construct.

If it is indeed the case that girls are less likely to use physically forceful overt persuasion yet do not differ from boys on verbal aggression, how exactly do girls manage their anger and assert their social goals in the face of conflict or disagreement? Let us now examine the small body of research investigating social aggression among preschool children.

Social Aggression

Just how early in childhood do children begin to use social aggression as a way of expressing anger and contempt to hurt their peers and maybe even to get what they want? Researchers have recently begun to investigate the early beginnings of social aggression, but only a handful of studies are available.

The evidence thus far indicates that preschool-age children do engage in social aggression, that these behaviors appear to be distinct from physical aggression, and that according to some sources preschool girls display more social aggression than do preschool boys. In one study, McNeilly-Choque and colleagues (1996) observed relational and physical aggression among 4- and 5-year-olds on playgrounds, both at a Head Start preschool for lower-income families and at a university preschool serving more middle- and upper-income families. Relational aggression of these preschoolers was coded by the above authors (p. 94) as follows:

1. Walking way from a peer when a peer tries to play with them
2. Telling other children not to play with someone
3. Whispering or saying mean things about other children
4. Telling a child to go away
5. Not listening to another child—covering ears
6. Telling another child he/she will stop liking them unless they do what they want
7. Telling other children they can't play with the group unless they do what the group wants them to do

Factor analyses showed that teacher raters, peer nominators, and adult observers could distinguish between relational and physical aggression;

relational and physical aggression items loaded on separate factors (McNeilly-Choque et al., 1996). However, interrater reliability was higher for overt than for relational aggression. Girls were observed to engage in more relational aggression than boys were, and girls were also described as more relationally aggressive by classmates and teachers. Children from the lower-income Head Start subsample were lower on relational aggression than were children from the more affluent university preschool subsample.

In another study, 3- to 5-year-olds were asked to nominate preschool classmates for the following specific behaviors related to relational aggression: "Kids who say they won't invite someone to their birthday party if they can't have their own way"; "Kids who won't let a kid play in the group if they are mad at the kid—they might tell the kid to go away"; "Kids who tell other kids they can't play with the group unless they do what the group wants them to do"; and "Kids who won't listen to someone when they are mad at them—they might even cover their ears" (Crick, Casas, & Mosher, 1997, p. 583). Teachers rated the preschoolers on similar items. Here again, factor analyses showed that for both peer ratings and teacher ratings, relational and physical aggression items loaded on separate factors. Although teachers described girls as more relationally aggressive than boys and boys as more overtly aggressive than girls, children's peer nominations showed no gender differences for relational or overt aggression. Crick, Casas, and Mosher (1997) suggested that the lack of gender differences for the peer nominations may have been due to inadequate statistical power or to young children's inability to distinguish between forms of aggressive behavior. However, another explanation seems possible. Perhaps girls and boys truly do not differ on relational aggression, but teachers perceive that they do because they are more conversant in stereotypes of girls as backbiting and manipulative. Gender differences aside, the results of this study for both boys and girls indicated that engaging in relational aggression was related to being disliked by peers.

Another study of relational aggression in preschool children examined how parenting style and marital conflict were related to overt and relational aggression for a sample of nursery school children in Russia (Hart et al., 1998). Teachers rated children on overt and relational aggression using measures similar to those developed by Crick, Casas, and Mosher (1997), and there were no gender differences for relational or for overt aggression. (The findings related to parenting variables are presented in a subsequent section of this chapter.)

Willoughby and colleagues (2001) examined the prevalence of antisocial behaviors in a large and diverse normal sample, and included some items assessing social aggression. Teachers rated preschool students on the frequency of overt and covert antisocial behaviors. Covert antisocial behaviors were defined as harmful actions that avoid confrontation, and specific items included the following: "Do sneaky things"; "Take things when others not looking"; "Play mean tricks"; "Tell other kids not to play"; "Tell lies about kids"; and "Say mean things behind back" (p. 181). (Note that covert aggression as measured here does not correspond perfectly to social aggression; the last three items seem the most closely related.)

The results of Willoughby and colleagues (2001) showed that overt and covert items loaded on separate factors. Test–retest reliability for teachers' ratings was acceptable for both dimensions. However, similar to the results of McNeilly-Choque and colleagues (1996) and Crick, Casas, and Mosher (1997) for relational aggression, interrater reliability between teachers and classroom aides was poor for the covert subscale (but good for overt antisocial behavior). Analyses of the data confirmed that individual teachers had characteristic styles of using the rating scales that seemed consistent across their students. The investigators examined the interclass correlations for teachers' ratings for all students in their classrooms and found that 10–50% of the variance in ratings was due to individual teachers' rating styles (and these interclass correlations were especially high for the covert items).

Because the items in this study asked teachers to rate frequencies as how many times per day each child engaged in particular behaviors, these results provide some of the first data on the frequency of covert antisocial behaviors for a normal preschool sample. The results indicated that 74% of preschool children did not engage in any covert antisocial behaviors on a daily basis but 10% did some two or three covert antisocial behaviors per day. These teacher ratings showed no gender differences in the frequency of overt and covert antisocial behaviors.

In a study using similar methods with Head Start and community preschool samples, once again there were no gender differences for relationally aggressive behaviors (Kupersmidt, Bryant, & Willoughby, 2000). Overall mean levels of physical aggression were higher for the Head Start group, although mean levels of verbal aggression were higher for the community sample. There were no group differences in person prevalence of highly antisocial behavior; about 10% of children were aggressing once or more per day in both samples.

What do young children understand about the moral acceptability of social aggression? In the only study to examine this question to date, 3- to 5-year-olds responded to vignettes describing overt and relational provocation (telling another child he or she could not play with blocks; Goldstein, Tisak, & Boxer, 2002). Both girls and boys judged relationally aggressive responses to this provocation to be more acceptable than physical and verbal aggression. For the relational provocation scenario, girls rated relational aggression as more wrong than did boys. This suggests that as early as the preschool years girls may be more bothered by social aggression than are boys.

Although studies of social aggression in preschool are just beginning, the evidence to date suggests that by the age of 3 years or so social aggression has become firmly established in at least some children's behavioral repertoires. Across studies, interrater reliability for social aggression is poor, suggesting that measuring social aggression in such young children may continue to be challenging. Some research suggests that levels of verbal and relational aggression may be higher in middle-income than in lower-income samples. The evidence for gender differences is mixed; therefore, it seems important not to characterize social aggression as "female aggression." Caution is warranted in considering gender and developmental differences in social aggression for the following reasons: (1) boys too engage in the behavior; (2) it may not be a developmental accomplishment because children engage in social aggression at such young ages; and (3) gender and age differences may depend on the cultural context (Dunn, 2001).

In summary, research to date suggests that preschool girls may express anger and aggression in less overt, more indirect ways than do boys. Preschool girls are less likely to vent when they are angry, more likely to use mitigating strategies for resolving conflicts, and by the end of the preschool period are clearly less likely to resort to physical aggression than are boys. As early as age 3 some girls (and boys) engage in social aggression, and some (not all) studies find that preschool girls are more socially aggressive than preschool boys are.

ORIGINS AND EXPLANATIONS FOR PRESCHOOL GIRLS' ANGER AND AGGRESSION

Almost no research has examined the early developmental origins of social aggression, whether particular types of temperaments and early relationships and social contexts are associated with some children becoming socially aggressive. In many ways, it is premature to speculate that girls learn social aggression sooner than boys and engage in it more frequently. However, studies converge in suggesting that during the preschool years girls become less angry and overtly aggressive than boys and perhaps more likely to express anger via indirect means. Why? The following discussion highlights possible explanations for preschool-age girls' anger and aggression from the research literatures on temperament, emotion regulation, parental socialization, gender stereotypes and segregation, and peer relations. Although few of these studies specifically examined the early origins of social aggression, they offer some intriguing clues.

Temperament and Biological Factors

Perhaps preschool girls begin to express anger differently than boys do because of innate differences in how they regulate arousal and cope with environmental challenges—that is, in their *temperament*. Temperament has been defined as "constitutionally based individual differences in emotional, motor, and attentional reactivity and self-regulation" (Rothbart & Bates, 1998, p. 109). Most models of temperament in infancy and early childhood include dimensions for negative emotionality, difficultness, flexibility in adapting to new situations, activity level, self-regulation, reactivity, and sociability (Bates, 1989).

Much research on temperament in young children either does not test or does not find gender differences (Chess & Thomas, 1984; Guérin & Gottfried, 1994; Rothbart, 1986). In one observational study with 2-year-olds, a measure of temperament combining observations and parent ratings showed no gender differences for emotion dysregulation (Rubin, Hastings, et al., 1998). A very few studies suggest that boys may be more likely than girls to have difficult temperaments. For example, mothers rated 3-year-old boys as more active and less adaptable than 3-year-old girls, although this gender difference disappeared by age 5 (Guérin & Gottfried, 1994). In one study, teachers rated preschool boys as higher on arousability than preschool girls (Fabes, Shepard, Guthrie, & Martin, 1997), but in another investigation there were no gender differences for ratings of arousability (Fabes, 1994). In another study with toddler and preschool age children, child-care providers rated boys as slightly higher than girls on anger proneness and activity level, and parents rated boys as higher on activity level and high pleasure (Goldsmith, Buss, & Lemery, 1997). The bulk of the evidence does not support dramatic gender differences in temperament (the thorough review by Rothbart & Bates, 1998, barely mentions gender).

Further examination of gender differences in young children's temperament will be important because early biological/temperamental factors seem related to particular types of angry, aggressive behavior. For example, preschool children who had been rated by parents as difficult and hard to manage showed more negative emotion and antisocial behavior with friends than did a control group (Hughes, White, Sharpen, & Dunn, 2000). Other evidence suggests that a possible biological marker for temperament, low resting heart rate, may predict aggressive behavior. For a large community sample on the island of Mauritius, low resting heart rate measured at age 3 predicted aggression at age 11 as measured by parent ratings on the Child Behavior Checklist (Raine, Venables, & Mednick, 1997). In one of the first studies to examine biological factors that may be related to relational aggression, Dettling, Gunnar, and Donzella (1999) found that children rated by teachers as higher on relational aggression were more likely to show elevations in blood levels of cortisol from morning to afternoon, which may indicate greater reactivity to stress.

Another biological factor that has been suggested as an explanation for gender differences in aggression is testosterone. Although some have argued that men are more physically aggressive than women because they are higher on testosterone, the evidence on this point is inconsistent and the relationship between hormones and aggression is complex (for interesting discussions of these issues, see Bjorkqvist, 1994; Brain & Susman, 1997). Overall, the link between testosterone and physical aggression seems stronger in animals than in humans (Benton, 1992). Also, the relation between hormones and aggression may not be specific to testosterone. Studies with rats show that early exposure to estrogen (Edwards & Herdon, 1970), as well as to androgens (Edwards, 1969), is related to subsequent aggression.

Finally, an often cited but rarely tested biological factor that may relate to girls' anger and aggression is physical size. Many suggest that women may refrain from physical aggression and resort to more indirect means of expressing anger because they are smaller than men, and therefore aggressing physically is less likely to be successful and more likely to be dangerous for them (Bjorkqvist, 1994). This intuitively appealing speculation has yet to be tested; it seems unlikely to be an important explanatory factor for girls' anger and aggression in preschool because differences in physical size are not large in this age range.

In summary, as yet there is no overwhelming evidence that temperamental and biological differences explain why girls may choose to express anger in particular ways, although these questions have rarely been tested directly. Perhaps young girls' anger and aggression are related to the development and regulation of other emotions, or shaped more by the responses they evoke in adults.

Emotion Regulation

Although anger is the emotion most often studied in concert with different forms of aggressive behavior, it is important to mention that perhaps especially for social aggression, other emotions may be involved. Zahn-Waxler (in press) proposed that to understand why some children harm others, it is necessary to examine not only anger but also emotions and behaviors that mitigate against hurting other people:

empathy, guilt, and prosocial behavior. In many different studies, girls have been shown to be more prone to empathy and guilt than boys are and more likely to engage in reparative behaviors (see Zahn-Waxler, in press, for a review). Girls' more frequent experience of these moral emotions likely contributes to their being less physically aggressive than boys are. How these moral emotions are related to social aggression is an important topic for future research.

Two moral emotions that seem especially likely to be related to social aggression are shame and envy. Shame and envy are both self-conscious emotions that require self-recognition, differentiating between others and self, and an ability to measure oneself against standards or goals (Denham, 1998; Lewis, 1993). Shame results from judging oneself unworthy as a result of failing to meet someone else's expectations, and it involves perceiving that one is "failing in the relationship" (Denham, 1998, p. 44). Shame could bear on social aggression in that when children feel ashamed about a problem in a relationship they might try to protect or defend themselves by excluding others or by spreading nasty rumors about them.

Research suggests that preschool girls are more prone to feeling shame than boys are (Lewis, Alessandri, & Sullivan, 1992; Stipek, Recchia, & McClintic, 1992). Although the relation between shame and social aggression has yet to be tested, perhaps girls are more sensitive than boys to the types of failures that might incite social aggression, namely, perceived failures in relationships.

Another emotion that may be relevant to social aggression is envy or jealousy—coveting something that someone else has, be it a desired object, social status, or a close relationship. Although there is very little research on envy or jealousy in preschool samples, investigations with older children suggest that self-reported jealousy in relationships may be positively related to social aggression (Parker & Low, 1999). Children who report feeling more jealous in their best friendships are nominated by peers as higher on relational aggression.

In addition to specific emotions that may be relevant to social aggression, it is important to consider how gender differences in emotion regulation may be related to anger and aggression. Overall, research suggests that preschool girls use "display rules" more than do boys (Cole, 1986). A *display rule* is a social convention for masking or expressing a particular emotion in keeping with norms of the culture. For example, when given a disappointing gift, preschool girls display more positive facial expressions in the presence of an experimenter than do preschool boys; in fact, the girls' smiles are just as intense as when they previously were given their most preferred prize (Cole, 1986). Interestingly, 3- to 4-year-old girls inhibited their negative expressions only when an adult was present; in the experimenter's absence they expressed more negative emotions. That preschool girls use display rules more than preschool boys do suggests that young girls might be more concerned with being socially appropriate and avoiding adults observing them hurting others' feelings, goals that also are consistent with fighting less and using social aggression more.

How might gender differences in emotion regulation develop? To answer this question for children so young requires careful consideration of interactions between children and caregivers.

Socialization by Parents and Teachers

Research evidence from diverse sources suggests that parents may differ in how they help preschool boys and girls learn to manage angry feelings, and that parents may work particularly hard to minimize girls' anger and overt aggression. Several studies indicate that parents are more likely to ignore angry behavior by daughters than by sons (see Zahn-Waxler, in press, for a review). In one classic study, mothers of preschoolers were trained to record carefully the details of their children's angry outbursts (Goodenough, 1931). The results showed that with their children's increasing age mothers tended more to ignore girls' anger and to respond to boys' anger with more assertive strategies. Similarly, in an observational study in which mothers and children interacted in a laboratory apartment, mothers tended to give boys attention when they were angry and even give in to them but to ignore angry girls or to tell them outright to stop (Radke-Yarrow & Kochanska, 1990). When asked to discuss a previous episode in which the child became angry, mothers of 32- to 35-month-old daughters, as compared to mothers of sons, spoke more briefly about the child's anger, were less accepting of the anger and of attempts to retaliate, and were more likely to encourage their daughters to reestablish the relationship to repair any harm done by the anger (Fivush, 1991). In a home observation study with 24- and 36-month-old children, mothers responded to girls' moral transgressions by urging them to consider others' welfare, whereas mothers were more likely to command boys to stop the behavior to maintain social control (Smetana, 1989). In another observational investigation of mothers interventions in object struggles between toddlers, mothers more often asserted their son's rights in disputes (three times as much as mothers of daughters), whereas mothers more often urged daughters to yield the object to the peer (Ross, Tesla, Kenyon, & Lollis, 1990). As Ross and colleagues (1990) summarized, "mothers are more likely to demand proper social behavior from [preschool-age] girls than from boys" (p. 1001).

Other research suggests that not only do parents tend to ignore or even squelch girls' anger more than that of boys, peers and teachers may do the same. When 18- to 36-month-old children interacted in experimental playgroups, peers and teachers alike tended to ignore girls' assertive and aggressive behaviors (Fagot & Hagan, 1985). Girls in this study received no response for more than 50% of their aggressive behaviors, whereas boys' aggression elicited a response more than 70% of the time, usually from other boys. In a naturalistic observation study of how disciplinary practices of day-care teachers related to children's misbehaviors, the teachers were more lax in response to boys' misbehavior and, not surprisingly, boys misbehaved more than did girls (Arnold, Williams, & Harvey-Arnold, 1998). In another study using laboratory play group methods, 21- to 25-month-old girls responded more readily to teacher directives than did boys (Fagot, 1985), despite the fact that teachers gave similar rates of guidance to both genders. These findings suggest that girls might be more sensitive to negative adult responses elicited by overtly aggressive behavior.

Although parents seem to respond more negatively to angry behavior by preschool girls than by preschool boys, other research suggests that parents engage in more expressive behavior and more discussion of emotions with girls (see Halberstadt, Crisp, & Eaton, 1999, for a review of research on family emotional expressiveness). In an observational study of 2-year-olds playing with mothers and reuniting with them after a brief separation, there were few gender differences in the children's emotional expressions (except that girls were slightly more angry than boys on reunion; Malatesta et al., 1989). Mothers' behaviors seemed to be influenced by the gender of the child; mothers showed more positive emotions and a wider range of emotions with daughters than with sons. In a follow-up study when the same sample was 3 years old, again there were few gender differences in the children's emotional expressions, but mothers responded differently to sons' and daughters' emotional expressions (Malatesta-Magai et al., 1994). Again, mothers of girls showed more positive affect toward their children than did mothers of boys. Interestingly, mothers of sons displayed more anger toward them.

Although investigators are only beginning to examine the specific processes by which parents socialize children's emotions, it seems that mothers might talk more about emotions with their preschool daughters than with their sons (Kuebli, Butler, & Fivush, 1995). Mothers were observed talking with children at ages 40, 58, and 70 months about three recent novel family events. Mothers' speech was coded for number and type of emotion words and how emotions were discussed. With daughters, discussions of emotions were longer than with sons, mothers used a larger number and greater variety of emotion words with daughters than with sons, and mothers used a larger number of negative emotion words with daughters. Kuebli and colleagues (1995) suggested that mothers' more extensive discussions of emotions with daughters may be teaching them that emotions matter and that an important way to cope with feelings is to talk about them.

How can the findings that mothers seem to be more expressive and more willing to discuss emotions with their daughters be reconciled with research showing that girls' actual angry and aggressive behaviors are more likely to be ignored? Mothers (and perhaps other adults and peers too) may be perturbed by girls' emotional behaviors in the heat of the moment but more willing to discuss emotions with them after the fact. As Denham (1998) aptly summarized, "Girls think of emotions as something to share with others, whereas boys learn to express anger directly, but not to talk about it to others as much" (p. 139). If this is indeed the case, girls may be learning that open expressions of anger are not particularly welcome in social interaction but that discussing angry feelings with third parties afterward might actually be encouraged.

One reason why girls may discuss emotions more with their young daughters might be that they are more emotionally connected with them than are mothers of sons. When observed during semistructured play with mothers, daughters stayed physically close to their mothers, maintained more eye contact, and expressed more enjoyment than did sons (Benenson, Morash, & Petrakos, 1998). Greater proximity and more focused attention might provide daughters with more opportunities to discuss and witness their mothers' emotions.

Young girls' exposure to their mothers' expressions of anger may strongly influence the girls' levels of anger and aggression. In a laboratory study in which 18- to 24-month-olds witnessed adults having a negative, emotionally charged interaction, the children ceased all activities and watched the adults showing extreme anger or sadness (Jenkins, Franco, Dokins, & Sevell, 1995). Research shows that 4-year-olds are quite adept at identifying the causes of anger not only for themselves but also for their mothers and friends; moreover, they understand that anger is frequently caused by interactions with friends (Dunn & Hughes, 1998).

Chronic exposure to parents' anger has negative consequences for preschool children, some of which persist long term. Research on marital conflict shows that children exposed to interparental anger have higher rates of physically aggressive behavior (an extensive discussion of this issue is beyond the scope of this chapter; see Cummings & Davies, 1994, for a thoughtful review). Even if parents are not divorced, exposure to their anger can have negative consequences. In a sample of 4- to 8-year-olds, children exposed to angry marital conflict were rated as more aggressive by peers, teachers, and mothers, and were observed to show more angry responses in peer interactions (Jenkins, 2000). In one longitudinal study of families (most of whom were intact), high levels of parental anger in early childhood predicted more behavior problems at middle childhood, even after controlling for high stability of children's behavior problems (Denham et al., 2000).

Only one study to date has investigated whether exposure to marital conflict is related to social aggression by preschool children (Hart et al., 1998). Russian parents completed questionnaires assessing marital conflict and parenting styles (responsiveness, coercion, and psychological control). Nursery school teachers rated children on overt and relational aggression. The results showed that, for boys, marital conflict was related to higher overt and relational aggression; for both genders, lower maternal and paternal responsiveness and maternal coercion were related to relational aggression. Although these intriguing findings await replication, these data suggest that the early origins of social aggression may include parenting and exposure to marital conflict.

Other research suggests that young girls may be more reactive than young boys to parents' negative emotions. For example, in one study, the ratio of parents' happiness to anger predicted daughters' positive emotions expressed at preschool but not those of sons (Denham, Mitchell-Copeland, Strandberg, Auerbach, & Blair, 1997). Also, parents' internalizing symptoms were negatively associated with daughters' expressing positive emotions at school but not with boys' positivity in the classroom. Even parents' marital dissatisfaction may have subtle effects on how they respond to their daughters and sons. For example, an observational study found that fathers low on marital satisfaction responded more negatively to daughters than to sons and that mothers low on marital satisfaction responded more negatively to assertions from daughters than to assertions from sons (Kerig, Cowan, & Cowan, 1993). Given that preschoolers with unhappily married parents may be witnessing discord and conflict, it is all the more worrisome that daughters especially are treated negatively by their fathers and discouraged from asserting themselves by their mothers. In her thoughtful and comprehensive book on emotional development during the preschool years, Denham concludes, "Little girls are exquisite barometers of their parents' emotions. This may be both a blessing and a curse!" (p. 224).

"Doing Gender": The Onset of Gender Labeling, Gender Segregation, and Gender Stereotypes

Some of the previous discussion might imply that children's role in the socialization of emotions is a fairly passive one in which they respond to their parents' behaviors and gender differences emerge because parents do things differently with girls and with boys. However, gender scholars have argued convincingly that gender is not simply something that one *is*, it is something that one *does*—"gender is something that one practices" (Shields, 2000, p. 6).

Parents are practicing gender with their preschool children when they hold and speak to male and female infants differently and when they respond differently to sons' and daughters' anger. Adults also "do gender" when they perceive rough-and-tumble play as more aggressive when they are told that children wearing snowsuits (making their gender indeterminable) are girls than when they are told they are boys (Condry & Ross, 1985). Teachers are "doing gender" when they use a "different frame of reference" when rating boys and girls on aggression in relation to the stereotype for each gender (Feshbach & Feshbach, 1969, p. 104). When do children themselves start to "do gender" in their social interactions?

Gender Labeling

Some extremely clever studies suggest that children may begin to practice gender at least by the time they learn to label gender, when they can reliably determine who is a boy and who is a girl. To assess when children begin to label gender, Fagot and colleagues developed a task in which children are presented with pairs of pictures in a notebook, one of a boy and one of a girl wearing similar clothing (Fagot et al., 1986; Fagot, Leinbach, & O'Boyle, 1992). When children correctly identify 10 or more of the 12 pairs, they are judged to be able to label gender. The age at which children develop this ability varies widely, from 18 to 36 months (Fagot et al., 1992).

Learning to label gender appears to be associated with increased knowledge of the many characteristics associated with our cultural notions of what is male and female (called gender schemas; see Bem, 1993), as well as with important changes in social behavior. Fagot and colleagues (1992) developed a creative method of measuring young children's knowledge of both the conventional associations (trucks are for boys) and the metaphorical associations (softness is feminine) to masculinity and femininity. Children were seated in front of two large pictures with a row of Velcro along the bottom, one of a woman and a girl and one of a man and a boy. They were then presented with Velcro blocks with pictures on them; they were asked, "Does this go with the mommy and the little girl or with the daddy and the little boy?" and instructed to place the block on one picture or the other. Children who had passed the gender-labeling task had more extensive and accurate knowledge of gender schemas than did children who could not yet label gender. Knowing who is male and who is female seems to foster rapid learning of the cultural stereotypes related to gender. Some evidence suggests that toddler girls might learn at least some aspects of gender stereotypes earlier than do boys—in particular, for household activities (Poulin-Dubois, Serbin, Eichstedt, Sen, & Beissel, 2002).

Four-year-olds understand many of the conventional and metaphorical associations for gender (Leinbach, Hort, & Fagot, 1997), and some of these may bear on anger and aggression. Fagot and Leinbach (1993) have argued convincingly that gender schemas likely involve emotion. For example, even children as young as 3–5 years seem to associate overt expressions of anger with the male gender schema; they reliably designate line drawings of animals with angry faces as associated with "Daddy" as opposed to "Mommy" (Leinbach & Hort, 1995).

Interestingly, learning to label gender also appears to influence girls' social behavior. One study observed 21- to 40-month-old children in play groups and found that whether boys could label gender was unrelated to their aggression with peers (Fagot et al., 1986); for girls, however, those who could label gender showed lower levels of aggression than girls who could not. These findings suggest that when girls learn to tell the genders apart, they may quickly learn that girls are not supposed to hit and they may adjust their behavior accordingly.

Gender Segregation

Yet another way in which preschool children may begin to "do gender" is that they prefer to play with members of their own gender group. Preferences for same-gender play partners emerge in the toddler period (Serbin et al., 1994), and cross-gender friendships are rare as late as the early adolescent years (Gottman & Mettetal, 1986). Researchers have proposed several reasons why young boys and girls seem to prefer same-gender interactions and why girls' same-gender preferences develop slightly earlier in the third year than do those of boys (see Maccoby, 1998, for a thorough discussion). Perhaps boys and girls develop different play styles as a result of important differences in physiological and emotional arousal (Fabes, 1994). Boys and girls might naturally prefer same-gender peers because their play styles are more compatible with their own (Serbin et al., 1994). Girls might well recoil from boys because of boys' higher levels of bossy, rough, aggressive behavior (Maccoby, 1998). Perhaps children are more rewarded by peers and teachers for same-gender social behavior (Fagot, 1994). Or maybe simply having the concept of gender leads children to prefer peers who are "like me" (C. L. Martin, 1994).

Whatever the reasons, the fact that girls begin to play mostly with other girls during the preschool period likely reinforces lessons they are learning from adults about how girls and boys ought to behave. Girls may socialize each other to refrain from physical fighting. In a study investigating the contributions of temperamental arousability and same-gender interaction to children's peer status, highly arousable girls who frequently played with other girls showed a decrease in problem behaviors whereas highly aggressive boys who engaged in frequent same-gender play showed an increase in behavior problems (Fabes et al., 1997).

Preferring same-gender playmates may also be an important way in which children begin to carve out their identities as male and female. Brody (2000) has suggested a differentiation model of gender role identity in which children must alter their behaviors to be similar to those of their own gender: "If males hit, to be a 'real' girl means not to hit" (p. 6). Girls may work toward this differentiated gender role by segregating themselves from boys, by refraining from physical fighting, and perhaps even by resorting to more indirect expressions of anger and aggression.

Peer Relations and Preschool Girls' Anger and Aggression

Although the relation between aggression and peer rejection is less well studied for preschoolers than for other age groups, overt angry behavior seems to have different peer consequences even for young girls and boys. Observational research shows that both coping with anger by venting and being angered by interpersonal rejection are negatively related to being liked by peers for girls but not for boys (Fabes & Eisenberg, 1992). In general, girls' aggressive behaviors are less likely to influence peers than boys' aggression (Fagot & Hagan, 1985). In light of these findings, it would not be surprising if girls chose to refrain from being openly angry and aggressive because such behaviors invite social rejection and do not work very well to accomplish their social goals anyway.

Here it seems important to note that for both girls and boys physical aggression seems to often result in immediately being the target of socially rejecting behaviors (Arnold, Hanrock, Ortiz, & Stave, 1999). In this study, preschool children were carefully observed in classrooms to examine the temporal relation between physical aggression and rejecting behaviors. "Rejecting behaviors" were defined as actions that convey dislike or exclusion, and the investigators acknowledged that this category corresponds to social or relational aggression (Arnold et al., 1999). This study is important because it suggests that even for preschool children social aggression and physical aggression are intimately intertwined. Overt aggression is likely to be met with overt aggression, with also more subtle forms of hurtful, rejecting behavior.

Although there is more to say about peer responses to particular types of aggression in subsequent chapters in Part II on older age groups, before we leave preschool it seems important to point out that even among preschoolers physically aggressive children tend to hang around together. When 4-year-olds were observed during free play at preschool, children who spent time together were similar in their levels of aggression (defined broadly as name-calling, teasing, physically hurting someone with the intent to harm, or physically hurting someone to gain access to a desired object; Farver, 1996). In another study with preschool (high-risk sample) children, those rated by teachers as highly aggressive spent time with peers who had similar levels of aggression, although they seemed to have more difficulty establishing peer contacts (J. Snyder, Horsch, & Childs, 1997).

Of course, the processes by which aggressive peers affiliate together are unknown and there are several possibilities. Perhaps aggressive children are attracted to each other because of similarity, or perhaps aggressive children socialize each other to become more aggressive as they spend more time together (Kindermann, 1993). Or possibly aggressive children might seek each other out because they are disliked by peers and have no one but each other with whom to affiliate (Ladd, 1983). Understanding which or how all of these mechanisms might be operating for preschool children awaits longitudinal studies of social networks with young samples. Still, given that physically aggressive children socialize with each other for whatever reasons, it is interesting to speculate as to whether socially aggressive children might do the same. What if children who hurt others by social exclusion and friendship manipulation are drawn to each other for reasons of similarity, and what if they develop a peer culture in which these behaviors are frequent and perhaps highly effective?

SUMMARY: WHY MIGHT PRESCHOOL GIRLS PREFER SOCIAL TO PHYSICAL AGGRESSION?

At the end of each of these large developmental chapters, I summarize briefly what research to date suggests about six major themes running throughout this book: how girls express anger and behave aggressively; how social aggression occurs among girls; developmental differences in forms and functions of social aggression; developmental consequences of girls' social aggression; and possibilities for intervention. These are offered as short synopses of material discussed in detail throughout the body of each chapter:

• *What does research evidence suggest about how preschool girls express anger and behave aggressively?* Overall, research suggests that although preschool girls are fully capable of expressing anger, asserting their positions in disputes, and defending their own interests, the manner in which they do so may differ in subtle ways from that of boys. It is important to remember that many findings suggest that gender differences are small or nonexistent: preschool girls and boys do not differ on overall frequency or intensity of anger expressed, both girls and boys are likely to resolve conflicts using moderate persuasion attempts, younger preschool girls do not differ from boys on physical or verbal aggression, and several studies show no gender differences for social aggression. Still, the data suggest that compared to boys, preschool girls—perhaps especially older preschool girls—are less likely to vent when angry, more likely to be unpopular if they vent and show anger in response to interpersonal rejection, more likely to respond to provocation by socially rejecting the provocateur, more likely to try to mitigate conflicts, less likely to be involved in rough-and-tumble play, more likely to desist from physical aggression as they move through the preschool years, and perhaps more likely than boys to engage in relational aggression (although this depends very much on the sample and the methods used).

Research to date suggests that as girls move through the preschool period, most become less physically aggressive and social aggression may become more prominent in their behavioral repertoires than physical fighting. Although it is tempting to extend this argument to suggest that preschool girls are more socially aggressive than preschool boys, it seems important to refrain from drawing this conclusion because the few studies available show inconsistent findings.

• *How does social aggression unfold among preschool girls, and might this differ from social aggression in boys?* Research to date has provided little evidence as to the processes by which social aggression unfolds among young girls and whether this might differ from social aggression among boys. There is some initial evidence that social aggression may have more social importance for girls than for boys. Remember that girls are more likely to socially reject those who provoke them to anger than are boys, older preschool girls are more angered by social rejection than are younger preschool girls, and—for girls only—responding angrily to social rejection is related to being disliked by peers. Also, girls view responding to relational provocation with relational aggression as more wrong than boys do.

Most of the few studies available have measured social aggression with teacher ratings or peer nominations, which treat social aggression as a personality trait rather than as a behavioral phenomenon arising in a particular social context. It would be fascinating to know in which social situations social aggression is most likely to occur, and whether young boys and young girls enact social aggression in different ways. Observational research could be helpful in illuminating these processes, especially studies that use microanalytic codes and sequential analyses to examine interaction sequences.

• *Are there developmental differences in the forms and functions of social aggression?* Although the most thoughtful analysis of this question awaits our consideration of other age groups, evidence to date suggests that social aggression in the preschool years tends to take fairly overt, straightforward forms (see Crick et al., 1999, for a detailed discussion). Whereas older children may be likely to practice friendship manipulation, social exclusion, and malicious gossip in fairly complex and subtle ways, preschoolers are more likely to engage in fairly direct behaviors such as threatening not to invite others to a birthday party if they do not comply with demands, or executing the silent treatment by putting hands over their ears and singing loudly when someone else tries to talk with them.

• *What are the developmental antecedents of social aggression among girls? How and why might girls come to express anger and aggression in this particular way?* The fact that preschool girls become more socially aggressive than physically aggressive demands an explanation, whether or not they are more socially aggressive than boys are. Although few published studies to date have examined the early origins of social aggression, the fact that girls' anger and aggression may begin to take this form fits in fascinating ways with the research described on emotion socialization, gender labeling and segregation, and peer relations. Girls may be more adept at emotion regulation than boys are, and more skilled in following social conventions to mask negative emotions in the heat of the moment. This suggests that girls may be able to refrain from open, angry displays and keep their composure while enacting a more indirect, subtle response. When young girls do behave angrily, their mothers and teachers are highly likely to ignore them or tell them to stop, but their mothers seem to welcome discussing emotions afterward and focus on relationships in these conversations. Young girls are more responsive than young boys are to teachers' directives, which suggests that they might be more sensitive to the danger of being punished for overt aggression and perhaps more likely to resort to indirect means. When young girls learn to label gender and begin to refrain from physical aggression but still feel anger, it is not hard to imagine that they might cope with their fury by more indirect means, perhaps in ways that involve talking with others and using relationships to inflict harm.

• *What are the developmental consequences of girls' anger and aggression?* Because we have only begun to study children's social aggression in the preschool years, there is still much to learn about the developmental consequences of engaging in social aggression at such a young age. There is some evidence that being nominated by preschool peers as high on relational aggression is related to peer rejection (Crick, Casas, & Mosher, 1997) and that for girls responding angrily to peer rejection is related to being disliked. Therefore, it seems that even among very young children, there is a social price paid for perpetrating social aggression and for being upset by victimization.

• *What does research on the processes involved in social aggression suggest for intervention?* Few studies to date have illuminated the processes by which social aggression occurs among preschoolers. One exception is an investigation showing that physically aggressive behavior is almost always followed by rejecting behavior by peers, including some forms of social aggression. If we knew even more about the settings and interpersonal contexts in which social aggression is likely, the responses it elicits, the conditions that prolong it or discourage it, we might have some clues that could be useful for interrupting these behaviors in prevention or intervention programs.

FUTURE RESEARCH

Additional studies with young children are desperately needed to understand the development of social aggression in the preschool years. Fascinating questions remain to be tested; the following is almost certainly an incomplete list:

• How normative and frequent is social aggression among preschoolers, and can gender differences be observed reliably?
• Is social aggression stable across the preschool years, as physical aggression seems to be for boys?
• Is early social aggression related to qualities of temperament?
• How are qualities of parent–child relationships related to social aggression? Are children with insecure attachments to parents

more likely to feel threatened and to respond with social aggression? How are parenting styles and practices related to social aggression?

- How do parents respond to young children's social aggression? Do parents perceive these behaviors to be hurtful and wrong, and do they try to discourage children from engaging in them? Do parents know whether their children engage in these behaviors with peers at school?

- How do preschool teachers perceive and respond to social aggression? Do they attempt to discipline children for this form of hurtful behavior? Can teachers structure preschool classroom environments to foster a sense of community and belongingness and to discourage social aggression?

- Are gender labeling and stereotyping related to social aggression? When girls learn to label gender, do they begin to engage in more social aggression? Are girls higher on knowledge of stereotyping more likely to be socially aggressive?

- Are the peer consequences of engaging in social aggression similar for girls and boys? Do girls who engage in social aggression tend to congregate together, or do girls' groups encourage this behavior in their members, or both? Does social aggression occur within preschool girls' friendships?

- How does social aggression develop during the transition from preschool to kindergarten? Are socially aggressive children or their victims likely to have more difficulty with this transition?

Perhaps most importantly, how might these early developments in girls' anger and aggression lay the groundwork for girls to engage in social aggression during childhood, and beyond?

Middle Childhood
Gossip, Gossip, Evil Thing?

I was always mean to people outside my group like Crystal, and Emily Fiore; they both moved schools. . . . I had this gummy bear necklace, with pearls around it, and gummy bears. She came up to me one day and pulled my necklace off. . . . [I]t was my favorite necklace, and I got all of my friends, and all of the guys even in the class, to revolt against her. No one liked her. That's why she moved schools, because she tore my gummy bear necklace off and everyone hated her. They were like, "That was mean. She didn't deserve that. We hate you."
  —HILARY, A FOURTH-GRADE CLIQUE LEADER (in Adler & Adler, 1995, p. 153)

In fifth grade I came into a new class and I knew nobody. None of my friends from the year before were in my class. So I get to school a week late, and Amy comes up to me and she was like, "Hi Julie, how are you? Where were you? You look so pretty." And I was like, wow, she's so nice. And she was being so nice for like, two weeks, kiss-ass major. And then she started pulling her bitch moves. Maybe it was for a month that she was nice. And then she had clawed me into her clique and her group, and so she won me over that way, but then she was a bitch to me once I was inside it, and I couldn't get out because I had no other friends. 'Cause I'd gone in there and already been accepted into the popular clique and her group, and so she won me over that way, but then was such a bitch to me once I was inside it, and I couldn't get out because I had no other friends. 'Cause I'd gone in there and already been accepted into the popular clique, so everyone else in the class didn't like me, so I had nowhere else to go.
—JULIE, FIFTH-GRADE MEMBER OF A POPULAR CLIQUE (in Adler & Adler, 1995, p. 149)

Gossip, gossip, evil thing.
Much unhappiness it brings.
If you can't say something nice,
Don't talk at all is my advice.

Gossip often breaks up friendships,
Even ruins somebody's life.
Do as much as any one thing can,
To separate a man from wife.

Wagging tongue abomination,
Self-control a precious jewel.
Even in your conversations,
You should practice Golden Rule.
—CHILDHOOD SONG, ORIGIN UNKNOWN

Social aggression may become even more prominent during middle
childhood (from about age 6 to age 12) because children strongly value
feeling accepted by their same-gender peer groups, seek to avoid embarrassment at all costs, and work hard to stay cool, calm, and collected
as they manage disagreements with peers (Gottman & Mettetal, 1986).
Social aggression might serve as an important strategy for acting on angry feelings without losing composure in the presence of the provocateur and without facing the threat of expulsion from the peer group
that direct anger expressions might bring. Social aggression might also
serve as a way for children, girls but perhaps also boys, to reassure
themselves about their own belongingness and acceptance by excluding others. Negative evaluation gossip about peers might serve as a
means of testing and confirming the boundaries of acceptable behavior
(Gottman & Mettetal, 1986). Spreading nasty rumors and excluding
others may also promote group cohesion (Adler & Adler, 1995).

For the best understanding of social aggression among girls in
middle childhood, it is important to consider research on the more
broad range of ways that girls express anger and pursue their social
goals: anger, conflict, rough-and-tumble play, physical aggression, and
verbal aggression. Most research to date on social aggression has focused on the middle-childhood age range. Social aggression in middle
childhood begins to take more subtle and complex forms as children
use indirect means (phone calls, online communication, and even old-
fashioned note passing) as well as face-to-face interactions to manipulate friendships and undermine others' social relationships. Whether
researchers find gender differences in social aggression in middle
childhood depends on the method used; gender differences are often
apparent in teacher ratings, less frequent in peer nomination studies,
and even less apparent in observational investigations.

Regardless of whether girls in middle childhood are more socially
aggressive than their male peers, they certainly are more socially aggressive than they are physically aggressive, and this demands an explanation. To explore why girls might engage in social aggression during
this developmental period, this chapter examines previous research on
temperament, emotion regulation, parental relationships, gender stereotypes, social information processing, and peer relationships. The
goal of the following sections is to point out clues from existing work
about why girls engage in social aggression and what it means to them.

FORMS OF ANGRY, AGGRESSIVE BEHAVIOR
AMONG GIRLS IN MIDDLE CHILDHOOD

Anger

Because children in this age range strive for emotional composure (Gottman & Mettetal, 1986), becoming angry with peers presents a challenge. Surprisingly, relatively little research has specifically examined the broad range of ways that school-age children manage anger with peers (although many more studies have focused on aggression; see Lemerise & Dodge, 2000).

Most studies of children's anger to date have utilized hypothetical vignettes or self-report measures, and a distinctive picture of girls' anger in this age range has yet to emerge. One such study explored children's understanding of display rules for anger—that is, social conventions about when it is appropriate to express anger and when it is not (Underwood, Coie, & Herbsman, 1992). We showed third-, fifth-, and seventh-grade children videotaped vignettes of anger-provoking situations, some with peers and some with teachers. We asked participants how they would feel, what they would do, and why. Both boys and girls reported they would express anger much more openly toward peers than teachers. The patterns of gender differences varied with age. Younger girls said they would mask anger more than boys would, but older girls said they would express anger more openly than boys would. For this African American sample, we speculated that older boys reported more masking because they were practiced in "playing the dozens," engaging in verbal banter, including ritual insults, in which being able to stay calm and "chill" is of premium importance. For girls, becoming more formidable in their assertiveness with age may come as a result of growing social confidence, or an increasing ability to assert their own needs as well as being considerate of others (Gilligan, 1982).

Although children may say they are more openly expressive of anger with peers than with teachers, they are still wary of expressing anger in interactions with other children. In another vignette study with a mostly European American sample in the northwestern United States, second-, fourth-, and sixth graders responded to hypothetical vignettes describing a variety of types of emotion-provoking situations, including anger (Underwood, 1997). Children said they would be much less expressive of anger, as compared to other emotions, and reported that all types of responses to anger would invite peer rejection (including masking anger by showing an opposite emotion, masking by showing no emotion, a moderated expression of anger, and a full, intense anger expression). There were no gender differences in endorsing anger expressions. In this study, older children reported that they would express emotions more openly than did younger children.

Girls and boys alike seem aware that the consequences of showing anger toward peers can be grave, that others may not like you no matter what you do, and that even showing anger to an observer (not the target) may be ill advised. Even in the presence of neutral observers, first, third, and fifth graders reported that they would be much more likely to mask anger in the presence of a "medium friend" than with either parent (Zeman & Garber, 1996). In another study, school-age children anticipated negative reactions to anger expressions regardless of whether the observer was a best friend or a medium friend (Zeman & Shipman, 1996).

Other research suggests that children respond differently when angry toward friends than when angry toward acquaintances and that girls might be more distressed than boys when a friend treats them badly. In one study, 11- and 12-year-olds and 13- to 15-year-olds read vignettes describing name-calling and indicated how they would respond to this behavior from a friend and from other classmates (Whitesell & Harter, 1996). As compared to their interactions with other classmates, participants said that with those who were friends they would feel more violated, more often feel blends of emotions (mostly anger and sadness), be more likely to share responsibility for the conflict (even though the precipitating event was name-calling), and try to restore the relationship by directly discussing the issue. Girls reported that they would feel more violated and experience more negative emotions as a result of the name-calling than did boys. In another study, when 7- to 11-year-olds were asked to describe recent angry experiences with peers, girls said that they more often felt anger related to social and control issues than did boys, and that they responded to provocation with more affiliative strategies (Murphy & Eisenberg, 1996).

Across this handful of investigations using questionnaires and hypothetical vignettes, some intriguing gender differences have been found in individual studies, but few of these have emerged consistently. Some studies find few gender differences for anger experiences or expressions (Underwood, 1997; Zeman & Shipman, 1996). Other evidence indicates that girls feel more hurt by name-calling (Whitesell & Harter, 1996), older school-age girls express anger more openly (Underwood et al., 1992), and girls report more affiliative responses when angry than do boys (Murphy & Eisenberg, 1996). One reason for these discrepant findings may be that questionnaires and hypothetical vignettes may be invalid because children respond in socially desirable ways or simply cannot accurately report how they manage anger in the heat of the moment.

To overcome some of these challenges and to learn more about how children actually behave when provoked, our research group developed a laboratory method for inducing a mild degree of anger toward a peer (Underwood, Hurley, Johanson, & Mosley, 1999). Children in the second, fourth, and sixth grades (approximately 8, 10, and 12 years old) participated in play sessions during which they played a computer game and interacted with a same-age, same-gender peer confederate. Participants experienced two types of provocation: repeatedly losing at a computer game they were playing for a desirable prize, and being taunted by the peer actor. Play sessions were videotaped and coded for facial expressions, verbalizations, and gestures in response to the provocation.

We chose this method to maximize ecological validity but also designed the procedures to adhere to our ethical responsibilities to protect children from harm and to ensure that their overall experience with us was positive. Clinical observations indicate that one of the most challenging types of provocation for children is teasing or taunting related to competence or achievement. When asked to describe what most makes them angry with peers or with siblings, sixth graders cite being disturbed in play, mockery, and bragging (Karniol & Heiman, 1987). Children anticipate that peer encounters will provide them with opportunities for learning, self-competence, sociability, developing relationships, and feeling a sense of belonging (Zarbatany, Hartmann, & Rankin, 1990). By violating these expectations by having children lose and be teased, we believed that we would be able to induce a mild degree of anger in most participants.

However, we were also very careful to embed the provoking segment in a larger, positive context. Children were with us for more than an hour; the provoking part of the experiment lasted 10 minutes at most. Children were repeatedly told how to stop participating if they wished, they were carefully and fully debriefed, they remained with us for 20–30 minutes of positive play with the peer actor after debriefing, they were given a prize and snack and payment for their help, and they were encouraged to contact us with concerns (and we contacted a subset of them to assess any negative effects of participating). We used these procedures with more than 600 families: no child or parent ever complained about any feature of our study, and more than 95% of participants were willing to take part in follow-up questionnaire studies.

Overall, the results of this large observational study indicated that most children remained remarkably composed when provoked, in keeping with the theory that school-age children strongly value emotional control (Gottman & Mettetal, 1986). Overall, older children were less expressive of anger or distress than younger children: they maintained more neutral facial expressions, made fewer gestures, were more likely to keep quiet when provoked, and made fewer negative comments when they did speak.

Although there were some significant gender differences, the magnitude of these was smaller than would be expected on the basis of previous questionnaire and vignettes studies. For example, for mean proportions of verbal responses, girls were more likely than boys to keep quiet (54% vs. 48%), less likely to make negative comments (10% vs. 13%), more likely to make self-negative statements (8% vs. 6%), less likely to talk about specifics of the game (7% vs. 9%), and less likely to make positive comments (3% vs. 4%).

Gender differences in anger expression might have been smaller here because the situation was structured, children knew they were being observed, and the peer was unfamiliar. Still, these modest gender differences suggest that caution is needed in interpreting the gender differences shown in the vignette/questionnaire studies. Caution is further warranted by the fact that in this same study children's observed responses to the provocation were only very modestly—if at all—related to self-reports of their own behavior immediately following the provocation (Underwood & Bjornstad, 2001).

In another recent pair of observational investigations, 8-year-old children were provoked by losing at a game and being cheated by a confederate actor (Hubbard, 2001; Hubbard et al., 2002). In the first study (Hubbard, 2001), boys responded more angrily than did girls in their facial expressions, gestures, and verbal intonation (the content of verbalizations was not coded). Aggressive and nonaggressive children did not differ in their anger expressions, although peer-rejected children showed more facial and verbal anger than did children with average peer status. In a subsequent study that used these same procedures with the addition of physiological measures (heart rate and skin conductance; Hubbard et al., 2002), reactive aggression as assessed by teacher ratings was related to skin conductance reactivity and to angry nonverbal behaviors, but proactive aggression was not related to physiological arousal or to anger expression in this context. Interestingly, in this second and larger study, no gender differences were evident in how children expressed or experienced anger in response to the provocation.

In summary, despite widespread beliefs that anger is the province of men and boys, observed gender differences in anger in particular social contexts are not always dramatic (Kring, 2000). With the exception of boys being more physically aggressive than girls, the bulk of the evidence so far indicates that boys and girls seem to experience and express anger in fairly similar ways. However, it is important to note that few observational data are available, and those that are were collected in competitive game situations with unfamiliar peers (Hubbard, 2001; Underwood et al., 1999). These situations were likely more compelling for boys, and not well suited for eliciting more social, subtle forms of anger expressions, perhaps because established relationships were less at stake. Existing data offer clues that girls may feel more distress when angered by peers, perhaps especially by close friends (Whitesell & Harter, 1996), and that girls' anger more often focuses on social concerns (Murphy & Eisenberg, 1996).

Conflict

Rather than focusing on overt displays of particular emotions, other research has addressed how children resolve disputes, regardless of the particular emotions or behaviors. Conflicts only sometimes feature anger and aggression, and focusing on conflict as the unit of analysis illuminates the broad range of both positive and negative ways that children resolve disagreements. Conflicts confront children with critical decisions, such as whether to resolve the conflict so as to preserve the relationship or to be so assertive or overbearing that they risk losing it (Laursen, Hartup, & Koplas, 1996).

Experts seem to disagree as to whether girls and boys resolve conflicts differently. Early investigators did not hypothesize gender differences. In one study, conflict episodes were observed during 10 hour-long sessions in same-gender play groups of a dozen first and second graders, with sociometric data collected before and after the 10 sessions to assess peer status (D. W. Shantz, 1986). Conflicts were coded according to a rigorous definition requiring that an initiator attempted to influence a target, the target resisted, and the initiator persisted. Rates of conflict were quite high; approximately 23 conflict episodes were coded per one-hour session with 12 children. Boys were observed to engage in higher rates of conflicts than did girls, but patterns of relationships between conflict and peer status did not differ by gender. Conflict participation was related to physical but not verbal aggression, and engaging in conflict was related to being disliked even when aggression was controlled statistically (the converse was not true).

Another observational study compared how 9- and 10-year-old friends and nonfriends resolved a conflict when they were told to play a board game by different rules; no gender differences were predicted (Hartup, French, Laursen, Johnston, & Ogawa, 1993). The results showed that, for both genders, conflicts between friends lasted longer and were more intense than conflicts between nonfriends. Interestingly, gender differences emerged only for conflicts with friends; girls used assertions with rationales more than did boys and boys used assertions without explanations more than did girls.

Reviewers of the conflict literature have differed in their emphasis of gender. One early and otherwise thorough review barely mentioned gender (C. U. Shantz, 1987). Another review of conflict and social competence considered conflict more broadly as occurring in situations involving group entry, limited resources, and provocation (Putallaz & Sheppard, 1992), and highlighted interesting gender differences. This review concluded that in resolving conflicts, girls are more likely than boys to focus on preserving relationships whereas boys are more likely to assert their power and status. Putallaz and Sheppard (1992) concluded that girls are more likely to struggle with conflict situations involving group entry whereas boys have more difficulty with provocation. Another thoughtful review discussed how conflicts can be understood in terms of social exchange and emotional investment, that individuals interact in relationships so as to preserve rewards and minimize costs. Because peer relationships are voluntary and can be highly rewarding, close peers often resolve conflicts in ways that preserve the relationship (Laursen et al., 1996). This review did not comment on whether girls and boys might differ in their goals and strategies for resolving conflicts with close friends.

Although the suggestion that girls are more likely than boys to resolve conflicts in ways that preserve relationships is intuitively appealing, evidence on this point is mixed. In one observational study with 5- and 7-year-olds described in full in Chapter 5, girls were more likely to try to diffuse conflicts whereas boys were more assertive and insistent (P. M. Miller et al., 1986). In another study in which 6-year-olds were observed as they interacted with unfamiliar same-gender peers, girls' disputes were briefer than boys' were, and girls with high peer status had fewer conflicts than all other groups and were also more likely to provide explanations when engaged in conflict (Putallaz, Hellstem, Sheppard, Grimes, & Glodis, 1995). But in another study with 6-year-olds, girls reported that they were involved in interpersonal, nonaggressive conflicts more than were boys, and there were no gender differences for resolving conflicts with coercion (Crockenberg & Laurie, 1996). Another recent vignette study showed that for both genders conflict goals and strategies are related in reasonable ways, and that girls and boys did not differ on their endorsement of relationship goals (Chung & Asher, 1996). However, girls were lower than boys on control goals and higher on avoidance, and for strategies, boys endorsed more hostile coercive tactics whereas girls advocated more prosocial/passive strategies.

Gender differences in conflict goals and strategies may be more apparent in the context of close friendships. When presented with hypothetical conflict scenarios with close friends, fourth- and fifth-grade girls more strongly endorsed goals of relationship maintenance whereas boys rated instrumental-control goals more highly than did girls (A. J. Rose & Asher, 1999). Girls were higher on their ratings of accommodation/compromise-type strategies, whereas boys said they were more likely to use self-interest assertion and hostile strategies (including verbal aggression, leaving, and threatening to end the friendship). For both boys and girls, revenge goals and hostile strategies were negatively related to the number of best friends each had and to conflicts with friends.

Just as for research on anger, the data on conflict to date do not suggest consistent large gender differences in how girls and boys respond to conflicts, but context may make all the difference. With friends, girls seem to be more prosocial and concerned with maintaining the relationship than do boys. However, note that here again the methods used so far may not be well suited to detecting gender differences in resolving conflicts that are less overt. Most studies involve observing conflicts in play groups of only casually acquainted peers, an approach that requires that a conflictual encounter be obvious enough to be detected by outside observers (P. M. Miller et al., 1986; D. W. Shantz, 1986) or occurs in situations involving games or competitions (Hartup et al., 1993). If girls have a distinctive style of resolving conflicts, this might be most apparent for group entry situations (Putallaz & Sheppard, 1992), or in disputes involving friendships and social status that might be difficult for outside observers to detect (Crick & Grotpeter, 1995). Research with adolescents suggests that conflicts are often resolved by disengagement—simply withdrawing from the interaction. This might be difficult to discern in observational studies, especially those with definitions of conflict that require resistance and persistence.

Rough-and-Tumble Play

Just as not all conflicts are angry, all physical play and even some forms of fighting are not angry or aggressive. As defined by Pellegrini and Smith (1998), "Rough-and-tumble play refers to vigorous behaviors such as wrestling, grappling, kicking, and tumbling that would appear to be aggressive except for the playful context" (p. 579). The frequency of rough-and-tumble play peaks in middle childhood; from 7 to 11 years of age, rough-and-tumble play constitutes about 10% of children's playground behavior (Humphreys & Smith, 1987).

The immediate consequences of rough-and-tumble play may differ depending on the social status of the child engaging in the behavior. An observational study with kindergarten, second-, and fourth-grade children found that rough-and-tumble play led to different proximal outcomes for children who were well liked and those who were disliked by peers (Pellegrini, 1988). Popular and rejected children did not differ in their overall rates of rough-and-tumble play. For rejected children rough-and-tumble play more often led to physical aggression, whereas for popular children rough-and-tumble play was more often followed by playing games with rules and was positively correlated with being able to generate a variety of solutions to social problems (gender was not examined in this study).

Other research indicates that across cultures and even other mammalian species, females engage in less rough-and-tumble play than do boys (Pellegrini & Smith, 1998). However, gender differences may depend on the particular form of rough-and-tumble play. For example, an observational study with 8- and 11-year-olds in Great Britain found that, although girls did less initiating of chasing and play boxing/hitting than boys, girls and boys did not differ on participating in chasing and wrestling (Boulton, 1996).

What might it mean that girls may engage in some forms of rough-and-tumble play less than do boys? Developmentalists have argued that rough-and-tumble play may serve important developmental functions: the opportunity to practice and develop fighting skills, a safe mechanism for establishing dominance, and perhaps even experience in emotion coding and emotion regulation (although the evidence is less clear on the this last point; see Pellegrini & Smith, 1998). That girls may be deprived of chances to practice fighting skills seems not to be surprising or worrisome given their overall lower levels of physical aggression, but it is interesting to speculate about other ways in which girls might seek to establish dominance.

For girls, might some forms of social aggression function similarly to rough-and-tumble play? Children in this age range seem to engage in some teasing forms of social exclusion, with positive affect evidenced by all. For example, one child might jokingly say to another approaching the lunch table, "Hey, let's be snobs. You're not cool enough to sit with us today," at which time all involved laugh. Still, the lesson about who has the higher status may be all too clear. Children's gossip may also at times be accompanied by positive affect, high glee, as children swap stories of great entertainment value but little real consequence. Although research has yet to explore this question, it seems possible that these types of behaviors might be ways that girls practice asserting dominance or confirming their own belongingness, in a manner similar to rough-and-tumble play for boys.

Physical Aggression

The bulk of the research evidence suggests that most children engage in less aggression as they move through middle childhood, though a few escalate and fight more (see Coie & Dodge, 1998, for a thorough review). However, developmental trends may depend on who reports the aggression. According to one large household survey of youth, levels of physical aggression increase across the childhood years, and peak just after middle childhood, around age 14, for both girls and boys (Lahey et al., 2000). In another study with a high-risk sample of the brothers and sisters of delinquent boys, maternal reports indicated no developmental differences in physical aggression for children ages 4–18 (Tiet, Wasserman, Loeber, McReynolds, & Miller, 2001).

If there is one point on which almost all experts agree, it is that girls engage in less physical fighting than do boys (for reviews, see Coie & Dodge, 1998; Hyde, 1984; Knight, Fabes, & Higgins, 1996; Maccoby, 1998; Maccoby & Jacklin, 1974). This pronounced gender difference seems apparent by the time children enter organized schooling and remains through the rest of the lifespan.

Some have argued that in modern times gender differences in aggression have been decreasing (Hyde, 1984), perhaps due to more egalitarian treatment of girls and boys. As intuitively appealing and even hopeful as this suggestion might seem, it is not supported by data.

A more recent meta-analysis suggests that gender differences in aggression have remained remarkably stable when the methods for measuring aggression are considered (Knight et al., 1996). For example, gender differences are typically smaller in experimental studies in the laboratory, and larger in naturalistic and correlational studies. The fact that more recent investigations are experimental accounts for the seeming decline in the magnitude of gender differences; in fact, study characteristics accounted for 65% of the variance in effect size. For gender differences in aggression, the median effect size for the more than 100 studies reviewed was around .5, usually considered to be a medium-sized effect (Cohen, 1988).

What does even more recent research suggest about gender differences in physical aggression? In a large survey of a nationally representative sample of more than 1,000 youth, boys engaged in more physical aggression than did girls according to both parent and youth reports (Lahey et al., 2000). However, other recent studies confirm the proposition that context as well as study characteristics influence the magnitude of the findings. For the longitudinal Child Development Project, growth analyses for externalizing behaviors from kindergarten through seventh grade showed that, whereas teachers perceived that boys were higher than girls on externalizing problems and had greater growth over time, mothers did not perceive gender differences (Keiley, Bates, Dodge, & Pettit, 2000). When a sample of aggressive children and a matched sample of nonaggressive children were observed on a playground by investigators using remote audiovisual recording, there were no gender differences in the frequency of physical aggression (Pepler, Craig, & Roberts, 1998). These results suggest that whether gender differences are evident may depend on the social context (Underwood et al., 2001b); even highly aggressive children may only fight in very particular circumstances (Wright, Zakriski, & Drinkwater, 1999).

Before moving on to discuss forms of aggression that may be more typical among girls, I should note that some girls do fight and that understanding how and why is important (Cairns & Cairns, 1994). Just as the lack of research on heart disease among women is unfortunate, the paucity of research on physical aggression among girls is lamentable. Recent statistics strongly suggest that the rates of physical violence among young women are increasing faster than the rates for young men. For example, from 1981 to 1997 the violent crime rate for juvenile males increased by 20%, whereas the comparable rate for juvenile females nearly doubled (H. N. Snyder & Sickmund, 1999). Other research suggests that for girls, engaging in physical aggression may be more strongly linked to depression (Obeidallah & Earls, 1999). Childhood aggression may predict different later outcomes for girls than for boys—for example, adolescent motherhood (Miller-Johnson et al., 1999; Underwood, Kupersmidt, & Coie, 1996). Physical aggression in girls and boys may follow different developmental trajectories (Loeber & Stouthamer-Loeber, 1998); longitudinal studies of physical aggression among girls are badly needed.

Verbal Aggression

Cross-cultural data suggest that, of the total aggressive behaviors engaged in by 8- and 11-year-olds, some 30–40% of these behaviors involve verbal aggression by both girls and boys (Osterman et al., 1998). Given that girls are often found to fight physically less than boys do, it has long been tempting to assume that girls are more verbally aggressive.

Remember from Chapter 5 that investigators have struggled with how to define verbal aggression (McCabe & Lipscomb, 1988), and this challenge has become all the more formidable since the other constructs for nonphysical aggression have been introduced. As discussed in Chapter 2, it may be helpful to conceive of verbal aggression as hurtful speech that does not specifically harm friendships or social status (such as some forms of insults, name-calling, and threats).

Experts disagree as to whether there are gender differences in verbal aggression. Many studies show no gender differences, and those that find a difference show that boys are more verbally aggressive than are girls (Maccoby & Jacklin, 1974; McCabe & Lipscomb, 1988). However, there is one notable exception. Classroom observations of 7- to 11-year-old children in Great Britain found that girls engaged in more verbal aggression than did boys (verbal aggression was defined as "insulting words or statements directed at another child"; Archer, Pearson, & Westeman, 1988, p. 384). Perhaps the contradictory evidence for gender differences in verbal aggression is due to the fact that many of these studies were observational, and verbal aggression may be difficult for observers to detect both because it can be subtle and more frequently deployed in settings to which observers may not have access (restrooms, school buses, and the like). Also, in the Archer and colleagues (1988) study, verbal aggression was defined broadly enough that social aggression may also have been involved, and this may have obscured gender differences in the more overt, direct forms of verbal aggression.

In an attempt to surmount these challenges, recently investigators have used peer ratings to measure verbal aggression, following the logic that peers are more able to observe each other across settings. One peer-rating measure developed primarily to assess indirect aggression includes a subscale for verbal aggression, the Direct and Indirect Aggression Scales (DIAS; Bjorkqvist, Lagerspetz, & Kaukiainen, 1992). In a study using this measure with five different cultural groups, peers consistently rated boys as more verbally aggressive than girls (Osterman et al., 1994). In another cross-cultural study examining the proportions of girls' and boys' aggressive behaviors that were direct, indirect, and verbal, there were no gender differences for the proportion of aggressive behaviors that were verbal (Osterman et al., 1998).

Most research to date suggests that there are no clear gender differences in verbal aggression. However, an unfortunate by-product of increasing focus on indirect/relational/social aggression has been decreasing attention to verbal aggression in recent years. Future research should continue to explore specific forms of verbal aggression (teasing, ritual insults, and name-calling), how these occur in particular social contexts, and how these might serve different functions for girls and for boys (for an interesting discussion of the scant research to date on teasing, see Lightner, Bollmer, Harris, Milich, & Scrambler, 2000).

Social Aggression

As children develop cognitively, the frequency of social aggression among children may increase from early to middle childhood because manipulating relationships requires complex thinking (Bjorkqvist, 1994;

Crick et al., 1999; Tremblay, 2000). To date, however, this interesting idea remains speculative because few cross-sectional or longitudinal studies are available to assess developmental differences in social aggression. Comparing across studies suggests that social aggression may take more sophisticated forms as children mature (Crick et al., 1999). For example, whereas preschoolers might baldly state, "Play what I want or you're not my best friend anymore!," older children may be more subtle, instead organizing others in the peer group to threaten or exclude a peer.

Chapter 2 discussed in detail the different constructs for understanding the less direct, more social forms of aggression (indirect/social/relational aggression) and the methods used to study them. Most research to date on indirect/social/relational aggression has been conducted with middle childhood samples, and the number of studies is rapidly increasing. The following subsections highlight the results of these investigations and, for clarity of presentation and because results depend heavily on methods, will be organized by type of method used: self-reports, semistructured interviews, parent and teacher reports, peer ratings, peer nominations, and observations.

Self-Report Questionnaires

Self-report measures of social aggression have included fairly direct questionnaires about perpetrating social aggression, questionnaires about how boys and girls generally respond when angry, measures that ask for children's responses to specific vignettes, and measures of victimization. Studies using direct self-report measures of social aggression have yielded inconsistent results. In one study, girls reported using less relational aggression than did boys (Crick & Grotpeter, 1995), but in another there were no gender differences for engaging in indirect aggression (Craig, 1998). Because self-reports are at best only weakly correlated with peer ratings of indirect aggression (Lagerspetz et al., 1988), Bjorkqvist, Lagerspetz, and Kaukiainen (1992) argued strongly that self-reports are not valid measures of indirect aggression. Children may be reluctant to disclose perpetrating indirect aggression, and some of these behaviors might be so subtle that they do not know they are engaging in them.

Other questionnaire measures ask children to report what boys and girls generally do when they are angry or mean to hurt someone. When asked, "What do boys/girls do when they are mad at someone?" 9- to 12-year-olds reported that the most likely behavior of girls is relational aggression and the most likely behavior of boys is physical aggression (Crick et al., 1996). When the same sample was asked what girls and boys do when they want to hurt someone, they reported relational and verbal aggression for girls and physical and verbal aggression for boys. These fascinating results support the claim that children view subtle harmful behaviors as aggressive (indicating anger and intent to harm). As interesting and intuitively appealing as the gender differences are, it is important to remember that the data were from self-report questionnaires and that children's responses may have been strongly influenced by stereotypes of girls as backbiting and manipulative and boys as fighters, stereotypes that may or may not have bases in fact.

Other researchers have studied indirect/relational/social aggression by asking children to respond to hypothetical vignettes. To investigate whether children perceive social aggression as harmful, fourth, seventh, and tenth graders responded to hypothetical vignettes describing social and physical aggression (Galen & Underwood, 1997). Whereas boys reported that social aggression hurts less than physical aggression, girls perceived social and physical aggression to be equally hurtful. When children were asked, "How often does this behavior happen in the group of people you hang around with?," there were no gender differences for frequency of social aggression for fourth or seventh graders, although tenth-grade girls reported more social aggression than did tenth-grade boys. There were no clear developmental differences for hurtfulness or frequency.

In another vignette study, fourth and sixth graders responded to a measure describing peer conflicts (adopted from Chung & Asher, 1996) and rated different types of goals and strategies, including relational aggression (Delveaux & Daniels, 2000). There were no gender differences in the endorsement of relationally aggressive strategies. Relationally aggressive strategies were related to particular types of social goals: avoiding trouble and preserving relationships with the larger peer group. Interestingly, endorsing relationally aggressive strategies was negatively related to the desire to maintain the relationship with the target peer, as if the children understood that they might risk an individual friendship to enhance their larger-group status.

Other studies using self-report measures have asked children to report on victimization, specifically how frequently they are the target of social aggression. Self-reported frequency of victimization by social aggression has been shown to be related to low self-concept, especially for girls (Paquette & Underwood, 1999), and to loneliness and depression (Crick & Grotpeter, 1996). Neither of these studies found gender differences, nor did another investigation using similar methods (Phelps, 2001).

Although there may not be clear gender differences in the reported frequency of experiencing victimization by social aggression, other evidence suggests that girls may be more troubled by social aggression than are boys. In response to hypothetical vignettes describing relational aggression, girls reported that they would be more upset than boys would (Crick, 1995; Galen & Underwood, 1997). Girls may also respond differently than boys when victims of social aggression. In another vignette study, girls were more likely to respond to relational aggression by problem solving and seeking support than were boys (Phelps, 2001; here note that the same gender difference was found for overt aggression).

Semistructured Interviews

Other investigators asked children to describe their experiences of social aggression in semistructured interviews. In their longitudinal study following children from fourth through ninth grades, Cairns, Cairns, Neckerman, and colleagues (1989) conducted yearly interviews about the specific peers in school who bothered them and two recent conflicts with peers. Conflicts were coded for physical aggression and social ostracism (defined as "including active rejection of persons from a clique, slander, and defamation of reputation by gossip, and alienation of affection"; p. 321). The results showed that with increasing age, whereas physical aggression remained prominent in boys' peer conflicts, social aggression became more evident in older girls' conflicts. Only 10% of the conflicts described by fourth-grade girls featured social aggression, but by seventh grade more than one-third of girls' conflicts involved social aggression (at both ages, boys reported no conflicts involving social aggression). That children offered these accounts of social alienation in response to an open-ended question about conflicts provides convincing evidence of the robustness of the phenomenon and its salience for girls. However, given that children were asked to describe only two conflicts over a whole year, these data tell us less about gender and developmental differences in the daily occurrence of social aggression.

Parent and Teacher Reports

In an effort to avoid biases inherent in self-reports, other investigators have asked parents or teachers to report on children's relational aggression. Adult reporters have the advantage of being sensitive informants who can discriminate among different forms of aggression (Crick, Casas, & Mosher, 1997). However, disadvantages of relying on adult reports are that adults may not be privy to subtle forms of social aggression enacted in private settings and they may also be more subject to influence by gender stereotypes of girls as catty and backbiting (Underwood et al., 2001b).

Adult reporter studies have yielded mixed reports for gender and developmental differences. One study with a high-risk sample (brothers and sisters of delinquent boys) found that mothers reported similar levels of relational aggression in sons and daughters ages 4–18 and that relational aggression was most frequent in early adolescence (Tiet et al., 2001). Whether these findings would be replicated for normative samples remains unknown. Another study with a large, normal sample found that teachers of third- through sixth-grade children report that girls are more relationally aggressive than boys are, with no developmental differences (Crick, 1996). In this study, correlations between teacher ratings and peer nominations for relational aggression were high ($r = .74$ for girls and $r = .69$ for boys), suggesting that teacher and peer informants might concur to a large degree in their judgments of relational aggression.

Peer Ratings

Because responses to various types of self-report questionnaires could easily be biased by social desirability, difficulty in accurately perceiving one's own behaviors, and gender stereotypes, investigators have argued that peers may be best suited for assessing indirect/relational/social aggression (Crick & Grotpeter, 1995; Lagerspetz et al., 1988). Peer assessments of social aggression have taken two forms: peer ratings (in which children rate each of their classmates on a Likert scale for particular behaviors) and peer nominations (in which children chose individual peers—usually limited to three—as being high on a particular behavior). As discussed in Chapter 2, peer ratings may be a more sensitive measure of most children's social aggression because each child receives multiple ratings; peer nominations may be a more expeditious method for identifying children extremely high on particular behaviors.

The leading peer rating instrument for assessing indirect/relational/social aggression is the DIAS (Bjorkqvist, Lagerspetz, & Osterman, 1992). This measure asks children to rate classmates on specific behaviors in response to the question, "When angry, does this person . . . ?" In the first study using a measure that was a precursor of the DIAS with 11- and 12-year-olds in Finland, peers rated girls as higher on indirect aggression than they rated boys (Lagerspetz et al., 1988). Also, as based on peer reports using methods developed by Cairns, Perrin, and Cairns (1985), girls' friendship groups were described as more tightly organized, which the authors speculated might make it easier for them to hurt others by relationship manipulation. In a subsequent study (Bjork-qvist, Lagerspetz, & Kaukiainen, 1992), the DIAS was administered to 8- and 15-year olds (and compared with the 11-year-old data from the Lagerspetz et al. [1988], study). For the 8-year-old group, there were no gender differences for indirect aggression, which the authors inter-preted as suggesting that indirect aggression may not be fully devel-oped in this age group. Another study using the DIAS examined the proportions of children's total aggressive behaviors that were of partic-ular types for 8-, 11-, and 15-year-olds in Finland, Israel, Italy, and Po-land (Osterman et al., 1998). Across cultures and age groups, the larg-est proportion of girls' aggressive behaviors were indirect; this was not the case for boys.

In more recent years, the DIAS has been used to begin to examine some of the positive and negative correlates of indirect aggression. In a study with 10-, 12-, and 14-year-olds, Kaukiainen and colleagues (1999) examined the relation between indirect aggression and peer ratings of empathy and social intelligence. In all three age groups, indirect ag-gression was positively correlated with social intelligence, confirming Bjorkqvist's (1994) suggestion that these behaviors require a sophisti-cated understanding of the social world. For the 10- and 14-year-olds, indirect aggression was negatively correlated with empathy, but not for the 12-year-olds.

Peer Nominations

In peer nomination studies of relational aggression, children are al-most always asked to nominate three peers who are high on particular relationally aggressive behaviors: friendship manipulation, ignoring, so-cial exclusion, and gossip (although in some studies the gossip item is dropped from analyses because it loads on both the overt and relation-al aggression factors; see Crick, 1996; Crick & Grotpeter, 1995). Almost all of the peer nomination studies to date have used Crick and Grotpeter's (1995) items, but sometimes with very different results.

In the first study that proposed the construct of relational aggres-sion, Crick and Grotpeter (1995) administered their peer nomination measure (including items for overt aggression, relational aggression, and prosocial behavior), a sociometric instrument, and other measures of psychological adjustment to a sample of third- through sixth-grade children in the midwestern United States. In this study, girls received more peer nominations for relational aggression whereas boys received more nominations for overt aggression. There were no developmental differences for relational aggression. Peer nominations for relational and physical aggression were highly correlated (r = .55). Exhibiting higher levels of relational aggression was associated with peer rejection, loneliness, depression, and social isolation.

In a subsequent study that investigated the short-term stability of relational aggression and its prediction to social adjustment, Crick (1996) administered measures of aggression and social adjustment to third through sixth graders during October, November, and April of the same academic year. For girls, the stability of peer nominations for relational aggression was r = .80 for 1 month and r = .68 for 6 months (for boys, the corresponding stabilities were r = .86 and r = .56). To assess interrater reliability, teachers completed a questionnaire to assess children's overt aggression, relational aggression, prosocial behavior, and peer status. Correlations between peer and teacher reports of relational aggression were .57 for boys and .63 for girls (as compared to .69 and .74 for overt aggression). Teacher ratings of relational and physical aggression were highly correlated (r = .77). The results for social adjustment showed that for girls peer nominations for relational aggression predicted 4% of the variance in future social adjustment above and beyond variance predicted by overt aggression. This study did not report whether there were gender differences in peer nominations for relational aggression.

In another study, Crick (1997) investigated whether gender-nonnormative aggression is more strongly related to maladjustment than is gender-normative aggression. Because physical aggression more severely violates social norms for girls than for boys, physically aggressive girls should be at higher risk for maladjustment. Because relational aggression may be a more serious norm violation for boys, relationally aggressive boys should be at greater risk. In this study with 9- to 12-year-olds, children responded to the same peer nomination measure and teachers rated their students on the internalizing and externalizing subscales of the Child Behavior Checklist (CBCL). Overall, the findings confirmed the hypotheses: relationally aggressive boys and physically aggressive girls were rated as having more problems than all other groups. Here again, girls were higher on peer nominations for relational aggression than were boys, and boys were higher on peer nominations for overt aggression than were girls. Again, there were no developmental differences for relational aggression, and peer nominations for relational and overt aggression were highly correlated (r = .63).

Whereas Crick and her research team have fairly consistently found that girls are nominated more as relationally aggressive than are boys, other research groups using this same peer nomination instrument have found no gender differences (Phillipsen, Deptula, & Cohen, 1999; Rys & Bear, 1997), or even that boys are higher on relational aggressiveness than girls are (David & Kistner, 2000; Henington, Hughes, Cavell, & Thompson, 1998; Tomada & Schneider, 1997). Rys and Bear (1997) investigated the relation between relational and overt aggression and peer acceptance and rejection with third and sixth graders in the U.S. mid-Atlantic region. Although they found no gender differences, relational aggression did explain variance (9%) in peer rejection beyond that predicted by overt aggression for girls but not for boys. In a study with third through sixth graders at a university-affiliated school, relational aggression was measured at the level of the dyad (Phillipsen et al., 1999). Girl–girl and boy–boy dyads did not differ on relational aggression, although mixed-gender dyads were higher than same-gender friends.

Peer nomination studies showing that boys are more relationally aggressive than are girls have been conducted both in and out of the United States. For a sample of second- and third-grade students from Mississippi, peer nominations indicated that boys were higher than girls on relational aggression, and that the relations between relational aggression and maladjustment were similar for both genders (although the proportions of the variance explained were small; Henington et al., 1998). In a study with third through fifth graders from suburban and rural Florida, again boys were higher than girls on both relational and overt aggression (David & Kistner, 2000). African American students were higher on peer nominations for both relational and overt aggression than European American children. After controlling for gender and ethnicity, relational and overt aggression were both related to children perceiving that they had higher peer status than indicated by peer reports. Another study indicating that boys are more relationally aggressive than girls was conducted with children in Italy (Tomada & Schneider, 1997). The investigators speculated that Italian boys may be more relationally aggressive than girls "because of exposure to the dense, close-knit relational networks of their parents, in which they might acquire relational aggression by means of observational learning" (Tomada & Schneider, 1997, p. 606). Why this exposure would be more potent for boys than for girls is not clear. Just as for the U.S. samples, relational and overt aggression were both related to peer rejection.

How can it be that using almost identical peer nomination items, one research group finds that girls are more relationally aggressive than boys are (see Crick et al., 1999, for a summary) and others do not? One reason may be that many of the studies of Crick's team involve questionnaires administered to large samples, such that even fairly small mean differences become statistically significant, whereas these do not achieve significance in smaller samples. As noted by Maccoby

(1998), the magnitude of the gender difference for relational aggression is almost always substantially smaller than the corresponding difference for physical aggression. Although this might explain why some studies find no gender difference, it does not account for why other investigations find that boys are higher on relational aggression than are girls. Perhaps this is due to cultural differences, or subcultural differences within the United States, or perhaps it is due to subtle differences in how data are analyzed.

For example, in some of the studies by the Crick group, gender differences for relational and overt aggression are presented only with the other type of aggression statistically controlled (following the argument that because the two forms of aggression are highly correlated it is more correct to examine differences in one form after controlling effects of the other; e.g., Grotpeter & Crick, 1996). Most studies indicate that relational and physical aggression are highly correlated, for example, .73 for girls and .76 for boys (Crick, 1997). Therefore, given that these forms of aggression often occur together in nature, it might be helpful to report both the raw means and the means adjusted for the other type of aggression (Underwood et al., 2001b).

Some have suggested another reason for the inconsistent gender differences found for relational aggression: that when these appear, they are due more to stereotypes than to actual differences in behavior (Underwood et al., 2001b). Children acquire complex knowledge of gender stereotypes as soon as they learn to label gender, by age 3 or so (Fagot et al., 1992), and even young children view strong expressions of anger as more "male" (Leinbach & Hort, 1995). Although research has not directly addressed this question, by middle childhood, youth are likely well versed in stereotypes of girls as backbiting and manipulative. Children no doubt use gender stereotypes to guide their social behaviors and perceptions of others (Maccoby, 1998), and these stereotypes may influence their peer nominations in subtle but important ways. The female gender stereotype may make some children just a bit more likely to think of a girl when pressed to nominate someone as relationally aggressive, and this alone could account for the small but sometimes significant gender difference.

Observations

One way of surmounting the fairly daunting challenge of bias from gender stereotypes might be to collect observational data. If observers detect gender differences using fairly strict microanalytic coding systems, that would be valuable information indeed. Note that still, though, gender bias could have an effect, because it is almost never possible to be blind to children's gender in observational studies (with the possible exception of children clothed in snowsuits in extremely cold climates; see Condry & Ross, 1985).

Some have argued that observing indirect/relational/social aggression is likely to be difficult or perhaps even invalid because these behaviors are subtle and may require prior knowledge of the peer group to be understood at anything beyond the most superficial level (Crick & Grotpeter, 1995; Lagerspetz et al., 1988). However, more recent evidence suggests that observational research may be possible. In one small study to detect elements of social exclusion, pairs of seventh-grade girls who were best friends were observed as they interacted with an annoying peer confederate (Galen & Underwood, 1997). Socially aggressive behaviors occurred at fairly high rates and were able to be coded reliably. For a large-scale investigation using this same method with more than 200 fourth-, sixth-, and eighth-grade boys and girls, data collection and coding have just been completed (Underwood, Moore, Bjornstad, Sexton, & Galperin, 2001). Preliminary analyses indicated that boys and girls are equally likely to engage in verbal forms of social aggression but girls showed more nonverbal social aggression than did boys (rolling eyes, exchanging hostile stares, turning away, and sneering between friends).

In more naturalistic settings, a promising method for collecting observational data is remote audiovisual recording. By use of remote cameras with zoom lenses, children are filmed on a playground while they wear portable wireless microphones that record their verbalizations (Pepler & Craig, 1995). Microphones are housed in "fanny packs" on individual children—packs that are identical to those worn by the entire class, so no one knows who is being recorded and who is not. Research using this method is still underway, but early results show that even indirect aggression can be coded reliably (Pepler & Craig, 1995).

Although very few observational studies are available, the data obtained so far indicate that gender differences in indirect/relational/social aggression may not be large. Using remote audiovisual recording with a small sample of aggressive and nonaggressive children in grades 1–6, researchers found that there were no gender differences in observed gossip, social rejection, or even verbal attacks (Pepler et al., 1998). However, findings from this small, specially selected sample must be interpreted with some caution; larger studies with normative samples are needed.

Ethnographic data collected by social psychologists who are also parent-participant-observers in their son's and daughter's peer cliques indicates that the dynamics of social exclusion may be similar for boys and girls (Adler & Adler, 1995). Adler and Adler (1995) concluded:

our research found few significant variations in clique dynamics by gender; the boys we interviewed and observed were no less skilled at intricate emotional woundings and manipulations than were the girls. Inclusionary and exclusionary clique dynamics seem to be a strong common element in both boys' and girls' culture, located in girls' equalitarian but emotionally vindictive relationships and in boys' conflict-filled but emotionally uninvolved worlds. Thus we reinforce Thorne's (1993) assertion of gender parallels, in contrast to the more conventional portrayal of gender differences. (p. 159)

Might it indeed be the case that girls and boys both engage in social aggression—but for different types of reasons and perhaps with different types of consequences? Answering these questions will require that future investigators use creative and diverse methods for understanding more specifically the processes by which social aggression unfolds among girls.

ORIGINS AND EXPLANATIONS FOR GIRLS' ANGER AND AGGRESSION IN MIDDLE CHILDHOOD

Although there has been an explosion of recent research describing forms of anger and aggression that may be more common among girls, much less evidence is available as to the developmental origins and possible causes of these behaviors. In light of the paucity of evidence for causal factors for social aggression, the discussion in the following subsections highlights clues from related literatures—but is clear about what is and what is not yet known.

Temperament

Recall that whereas most experts agree that there are not prominent gender differences in infant temperament, these may emerge during the preschool period (Goldsmith et al., 1997). Even small differences in boys' and girls' temperaments may influence parents' socialization in subtle ways (Brody, 1999).

Very few studies have examined temperament with middle-childhood samples, but the available evidence suggests that there may be some important gender differences in temperament that could relate to girls' predilections for indirect expressions of anger and aggression. For a large birth cohort of 5-year-olds from Finland, mothers rated girls as lower than boys on activity level, nonadaptability, and stimulation threshold (the latter meaning that girls were more sensitive to bodily discomfort; Martin, Weisenbaker, Baker, & Huttenen, 1997). In a longitudinal study with children whose emotionality was rated by parents and teachers at ages 4–6, 6–8, 8–10, and 12–14, overall girls were higher on attentional and inhibitory control (Murphy, Eisenberg, Fabes, Shepard, & Gurthrie, 1999). With increasing age, intensity of emotion declined and regulation increased for both genders, and for girls impulsivity declined.

Researchers have yet to explore the relationship between temperament and emotionality and engaging in social aggression. Still, the fact that girls may be temperamentally more controlled and inhibited fits with their ability to refrain from the more immediate, overt forms of aggression. It would be interesting to examine whether more dysregulated girls are more likely to be physically rather than socially aggressive or whether more reactive forms of social aggression are more strongly associated with temperamental dysregulation.

Emotion Regulation

The first section of this chapter discussed girls' expressions of anger. Are there gender and developmental differences in the regulation of other emotions that might inform our understanding of why girls engage in more social aggression than physical aggression? Overall, much less is known about emotion regulation in the age range of middle childhood than for younger age groups (Denham, von Salisch, Olthof, Kochanoff, & Caverly, 2002). One major reason for this lack of information may be that children in this age range insist on maintaining an "emotional front" (Saarni, 1999) even when provoked (Underwood et al., 1999). Overall, research to date suggests that during middle childhood children need less assistance from caregivers in regulating their emotions and rely more on cognitive and problem-solving strategies (Denham et al., 2002). Also, perhaps in keeping with their goal of controlling emotions at all costs, older children seem to benefit from engaging in distraction when coping with negative affect (Denton & Zarbatany, 1996).

Perhaps because older children are verbally sophisticated as well as skilled at dissemblance, it has been tempting to study emotion regulation in this age group using hypothetical vignettes or other questionnaire measures. School-age children are capable of responding to fairly lengthy questionnaires, and given that they can be suave enough to mask emotional expressions, asking them about their inner emotional experiences may provide valuable information indeed. As discussed for research on anger, gender differences for the vignette studies are inconsistent. Some studies find no systematic gender differences in display rule knowledge for this age range (e.g., Jones, Abbey, & Cumberland, 1998) or in perceptions and responses to negative affect (Jenkins & Ball, 2000); others find that boys report controlling some negative emotions more than do girls (sadness and pain, but not anger; Zeman & Shipman, 1996).

A variety of types of evidence suggest that girls may mask negative emotions more than boys do (see Saarni & Weber, 1999, for a thoughtful discussion). With the exception of the work on anger described earlier in this chapter, almost all observational research on older children's emotion regulation has focused on disappointment. In a clever laboratory method developed by Saarni (1984), children are given a desirable toy for completing some task, which leads them to expect that other prizes given will also be attractive. After completing another task, the children are given a prize that is undesirable: a plastic key ring that is a baby toy (Saarni, 1984), toddler socks (McDowell, O'Neil, & Parke, 2000), or plastic spoons (Davis, 1995). By observing children's reactions to the disappointing gift, it is possible to measure their use of the display rule "to look pleased and smile when someone gives you something they expect you to like—even if you don't" (Saarni, 1984, p. 1505). In the original study using this method, older children were more likely than younger children to mask their disappointment, and girls were more likely than boys to mask disappointment.

Several subsequent studies using this method confirmed that girls mask disappointment more than do boys when given a disappointing gift. In one study, girls maintained equally positive facial expressions when given attractive and undesirable gifts whereas boys' faces became more negative when receiving the disappointing toy (Cole, 1986). In another study with third graders, girls showed less disappointment when receiving a disappointing gift, and girls' observed use of display rules in this situation explained more of the variance in their social competence than for boys (McDowell, O'Neil, & Parke, 2000). To explore whether gender differences in masking disappointment were due to ability or motivation, first and third graders engaged in two types of tasks: the above traditional disappointing gift method, and a highly motivating game that required children to mask disappointment from an adult so as to win a prize (Davis, 1995). For both genders, masking of disappointment was greater for the game task, where the reward for dissembling was explicit, but in both situations girls still masked disappointment better than boys did. Davis (1995) interpreted these findings as suggesting that girls may be more adept than boys at hiding negative emotions.

Here again, although no research has explored the relation between use and understanding of display rules and social aggression, it seems reasonable to imagine that girls' ability to dissemble negative emotions may be related to their preference for social aggression. Being able to hide irritation to someone's face seems to be a requirement of some kinds of nasty, backbiting behavior, perhaps especially relationship manipulation and malicious gossip. Girls' ability to mask negative emotions may enable them to express anger and pursue their social goals in covert ways that risk less punishment from peers and adults, reducing the effect/danger ratio (Bjorkqvist, 1994).

In addition to anger and more general emotion regulation, social aggression may be associated with specific, complex emotions such as shame and jealousy. Some experiences of shame may prominently feature perceived failures in relationships (Denham, 1998), and this type of shame may be particularly painful during middle childhood when children care so deeply about belonging and fitting in. Although no research has addressed shame in relation to social aggression for this age group, it seems that one way of coping with shame may be to retaliate or to attempt to regain one's relationship status via social aggression. In a large-scale cross-sectional study of children's and adults' responses to hypothetical anger-provoking scenarios (see Tangney, Hill-Barlow, et al., 1996, for a full description of the measures), self-reports of direct and indirect aggression were both related to proneness to shame (also measured by responses to hypothetical scenarios; see Tangney, Wagner, Hill-Barlow, Marschall, & Gramzow, 1996).

Another strong negative emotion likely related to social aggression is jealousy (Parker & Low, 1999). Jealousy has been defined as "a protective reaction to a perceived threat to a valued relationship or to its quality" (Clanton & Kosins, 1991, p. 133). Jealousy may take two forms: (1) *social comparison jealousy*, for which the challenge is to superiority or equality in a relationship, or (2) *social relations jealousy*, in which the exclusivity of the relationship is in jeopardy (Bers & Rodin, 1984). Almost all research to date on jealousy has focused on romantic jealousy among adults (White & Mullen, 1989); the few available studies with children have investigated social comparison jealousy (Bers & Rodin, 1984; Masciuch & Kienapple, 1993). Social relations jealousy in the context of children's friendships likely motivates social aggression. If a child feels that the exclusivity of a friendship is threatened, what better way to retaliate or protect the relationship than to exclude the interloper? Recently, a reliable measure of children's friendship jealousy has been developed (Parker & Low, 1999), and preliminary evidence suggests that friendship jealousy is related to peer reputations for socially aggressive behavior (as well as unrelated to children's tendencies for socially desirable responding, negatively associated with global self-esteem, and positively related to friendship conflict, sensitivity to rejection, and problematic peer group acceptance).

Additional research is needed to examine carefully the role of shame and jealousy in social aggression, as well as to explore the role of empathy and prosocial behavior.

Parental Relationships

Might girls experience and express emotions differently than boys because of particular qualities of their relationships with their mothers and fathers? Very few studies have addressed the family origins of social aggression (however, for exceptions, see Crick et al., 1999; Hart et al., 1998). What does research on parenting of school-age children suggest about anger and aggression among girls? A comprehensive review of the enormous number of studies on socialization and parent–child relationships is not possible here (see Bugental & Goodnow, 1998, and Parke & Buriel, 1998, for recent large-scale reviews). The discussion in the following subsections highlights three features of parent–child relations that seem likely to relate to social aggression among girls for theoretical and conceptual reasons: security of attachment, differential socialization of girls and boys by mothers and fathers, and children's exposure to marital conflict.

Attachment

Because one motivation for social aggression may be to preserve one's own sense of belonging and acceptance (Adler & Adler, 1995; Paquette & Underwood, 1999), it seems reasonable to wonder whether engaging in social aggression may be related to insecure parental attachment. Attachment theory proposes that when children have sensitive, responsive caregivers, they develop working models of others as available, reliable, and supportive (Bowlby, 1969). When caregivers are insensitive or rejecting, the theory suggests that children develop more negative expectations of others, such that they may be more sensitive to rejection, more likely to attribute hostility in the face of ambiguous social information, and perhaps more likely to respond to feeling threatened by engaging in social aggression.

Although no published research has addressed the relation between parental attachment and social aggression, a recent meta-analysis explored the relation between child–parent attachment and children's friendships and peer status (Schneider, Atkinson, & Tardif, 2001). Overall, the results suggested the effects of attachment on children's peer relations are in the small-to-moderate range. There were no gender differences for effect sizes. Effects of parent–child attachment were larger for peer relations in middle childhood than for younger or older children, and larger for friendship than for measures of peer status. Attachment relationships likely influence how children manage emotions and balance others' interests with their own (van IJzendoorn, 1997). Maternal attachment may be especially important for understanding children's social development and intergenerational continuities in social behavior (Putallaz, Costanzo, Grimes, & Sherman, 1998). The connection between parent–child attachment and engaging in social aggression merits empirical investigation.

Differential Socialization of Girls and Boys

Another intuitively appealing explanation for girls preferring social to physical aggression is that parents socialize girls and boys differently. As discussed in Chapter 5 on preschoolers, some studies suggest that adults' ignoring girls' anger and aggression may lead to this behavior declining dramatically, perhaps forcing girls to find other means by which to express anger and contempt.

For the middle childhood age range, just how compelling is the evidence for differential socialization of girls and boys? In an early review, Maccoby and Jacklin (1974) concluded that differences in how parents socialize boys and girls are small at best. However, their review was criticized for grouping parental behaviors into overly broad categories, perhaps masking gender of child effects for more specific dimensions (Block, 1983). In a more recent review, Lytton and Romney (1991) conducted a meta-analysis of 172 studies to determine whether parents socialize boys and girls differently both on 19 specific socialization areas (including "discouragement of aggression"; p. 270) and on eight more broad categories ("interaction, encourage achievement, warmth, encourage dependency, restrictiveness, discipline, encourage sex-typed activities, and clarity/reasoning"; p. 283). Of all of the areas they examined, the only dimension for which there was a significant effect of child gender was encouragement of sex-typed activities. For all other dimensions, specific and broad, including discouragement of aggression, effect sizes were small and nonsignificant. In this meta-analysis, there were not enough studies to examine whether the gender of the parent interacts with the gender of the child to affect socialization processes.

A more recent focused meta-analysis suggests that mothers and fathers may use language differently with their sons than with their daughters (Leaper, Anderson, & Sanders, 1998). Across investigations, as compared to fathers, mothers talked more, engaged in both more supportive and more negative speech, and used less directive and less informing speech. Although there were not enough studies to examine how fathers might speak to sons and daughters differently, the analysis for mothers indicated that with daughters as compared to sons, mothers talk more and use more supportive speech. Overall, these results suggest that mothers are engaging in more socioemotional dialogue than fathers, perhaps especially with their daughters. This may give girls more experience with discussing relationship issues, perhaps with third parties.

How can these results be reconciled with the findings of Lytton and Romney (1991) that provided less support for differential socialization? Leaper and colleagues (1998) argue that their review found more evidence for gender-of-child effects because they were also able to examine gender-of-parent effects and because they focused on more specific dimensions.

In the spirit of focusing on specific features of parent–child relationships, it seems worthwhile to examine the evidence for differential socialization in the few studies that have investigated the relation between parent–child relationship qualities and children's emotion regulation. Although the results are often not consistent across studies, evidence is mounting that at the very least some aspects of parents' beliefs about and responses to children influence some features of children's emotion regulation in some contexts (see, e.g., Jones et al., 1998).

Parents' beliefs about the gender appropriateness of specific types of aggression likely shape their socialization efforts with sons and daughters. For example, from early to middle childhood, mothers' responses to hypothetical aggression in girls become more negative whereas mothers' responses to aggression become more positive for boys (Mills & Rubin, 1992), which suggests that parents may respond to sons' and daughters' aggression differently. Future research should explore parents' beliefs about and responses to social aggression in their children.

Other research suggests that parental expressiveness of emotions may be related to children's capacity for emotion regulation and to their social competence with peers. A child likely learns a great deal about coping with strong feelings by observing his or her parents and from their responses to his or her emotional expressions. Lessons learned at home are highly likely to be imported to peer relationships. This relation seems evident for both genders, across middle childhood age groups, and whether parental expressiveness is measured by self-report questionnaires (Cassidy, Parke, Butkovsky, & Braungart, 1992) or by observations (Boyum & Parke, 1995).

Other research has focused on parents' control of children's emotions rather than on parental expressiveness and has found that parental control is negatively related to children's skills in emotion regulation for boys but not for girls. A study of third graders and their parents found that parental control of children's emotions was negatively related to children's knowledge of display rules for boys but not for girls (McDowell & Parke, 2000). Similarly, in a longitudinal study, parents' self-reported negative responses to children's emotions were related to children's poor social adjustment as rated by teachers and parents, but these relations were stronger for boys than for girls (Eisenberg, Fabes, Shepard, et al., 1999).

Although overall parents' negative expressiveness and attempts to control children's emotions seem related to peer problems for children, gender-specific findings are not consistent. One reason for this inconsistency in findings may be that many of these studies necessarily have small samples and therefore low statistical power to detect effects. Imagine the complexity of doing research in this area: examining the effects of both gender of the parent and gender of the child requires large samples; finding families where both parents are willing to be involved can be challenging; measuring emotions and emotion regulation requires complex observational coding systems and sometimes also questionnaires; and the context in which families are observed may influence the magnitude of the effects found (Leaper et al., 1998). Still, the bulk of the evidence suggests fascinating links between the emotional dimensions of parental and peer relationships. How parental socialization of emotion might influence social aggression merits research attention.

Exposure to Marital Conflict

Another feature of family life that has been suggested as a possible causal factor for social aggression is children's exposure to parents' marital conflicts (Crick et al., 1999). Exposure to marital conflict has been shown to be related to physical aggression, especially for boys (Cummings & Davies, 1994; Emery, 1982; Grych & Fincham, 1990). Social learning theory suggests that children may learn a wide variety of conflict behaviors from observing their parents arguing, and these may well include social as well as physical aggression. Cognitive contextual theories suggest that watching parents engage in heated, intense, unresolved conflict may be disorganizing and distressing for youth, causing them to have poor social adjustment and to behave aggressively with peers (Grych & Fincham, 1990).

Because social aggression involves damaging relationships, social learning theory suggests that children may learn social aggression by observing their parents resolving conflicts in ways that harm relationships: giving one another the silent treatment when angry, enlisting other family members or friends to support their point of view in an argument, threatening to end the relationship, withdrawing love or affection, and in particular involving the child in arguments or conflicts. Whether they are mediating, intervening, or even becoming triangulated in their parents' conflicts, children may begin to practice and to learn the power of social aggression. In an observational study of third parties intervening in naturally occurring family conflicts at the dinner table, daughters intervened in disputes more than did sons (Vuchinich, Emery, & Cassidy, 1988). If daughters indeed have more involvement in parental disputes than sons do, girls may have more opportunities to learn social aggression from triangulation in parents' conflicts than do boys.

Although the relation between marital conflict and child triangulation and social aggression has only begun to be explored, early results are fascinating. A review chapter includes as yet unpublished findings that children high on relational aggression report that their parents are more physically and relationally aggressive to each other than do nonrelationally aggressive children (Grotpeter & Crick, 1996, cited in Crick et al., 1999). In addition, relationally aggressive children tend to blame themselves for their parents' conflicts. In another recent study, divorced parents' triangulation of children in conflicts mediated the relation between postdivorce conflict and relational aggression in daughters (Kerig, Brown, & Patenaude, 2001).

Gender Stereotypes

Another legacy of family relationships may be children's adherence to gender stereotypes (Fagot et al., 1992). We know from research with preschoolers that young children are highly conversant in both the conventional and metaphorical associations that make up gender schemas (Leinbach et al., 1997), and that young children with more feminine sex-typed mothers label gender earlier and have more extensive stereotype knowledge (Fagot et al., 1992). Beginning in toddlerhood, children prefer to interact with peers of their own gender (Serbin et al., 1994). How do gender segregation and gender stereotypes continue to develop during middle childhood?

A variety of types of evidence suggest that, at least at school, children congregate primarily with peers of their own gender (Gottman, 1986). The strength of children's same-sex peer preferences increases from early to middle childhood according to children's own reports on questionnaires (Serbin, Powlishta, & Gulko, 1993) and mother's reports of children's preferences (Feiring & Lewis, 1987). Children's preferences for interacting with same-sex peers are strong in this age range and seemingly unaffected by features of the family context such as parents' traditionality or gender of siblings (McHale, Crowter, & Tucker, 1999). Still, it is important to remember that other-gender interactions do occur. Children in the elementary grades play in mixed-gender groups about 25% of the time (Crombie & Desjardins, 1993). When children are asked to provide unlimited friendship nominations, one-fifth of mutual friendships are mixed gender (Phillipsen et al., 1999). That these same-gender preferences persist even in the face of considerable other-gender interaction make them all the more striking.

Although children seem to remain fairly strident in their personal preferences for same-gender interactions, other research suggests that during middle childhood they become more flexible in their gender stereotypes. For example, from kindergarten to grade 6, children's knowledge of gender stereotypes increased, but so did their flexibility (Serbin, Powlishta, & Gulko, 1993). Serbin, Powlishta, and Gulko (1993) defined flexibility as "the child's resistance to stereotypes: that is, the extent to which a child believes that a culturally sex-stereotypes attribute, activity, or role is equally appropriate for males and females" (p. 26). Katz and Ksansnak (1994) proposed that there are two important components of flexibility: one's own degree of adherence to stereotypes, and tolerance of stereotype violations in others. In a study with children in grades 3–5, 7–9, and 10–12, Katz and Ksansnak found that both self-flexibility and tolerance of others' violating stereotypes increased with age, and that girls were higher than boys on both.

What do these developmental changes for gender stereotypes and the lack thereof for gender segregation suggest for the development of social aggression? First, the fact that girls are congregating primarily with other girls might reinforce their mostly giving up physical aggression and allow them more opportunities to practice and observe the power of social aggression with their female peers. Second, that their gender stereotypes are becoming more flexible may allow them to become more socially self-confident and more likely to assert their own needs in addition to being concerned about others (Gilligan, 1982). Girls must navigate between their increasing sense of "girl power!" and their powerful understanding that negative emotions are unwelcome in social interaction (Saarni & von Salisch, 1993). One way in which girls do this may be by being overtly nice but using social manipulation to inflict harm or achieve status or power. It would be interesting to examine whether girls who adhere more to gender stereotypes engage in more social aggression.

Social Cognition

Another group of cognitive factors that may be related to social aggression is social information processing—how children think about particular social encounters (Crick, 1995; Crick et al., 2002; Crick & Werner, 1999). One recent model of children's social information processing includes six steps, all of which interact with a database of social schemas: (1) encoding, (2) interpretation, (3) clarification of goals, (4) response access or construction, (5) response decision, and (6) behavioral enactment (Crick & Dodge, 1994). Research has demonstrated that children (most often boys) who are highly physically aggressive make errors at several steps of this process: they focus more on aggressive than on nonaggressive social cues (Gouze, 1987), they overattribute hostility in the face of ambiguity (Dodge, Pettit, McClaskey, & Brown, 1986; Guerra & Slaby, 1989), they access more aggressive responses (e.g., Dodge et al., 1986), and they evaluate aggressive responses more positively (Crick & Ladd, 1990) and expect more favorable outcomes for aggression (Perry, Perry, & Rasmussen, 1986).

Some research suggests that girls' social information processing may differ from that of boys in ways that might relate to aggression. For example, when responding to hypothetical vignettes describing physical aggression, school-age girls reported that as compared to boys they expected to experience more negative self-appraisals and more parental disapproval as a result of behaving aggressively (Perry, Perry, & Weiss, 1989). However, note that there were no significant gender differences for other types of outcome expectations: suffering by the victim, peer disapproval, and tangible rewards.

Researchers have only begun to examine the relation between social information processing and social aggression, but the early results are promising. In two studies, third through sixth graders responded to hypothetical vignettes describing relational and overt aggression, and reported their attributions of intent and distress levels (Crick, 1995; Crick et al., 2002). Children rated by peers as high on relational aggression were more likely to attribute hostility for relational provocation and said they would be more distressed by relational provocation than did nonaggressive peers. Girls said they would feel more distressed by relational aggression than did boys.

Other research suggests that children who endorse social aggression as a strategy in conflict situations may be pursuing particular types of social goals. In response to scenarios describing conflicts with friends, fourth and sixth graders reported use of relationally aggressive strategies was positively related to endorsing the goals of avoiding trouble and maintaining relationships with the larger group but negatively associated with the goal of maintaining good relations with the target peer (Delveaux & Daniels, 2000).

Another study examined whether relationally aggressive children (as rated by peers) evaluate responses differently than do nonaggressive children (Crick & Werner, 1999). Again, third through sixth graders responded to hypothetical vignettes describing relational and instrumental conflicts, and reported their outcome expectations ("What would happen if . . . ?"), self-efficacy ("How easy or hard would it be to . . . ?"), response decisions ("How often would you . . . ?"), and response evaluations ("How good or bad is it . . . ?"). For relational conflicts, girls evaluated relationally aggressive strategies more positively than did boys. However, there were no clear differences in how children high and low on relational aggression evaluated relationally aggressive vignettes.

Peer Relations

Chapter 3 includes an extensive discussion of gender differences in children's peer relationships. The following subsections briefly highlight specific features of middle-childhood girls' friendships, networks, and peer status that may relate to their preference for social over physical aggression.

Friendships

In the middle childhood age range, both boys and girls reported that they rely on close same-gender friends for companionship more than on siblings, mothers, fathers, and teachers (Lempers & Clark-Lempers, 1992). Girls and boys named similar numbers of classmates as friends (Berndt, 1982; A. J. Rose & Asher, 1999). In studies using time sampling methods, fifth through eighth-grade girls and boys report spending similar proportions of their time with same-gender peers, approximately 10% of their waking nonschool time (Richards et al., 1998). However, girls reported thinking more about same-gender peers than did boys.

Although Two Worlds theorists have proposed that girls' friendships are more intimate and exclusive than are those of boys (Maccoby, 1998), evidence on this point is mixed (see Chapter 3 for a more extensive discussion). When girls' report more intimacy in their close friendships, it may be due to their spending more time in activities and contexts in which intimacy is more likely. For instance, in a study with fifth and sixth graders, both girls' and boys' ratings of friendship intimacy were related to participating more in communal activities, such as telling secrets and eating at restaurants with friends (Zarbatany et al., 2000). Although Feshbach's early studies (1969; Feshbach & Sones, 1971) found that girls were more likely to exclude newcomers than were boys, in more recent investigations girls were more welcoming to guests than were boys (Borja-Alvarez et al., 1991; Zarbatany et al., 1996). Overall, gender differences in friendship variables are larger for questionnaire studies than for observational studies. Both girls and boys seem to strongly value friendships and intimacy.

Perhaps girls engage in social aggression rather than more overt forms of aggression because they experience greater discomfort when competing with friends (Benenson et al., 2002). In laboratory studies, groups of female friends (ages 6 and 10) showed more discomfort than boys in choosing a leader and when hearing the results of a competitive game. Discomfort was coded as nonverbal expressions of worry or tension (furrowed brows, crossed arms, and the like). Interestingly, girls were just as involved in the process of choosing leaders and seemed equally comfortable as boys while competing when separated by a barrier. However, despite their involvement in the tasks, girls were more distressed by competing directly with their friends. Benenson and colleagues (2002) interpreted this as one possible reason that girls engage in relational aggression rather than physical aggression (although relational aggression was not assessed in this study).

In the only study to date to examine specific features of friendship in relation to social aggression, Grotpeter and Crick (1996) asked third through sixth graders to respond to a detailed Friendship Qualities Measure and also collected peer nomination data for relational and overt aggression. They did not report gender differences for friendship qualities or for relational aggression. The results showed that friendships of children high on relational aggression were high on intimacy, exclusivity/jealousy, and relational aggression between the friends. In future research, it might well be fruitful to examine further the relations between social aggression and jealousy and exclusivity.

Networks

Although some Two Worlds theorists claim that girls' social networks are smaller and more tightly knit than are those of boys (see Maccoby, 1998, for a summary), evidence from peer relations research suggests that girls' and boys' social networks are equal in size and that girls and boys are equally likely to be central members of networks (Bagwell et al., 2000; Cairns & Cairns, 1994).

Ethnographic studies of children's networks in middle childhood confirm that girls' and boys' networks appear to operate similarly, using comparable techniques of inclusion and exclusion (Adler & Adler, 1995). Techniques of inclusion are recruitment (being invited to join), application (asking to join), realignment of friendships (working to become more strongly affiliated with the group leader), and ingratiation (currying favor with central members of the group). Inclusion strategies serve to attract group members and to keep them bound to one another by continually maneuvering for affiliation with the leaders. Techniques of exclusion include rejection of the outgroup (maligning lower-status peers), compliance (going along with the leader's subjugation of others), stigmatization (directing severe ridicule toward an individual for a long period of time), and expulsion (kicking someone out of the group). These exclusion strategies make groups cohere as they join in disparaging others and maintain group boundaries by ousting members. Within this framework, social aggression is a naturally occurring element of both girls' and boys' continual cycles of inclusion and exclusion.

Peer Status

Previous research suggests contradictory hypotheses for the relation between social aggression and peer status. Some studies indicate that engaging in relational aggression is related to peer rejection, both concurrently (Crick & Grotpeter, 1995), perhaps especially for girls (Rys & Bear, 1997), and predicts rejection 6 months later (although the proportion of variance explained was small, 4%; Crick, 1996). However, other research shows that social aggression may also relate to high peer regard. The sociometric group highest on relational aggression is the controversial group (Crick & Grotpeter, 1995), those children who are both intensely liked and disliked. Engaging in social aggression has also been found to relate to being a central member of a social network (Xie et al., 2002).

In other studies, children have been asked to report what makes them dislike someone, and girls reported social exclusion and relational aggression more than did boys. In one study, second-, fifth-, and eighth-grade girls and boys were asked to describe two events that made them like a peer more and two events that made them like a peer less (Foster, DeLawyer, & Guervremont, 1986). For events leading to dislike, older girls reported more social exclusion than did boys (at grade 2, 3% of boys' and 3% of girls' incidents; at grade 5, 0% of boys' and 22% of girls' accounts, and at grade 8, 7% of boys' and 15% of girls' episodes). In a cross-cultural study with 11- and 14-year-olds from the United States and Indonesia, children named two disliked peers and then responded to open-ended questions about why they disliked the person (French, Jansen, & Pidada, 2002). Responses were coded for physical aggression, verbal aggression, and three types of relational aggression (relationship manipulation, social ostracism, and malicious rumors). In both cultures, girls mentioned each type of relational aggression more than did boys: relationship manipulation (20% of girls vs. 4.8% of boys), social ostracism (31% of girls and 6% of boys), and malicious rumors (27% of girls and 11% of boys). Together, these interview studies suggest that, across age groups and cultures, social aggression is more salient in girls' conceptions of why they dislike peers than in those of boys.

SUMMARY

We know more about girls' social aggression in middle childhood than for any other age range. Examining this body of work in light of the major questions explored in this book shows how far we have come and how much remains to be learned.

• *What does research evidence suggest about how girls in middle childhood express anger and behave aggressively?* Overall, research to date on middle-childhood girls' anger and aggression suggests a more rich, complex picture of girls' anger and aggression than the stereotypes that only girls manipulate relationships and only boys fight physically. Clearly, girls engage in less physical aggression than boys do, but some girls do fight and many studies show that social/relational and physical aggression are highly correlated for both genders. Gender differences in the frequency of other forms of anger and aggression are much less clear. The evidence so far suggests that girls may be more distressed by anger, conflict, and aggression than are boys. Girls report being more upset by peer provocation than do boys, especially involving close friends, and girls' anger more often concerns relationship issues. In some studies of conflict behavior, girls are found to be more concerned with mitigating and preserving the relationship than are boys, and for girls in particular engaging in fewer conflicts and resolving them more prosocially may be related to being well liked by peers. Whether gender differences are found for social/relational aggression depends heavily on the methods used, the samples studied, and the social contexts observed. However, the evidence so far suggests there may be subtle differences in the forms and functions of these behaviors in girls and boys.

• *How does social aggression unfold among middle-childhood girls, and how might this differ from that in boys of the same age group?* Research on social aggression with this age group has relied heavily on peer ratings and nominations, which have been useful for identifying children extremely high on these behaviors but have been less illuminating as to the specific processes by which these behaviors unfold among girls and boys. Most peer nomination and teacher rating measures implicitly treat social aggression as a personality trait, and do not help in understanding the specific social contexts that elicit social aggression and how girls and boys might engage in social aggression differently within their peer groups. The little ethnographic evidence available suggests that girls might engage in social aggression in a manner that is more emotionally vindictive than boys do (Adler & Adler, 1995), and anecdotal evidence from extensive interviews with girls suggests that they might be more likely to deploy social aggression against close friends than boys are (Simmons, 2002). Still, much more research is needed to investigate whether episodes of social aggression among girls are somehow different than those among boys (perhaps more lengthy, emotionally painful, threatening, involving more participants, or occurring more often in intimate relationships).

• *Are there developmental differences in the forms and functions of social aggression?* Although few existing studies directly compare social aggression among preschool and middle childhood age groups, results of different studies and developmental theory together suggest that social aggression becomes more complex and sophisticated during middle childhood. Children in this age range are more capable of extensive conversation, care more deeply about fitting in with their same-gender peer groups, and are more skilled at emotional dissemblance, all of which might make them more capable of more complex forms of social exclusion, malicious gossip, and friendship manipulation.

• *What are the developmental antecedents of social aggression among girls? How and why might girls come to express anger and aggression in this particular way?* Although research specifically focused on the developmental origins of social aggression is only beginning, related literatures suggest intriguing hints as to why social aggression becomes prominent in girls' behavioral repertoires. Girls may have more temperamental capacity for inhibition, which might relate to their propensity to refrain from the more overt, impulsive forms of aggression. Research suggests that girls are especially adept at masking negative emotions, and this capacity for masking irritation or even fury might allow them to suppress immediate, overt expressions of anger and instead retaliate or pursue their social goals in a more delayed, covert, behind-the-back manner. Although differences in how parents socialize boys and girls are unclear for many variables, mothers engage in more relationship dialogue than fathers do, especially with their daughters, and this greater experience with talking about relationships may contribute to girls' propensity for social rather than physical aggression. Girls may also learn social aggression from their involvement in parents' marital disputes, particularly by being triangulated in parents' conflicts. Girls' social cognition may also influence their social aggression; they expect more negative interpersonal consequences for engaging in physical aggression than boys do, and they report being more distressed by relational aggression than boys do. Several distinctive features of girls' peer relationships may contribute to social aggression being prominent for girls: their greater time spent thinking about same-gender friends, perhaps a greater propensity for jealousy and exclusivity in friendships, and their greater distaste for social exclusion.

• *What are the developmental consequences of girls' anger and aggression?* Although both girls and boys may engage in social aggression, evidence is mounting to suggest that social aggression may be more salient and worrisome for girls. Girls may be more distressed by social aggression, more hurt by social victimization, and more likely to view social aggression as grounds for social rejection. Given that social aggression might be a more prominent feature of girls' behavioral repertoires, it would hardly be surprising if their social adjustment were more strongly related to perpetrating and being the victim of social aggression than boys'. As discussed at length in Chapter 8, additional longitudinal research is needed to understand more fully the long-term developmental consequences of social aggression.

• *What does research on the processes involved in social aggression suggest for intervention?* As extensive as the research on social/relational aggression is for this age range, most studies offer few clues as to how this behavior might be interrupted, reduced, or even prevented. Additional observational studies in different social contexts could be helpful in this regard; knowing more about exactly how the behavior unfolds will enhance the likelihood of effective intervention. Still, existing work suggests some promising avenues. If social aggression is related to girls' desire to be nice and dissemble negative emotions, then assertiveness training might be useful in providing girls more straightforward strategies for pursuing their social goals. If girls learn social aggression from being triangulated in parents' marital conflicts, perhaps parents might be educated about the possible harmful effects of involving their daughters in their disputes. If indeed social aggression is related to errors in social information processing, perhaps social cognitive interventions might be helpful. If social aggression serves important functions in how children confirm their own belongingness, then perhaps parents and teachers might devise creative strategies and structures for more children to be able to feel included without having to shut other people out. If girls indeed reject other girls because of relational/social aggression, perhaps this distaste for friendship manipulation might be harnessed by training peers to intervene with each other to reduce this behavior.

FUTURE RESEARCH

As in all of science, describing social aggression has preceded explaining it, and rightly so. However, as we begin to build on this first generation of studies, it will be critically important that we refine our methods for observing social aggression as well as move on to examining its developmental origins. The following questions seem especially important:

- How might temperamental qualities relate to social and physical aggression among girls?
- Does jealousy within friendships cause or result from social aggression?
- How might qualities of parent–child relationships, perhaps especially attachment, be related to the development of social aggression?
- Do parents view social aggression as worthy of socialization and discipline? Do parents respond differently to social aggression by sons or daughters?
- What might children learn from observing or becoming involved in their parents' marital conflicts?
- Does gender segregation foster social aggression among girls or at least increase its impact?
- Are girls who adhere to feminine gender stereotypes more likely to engage in social aggression?
- Is social aggression more or less intense in the context of particular types of friendships or social groups? Does engaging in social aggression require or interfere with high peer regard? Might popular girls actually be more likely to engage in social aggression?
- Might social aggression serve some positive functions for children? Might children sometimes exclude others as a way of confirming their own sense of belonging and acceptance? Might children engage in negative evaluation gossip for its entertainment value, or perhaps also as a way of testing social boundaries

and norms? Might social aggression serve important functions in helping children to maintain the cohesiveness and integrity of their social groups?

Most of the research on social aggression to date has investigated children in the elementary school years. However, many parents and teachers believe that these behaviors become even more prominent as children enter early adolescence and begin junior high school.

Chapter 7

Adolescence

Girl Talk, Moral Negotiation, and Strategic Interactions to Inflict Social Harm

Think back to when you were in middle or junior high school. Remember a time that another kid, or group of kids, did something that really hurt you.

I had not seen my best friend from elementary school for years because her parents had moved her to another school. When she came back at the end of seventh grade I was overjoyed. We got back to being really good friends, and the night before a school dance, she spent the night at my house. I gave her a headband that matched one that I had. We had a great time and I thought we were best friends again. Then, next week at school I heard that she had thrown the headband in a dirty creek while she and her new best friend laughed and made fun of me.

Even now I can't think about this without crying. I already felt terrible about myself, like I was an outsider, and then she hurt me like nothing else could.

What did you do when this happened?

I was really depressed—I cried for weeks. I tried to get my parents to move me to a different school but they refused.

Why do you think this person did that to you?

I thought it was because I was uncool and ugly. I felt stupid for thinking that she liked me again.

—A COLLEGE WOMAN'S MEMORY OF HER EXPERIENCE AT AGE 13, WRITTEN FOR
OUR RECENT STUDY OF ADULT MEMORIES OF CHILDHOOD VICTIMIZATION

At the beginning of the year, when I was into cheerleading, everything was fun. But after Christmas vacation, people started thinking I was stuck up...they started writing on the walls, "Melissa Martin is stuck-up. . . . " [T]hat got me pretty upset. . . .

See, sometimes they wanted to do things to make me look bad. Like that was after they started liking me again. Like they wanted me to act like a baby and get all scared. Like they told Mike to break up with me, and they got a

134

whole bunch of people not to like me. I was really upset. After they did not like me, they started acting like, "If we wanted to hate you, anything that we want, we have the power over you." I was sitting there like a baby. I wasn't speaking up or anything. Like I was so glad to have them back as friends.

—A 13-YEAR-OLD GIRL DESCRIBING THE RECENT MEANNESS
OF HER PEER CLIQUE (in Merten, 1997, p. 184)

Laura, an 18-year-old college student, is conversing with Bev and Toni, two 16-year-old friends.

LAURA: Will you explain to me who Debby Dicklick is?

BEV: Debby Dicklick is . . .

TONI: Debby Norton is the big fat one (*says in an exaggerated, high pitched voice*) Hi.

BEV: (*Says in a deep masculine voice*) Debby sucked me off. (*All laugh*) What a winning name.

TONI: Debby Norton.

LAURA: Debby Norton

TONI: Yeah.

LAURA: That name's familiar.

TONI: She's the one . . .

BEV: that was supposed to be pregnant in [*sixth*] grade.

TONI: By Ken Benson's dad.

LAURA: That's right.

—FINE (1986, p. 415)

Think of the most recent occasion in which a friend or acquaintance did something to hurt you.

The woman I thought was my best friend got mad at me—I had a new boyfriend and she said I didn't care about her anymore. She sent me nasty e-mails, put me down, and betrayed me by telling other people really personal things that I had told her were confidential. She tried to make other people not like me by telling lies and she made me miserable.

How did it make you feel?

I was crushed. I had trusted her and she used everything I told her to hurt me. She manipulated me, and made me feel crazy like there was nothing I could do.

What did you do when this happened?

I got so depressed that I cried for days and even stopped eating. I had to drop out of my courses that semester.

Why do you think this person did this to you?

She was mad that I had a boyfriend and she didn't. She felt neglected.

—ANOTHER COLLEGE WOMAN RECOUNTING A RECENT VICTIMIZATION EXPERIENCE

As the above episodes so clearly demonstrate, girls continue to perpetrate and feel devastated by social aggression throughout their teenage years. As children move through adolescence, they develop increasingly sophisticated cognitive and social skills, skills that might help them cope with social difficulties but that also enable them to engage in more complicated means of hurting one another. Adolescents also encounter the considerable challenges of entering new and often much larger schools, going through puberty, beginning to separate from their parents, developing an independent identity, and for many, developing romantic and sometimes sexual relationships.

Developmental theory suggests that adolescents become more skilled in resolving conflicts with peers, more able to honestly discuss their thoughts and feelings with one another, and more likely to use both positive and negative gossip in the service of self-exploration (Gottman & Mettetal, 1986). However, relatively little empirical research has been conducted to test these claims.

Although girls and women and parents and teachers widely view early adolescence as a time of heightened socially manipulative behavior, much less research has examined social or relational aggression per se in this age range. However, research on related issues can inform our understanding of anger among adolescent girls.

In describing forms of anger and aggression among teenage girls, this chapter reviews the related literatures on anger regulation, conflict resolution, physical aggression, verbal aggression, and the few available studies of social and indirect aggression. This chapter also includes several ethnographic studies of gossip and the cycle of popularity. Although these studies do not invoke the terms "social aggression" or "relational aggression," they describe these phenomena exquisitely and suggest fascinating hypotheses for future empirical research. This chapter focuses on girls of ages 13–18 because most girls in this age range operate within the social ecology of junior high and high school. Research with college and older samples is discussed in the section of Chapter 9 on social aggression in adulthood.

FORMS OF ANGRY, AGGRESSIVE
BEHAVIOR AMONG ADOLESCENT GIRLS

Anger

Although relatively few studies have investigated the experience and regulation of anger with adolescent samples, the evidence available suggests that a significant proportion of girls' anger experiences in this age range may occur in peer contexts. In one study, researchers used time-sampling methods to measure children's daily experience of emotions (R. Larson & Asmussen, 1991). Youth in the fifth through ninth grades for a week carried pagers that went off at a randomly selected time within each 2-hour interval of the participants' waking hours. When the pagers sounded, participants completed some brief rating forms about what they were doing, whom they were with, how they were feeling, and why. The results showed that, with increasing age, youth reported more frequent experiences of anger, worry, and hurt (analyses were conducted for negative emotions together). For both genders, there was a developmental increase in both positive and negative feelings related to their friends. Adolescent girls reported a larger proportion of negative feelings related to friend interactions than did boys (25% and 11%, respectively). For girls, the developmental increase seemed to be due mainly to an increase in negative feelings about boys. As R. Larson and Asmussen (1991) so eloquently argued, adolescents, perhaps especially girls, "have acquired a new area of concern, a new area of 'what matters,' and along with this, they have a new source of vulnerability to hurt" (p. 29).

A few studies have measured adolescents' anger with self-report or vignette questionnaires, with mixed results. In response to a self-report measure of anger expression, a large sample of mostly European American 13- to 20-year-old young women reported they would suppress their anger more than their male agemates (Musante & Treiber, 2000). Remember that a vignette study of children's reactions to name-calling by friends and nonfriends found that both preadolescent (ages 11–12) and adolescent (ages 13–15) groups reported more complex emotional responses and more direct confrontation with friends than with non-friends (Whitesell & Harter, 1996). For this mostly European American middle-class sample, girls reported feeling more indignation than boys and reported more negative emotions. This study found few developmental differences for anger experience and expression, except that adolescents only reported a stronger sense of violation when provoked by friends than by nonfriends. In a study with an African American sample in which 9-, 11-, and 13-year-olds responded to anger-provoking vignettes, with increasing age girls said they would express anger more openly whereas boys said they would suppress anger more (Underwood et al., 1992). Thus, we have one study suggesting that adolescent girls feel more hurt and angry than boys do in response to peer provocation, one study that suggests girls mask anger more, and one study finding that girls express anger more openly than boys do. These conflicting findings may be due to sample differences or to the fact that adolescents may be well aware of social prohibitions against anger expression and may not respond honestly to questionnaires.

One of the few observational studies of anger expression with adolescents suggests that girls may be less openly angry when discussing problems with friends (Brendgen, Markiewicz, Doyle, & Bukowski, 2001). Pairs of 15- and 16-year-old best friends were observed as they discussed what each does that angers the other and then other peers known to them both. The interactions were coded for responsiveness, self-disclosure, assertiveness, conflict, and criticism, and well as positive and negative nonverbal behavior. The results showed that, as compared to boys, girls talking with friends disclosed more, were more responsive, engaged in less conflict, and were less critical and negative.

Taken together, these studies suggest that for girls difficult interactions with peers may be a significant source of negative affect. However, girls seem to refrain from expressing anger openly, perhaps especially with their close friends.

Conflict

Given that adolescents may be so capable of masking and dissembling when they feel anger, it may be especially important with this age group for researchers to focus instead on conflict, how teenagers resolve disputes, regardless of whether negative affect is openly expressed. Teenagers report being involved in approximately seven or eight disagreements per day, though only one or two of these are with friends or other peers (Laursen, 1995). Adolescents perceive most conflicts as relatively benign—as involving minimal negative affect and little disruption to ongoing relationships (Laursen, 1993). As compared to conflicts with family members, adolescents report that conflicts with friends more often concern relationship issues (such as honesty and intimacy between friends; Adams & Laursen, 2001), are less negative emotionally, and are more often followed by continued social interaction and improvement in the relationship (Laursen, 1993).

In a thoughtful review of research on adolescent conflict, Laursen (1996) surmised that, with increasing age, adolescents use less coercion and more negotiation in conflicts with close peers and understand that conflict may be related to relationship costs such as negative affect, decreased interaction, and relationship harm. Some evidence suggests that girls may be especially sensitive to the potential of conflict to harm relationships; they are more likely than boys are to resolve disputes with compromise (Collins & Laursen, 1992). This seems particularly interesting in light of the fact that in at least one study girls reported more negative affect during conflicts than did boys, though there were no gender differences in reported negative emotion after conflicts (Laursen, 1993). If girls indeed strongly value relationships, it seems sensible that they might feel more distress than boys in the face of conflict, seek to reduce their own upset by using more relationship-protective strategies, and then feel better afterward as a result.

Regardless of gender, adolescents report in telephone interviews that they resolve most of their conflicts by submission and disengagement (Laursen & Koplas, 1995), confirming that protecting relationships may be paramount during this developmental period. It would be interesting to examine disengagement more carefully to see whether it is always followed by cessation of the conflict or whether other events ensue later. What looks like disengagement in a shorter time frame may be related to engaging in more covert retaliation in the longer term. For example, an adolescent may choose not to pursue a conflict directly with a friend but may engage in social aggression at a later point in time, perhaps behind the person's back.

Ethnographic research suggests that at least sometimes with friends, girls engage in direct strategies for conflict resolution (Eder, 1990). In a longitudinal observational study that followed a cohort of youth as they moved through junior high school, Eder (1990) observed students at lunchtime and during activities such as sports and cheerleading. She noted that direct conflicts among girls became more common during the later junior high school years when more stable social groups had formed. Girls' conflicts often began with claims that others were violating important peer norms, and some of these conflicts remained unresolved. When girls did resolve conflicts, they did so by outright denial, explanation, defending themselves, and sometimes by laughter and humor. Eder (1990) concluded that, "disputes are an important way for females to resolve and communicate normative concerns" (p. 83) about what types of social behaviors are and are not acceptable.

Physical Aggression

Perhaps because physical aggression so strongly violates social norms for appropriate behavior for both genders, for most youth physical aggression is quite rare and declines during adolescence (Coie & Dodge, 1998; Loeber, 1982). Even for youth considered to be chronically aggressive, fighting is quite rare (Tremblay, 2001). However, in some subcultural contexts, for example, among lower-income African American youth, aggression might become more socially accepted during the adolescent years (Coie, Terry, Zakriski, & Lochman, 1995). Some youth greatly accelerate their rates of violent behavior in adolescence; hence, this is when many violent offenses occur (Coie & Dodge, 1998).

Throughout adolescence, the gender difference in physical aggression remains large (Silverthorn & Frick, 1999). In response to the National Youth Survey (Elliott, 1994), only 16% of girls reported having committed a serious violent offense as compared to 42% of boys (serious violent offenses included assault, robbery, and rape). However, girls may begin engaging in violence earlier than do boys (for girls, the peak age of onset is 14 as compared to age 16 for boys). Other evidence suggests that more recently rates of violent offending are increasing more rapidly for girls than for boys (H. N. Snyder & Sickmund, 1999).

Although most adolescent girls may engage in less physical aggression with peers than boys do, there may be one context in which they are developing the capacity for violence—relationships with romantic partners. In an investigation with the New Zealand community sample from the Dunedin longitudinal study when participants were 21 years of age, 37.2% of men and 21.8% of women reported perpetrating physical violence with partners (Magdol et al., 1997). Of 21-year-old couples in which the men had been part of the Oregon Youth Study of high-risk boys, 43% of men and 34% of women reported engaging in physical aggression toward romantic partners in young adulthood (Capaldi & Owen, 2001). Much additional research is needed to understand why such significant proportions of young women physically aggress in romantic relationships. Do developmental processes during adolescence account for girls fighting with their boyfriends in young adulthood, or are girls fighting with boyfriends due to specific qualities of the relationship context or even in self-defense? We return to these issues later in this chapter in the section on adolescent romance and also in Chapter 8 on developmental and clinical outcomes of aggression.

Although some teen girls may become physically violent with romantic partners, the fact remains that most girls in this age range do not fight physically with other girls. Understanding how most adolescent girls respond when angry or when they seek to hurt peers requires considering other forms of hurtful behavior.

Verbal Aggression

As tempting as it may be to believe that girls hurt each other with words more than boys do, the evidence for gender differences in verbal aggression is just as mixed for adolescents as for other age groups. Relatively few studies have examined verbal aggression among adolescents. In a study with 15- and 16-year-old students in Finland using the DIAS (Direct and Indirect Aggression Scales) peer-rating measure (Salmivalli, Kaukiainen, & Lagerspetz, 2000), boys were rated by peers as higher on verbal aggression than were girls (verbal aggression items included yelling, insulting, threatening harm, name-calling, and teasing). However, Kashani and Shepperd (1990) found that when 14- to 16-year-olds responded to the Conflict Tactics Scale (Straus, 1979), there were no gender differences for the verbal aggression subscale (which included items for shouting, threatening, and sulking to resolve conflicts). And, with a large sample of Finnish 15- and 16-year-olds using a semistructured interview about verbal and physical aggression, there were no gender differences in the reported frequency of verbal aggression (Rauste–von Wright, 1989).

Although the bulk of the evidence does not suggest clear gender differences in verbal aggression during adolescence, such aggression may take different forms and serve different functions for girls and for boys. Girls report being the target of verbal aggression related to their appearance and to their social relationships more than do boys, whereas boys report more teasing about sports and school achievement (Rauste–von Wright, 1989). In her ethnographic work with junior high school students in the United States, Eder (1990) noted that for girls ritual teasing and insulting was more related to communicating about norms for behaviors, whereas for boys ritual insults seemed more often to be related to status.

Other evidence suggests that during adolescence girls and boys begin to direct verbal aggression toward the other gender (Craig, Pepler, & Connolly, 2002). In a longitudinal study of children's other gender interactions during sixth and seventh grades, teasing increased for both genders during the transition to middle school and boys increasingly targeted girls in their rough play and their teasing (Pellegrini, 2001). As we continue to work toward understanding social aggression, it will be important also to investigate more about what verbal aggression means for girls and for boys.

Social Aggression

Adolescent girls are prone to feeling distress about friendships (R. Larson & Asmussen, 1991), but they are less likely than boys to engage in physical and perhaps even verbal aggression. One powerful strategy for girls who are expressing anger or pursuing social goals such as dominance or status might be harming others covertly by damaging their relationships. When adolescent girls engage in social aggression, they are enacting their wrath by hurting what other girls strongly value (Crick & Grotpeter, 1995) within the very domain that is often their own focus of concern. When seeking revenge, nothing may satisfy more than hurting someone in the arena in which you yourself feel most threatened. In addition, social aggression is covert, thereby maximizing the effect/danger ratio (Bjorkqvist, 1994) and complying with strong gender stereotypes dictating that girls do not fight and that women's anger is something that must be managed and controlled (Lutz, 1990).

The evidence to date suggests both that social aggression is fairly widespread among adolescent girls and that it is perceived as extremely hurtful. In a large-scale survey with more than 6,000 secondary students in Great Britain, 20% of youth reported having been bullied by others spreading rumors about them (Sharp, 1995). Regardless of gender or age, youth reported that the most stressful type of bullying for them was being the target of malicious rumors.

Despite the fact that social aggression appears to be frequent and hurtful for this age group, important questions about social aggression remain to be addressed in empirical research. Much of the recent work on relational aggression has focused on middle-childhood samples (see, e.g., Crick & Grotpeter, 1995; Crick et al., 1999). A few of the early studies of indirect aggression included young adolescent samples and a few recent studies of victimization by social aggression included adolescents; these are discussed below. However, as the constructs of indirect, relational, and social aggression emerged, ethnographic researchers were observing these very same phenomena, although they called them by different names such as "gossip," "meanness," and "the cycle of popularity." This review of research on social aggression begins with the ethnographic evidence (in the following subsection) and then moves on to discuss more quantitative research specifically focused on indirect and social aggression.

Ethnographic Studies of Gossip and the Cycle of Popularity

Several ethnographers have offered vivid portraits of aggression among girls in their research on interpersonal relations in adolescence, including popularity, gossip, discourse, and gender segregation. A comprehensive discussion of these detailed portraits is prohibited by space limitations here; the studies and their details highlighted below were selected because they connect with some of the more recent research on social aggression.

In the early-to-middle 1980s, Eder (1985) conducted a longitudinal ethnographic study of how social stratification develops among girls over the course of junior high school. On the basis of earlier research, Eder began with the premise that the transition to junior high school might be more difficult for girls than for boys, that girls become increasingly concerned about peer relationships during junior high school, and more generally preoccupied with popularity and peer status. Eder hypothesized that these concerns intensified during early adolescence because students entering larger schools had more people with whom to form stable cliques and because extracurricular activities offered new avenues for status. For boys organized sports allowed a fairly large number of males the opportunity for peer status, whereas for girls the primary status-enhancing activity was cheerleading, in which very few girls could participate. Eder followed girls from sixth through eighth grades at a midwestern U.S. junior high school of about 750 students from diverse socioeconomic backgrounds but most of whom were European American. She observed them during lunch and during after-school activities (primarily sports and cheerleading), and also conducted semistructured interviews.

As girls moved through junior high school, social groups became more stable and exclusive, such that by eighth grade an obvious, stable hierarchy had been established. This was particularly evident in girls' seating arrangements at lunch: sixth graders had options as to where to sit, but by eighth grade girls seemed to follow strict social rules allowing them to sit only with their groups.

Popularity began to take on multiple meanings. Most girls agreed that popularity meant being prominently visible and getting a lot of attention. For girls, the most direct avenues to this type of popularity seemed to be physical attractiveness and cheerleading. Fewer girls agreed that popular people were always well liked; some described popular girls as nice and friendly, some described them as snobby and "stuck up," and some expressed mixed views, as illustrated by the following example (in all excerpts from Eder's work, capital letters refer to the first initial of different individuals speaking):

R—You say that everybody likes popular people, but actually you say you don't like them.

O—It depends, actually, on what kind of mood you're in, whether you like them or whether you—

N—Whether you're in the mood to put up with them.
(Interview, spring of eighth grade, from Eder, 1985, p. 159)

Regardless of whether popular girls were perceived as likable or not, friendships with popular girls were widely viewed as an important route for enhancing one's own peer status.

Eder (1985) observed that, not surprisingly, many lower-status girls were motivated to try to affiliate with their more popular peers but popular girls often avoided lower-status girls. These opponent processes created resentment that generated what Eder called "the cycle of popularity." Girls became popular because of their attractiveness, social skills, or status as cheerleaders and initially peers felt positively toward them and wanted to be their friends. However, popular girls often did not wish to associate with others less popular. At the same time, others held them to particularly high standards of friendliness and niceness, such that even acts of omission, such as ignoring or not paying adequate attention, were perceived as grave insults. As a result, feelings toward popular girls moved from extremely positive to negative. As resentment brewed, some popular girls were contemptuously labeled as "stuck up" and became subject to behaviors that we would now designate as social or relational aggression. Consider the following example:

> R—You say a lot of girls envy cheerleaders.
>
> D—Yeah. A lot of 'em get close friends. But then others, they think that they're stuck up and they get to hate us (*nervous giggle*) and say all this stuff.
>
> C—They start rumors and stuff. And say they don't like us and stuff.
>
> D—And in slambooks, "Who are your enemies? Cheerleaders, Number 21, or something" (*laughs*).
>
> R—Is that really hard on you when that happens?
>
> D—Well it makes us feel bad because, well, we really don't think that we're stuck-up. But like we have one big group, you know, that we're all good friends with. And then the others, I guess they just feel that the cheerleaders and the basketball and football players all just kind of hang around together. And then if you're not in something like that or you don't make it, then you just think that, you know, well, that we're stuck-ups (*embarrassed emphasis on the last word, then laughs*) or something.
>
> (Interview, spring of seventh grade, from Eder, 1985, p. 162)

Note how these girls firmly believe that they are victimized by peers because others resent and envy their status, and how they seem to take solace in their relationships with others who face the same risk.

A subsequent paper related to this same longitudinal study closely analyzed the structure and sequence of gossip in the lunchtime conversations of 16 adolescents (mostly girls), for whom there was also information about sociometric status (Eder & Enke, 1991). Gossip was defined as "evaluative talk about a person who is not present" (p. 494). It typically began with an explicitly evaluative statement, and unless this statement was immediately challenged, others present were likely to concur with and elaborate on the negative evaluation. Consider this example (from Eder & Enke, 1991, p. 501) of a conversation among eighth-grade girls:

> PENNY: In choir, that girl was sitting in front of us and we kept going "Moo."
>
> KAREN: We were going, "Come here cow. Come here cow."
>
> PENNY: And that girl kept going.

BONNIE: I know. She is one.

PENNY: She looks like a big fat cow.

JULIE: Who is that?

BONNIE: That girl on the basketball team.

PENNY: That big redheaded cow.

BONNIE: From Clintonville.

JULIE: Oh, yeah. I know. She is a cow.

Although these girls began by discussing their own previous behavior, they quickly moved on to elaborating on the basic theme that the girl they were discussing is large. As this example so clearly demonstrates, the structure of gossip most often fosters a predominantly negative tone (Eder & Enke, 1991). Although the structure of gossip is flexible in that challenges to negative evaluations can occur, these are rare and unless they occur immediately after the initial evaluative statement they are unlikely to persuade others. If the initial response to a negative evaluative comment is also negative, it is highly likely that subsequent comments by others will also be negative. Gossip was typically initiated by medium- or high-status youth, challenges were typically offered only by those of equal or higher status, while supportive comments were made by even the lowest-status students. Interestingly, challenges even by lower-status group members were observed to be effective if they were offered immediately in response to a negative comment, but this sequence of events was all too rare. The option most easily available to most youth present was to support another's negative evaluation, contributing to gossip becoming more and more negative.

In another ethnographic paper, Fine (1986) offered a different understanding of gossip among adolescent girls as "a continual thematic variation of blame, justification, excuse, and reputation" (p. 419). Fine began with the premises that "all talk is evaluative" (p. 405), an important goal of talk is involvement, and that group conversations are an impressive form of collective behavior. He examined a 90-minute interaction among three teenage girls "cruising" and "shooting the breeze" in a small midwestern U.S. town (one of the three was a first-year student in a college course, who was observing and talking with two 16-year-old best friends for a course assignment). In engaging in gossip, these girls seemed to be establishing moral consensus by testing out the boundaries of various stances. In gossiping, girls may blame themselves or others for moral defects, negligence, or moral blindness, and they may absolve themselves or others by justification or excuses. Consider the following example (from Fine, 1986, p. 416):

TONI: Oh . . . an' then you know how Jim Rollins is goin' with Susie
O'Dell, heavy.

LAURA: Real heavy . . . Oh . . .

TONI: Well . . .

LAURA: Well . . .

TONI: No, it's not very cool or nothin' but

BEV: (*Loud, deep, mocking voice to Toni*) Second woman.

LAURA: (*to Toni*) You?

TONI: You know it's not . . . we've never really done nothing . . . you
know, like we were at that party, and he comes up five . . . or fifteen
minutes, and tells Susie he's got to piss . . . comes up to talk to me.
(*Toni laughs.*)

LAURA: (*In a mocking, sarcastic voice*) You're a real homewrecker,
arncha Toni?

TONI: First time I've ever done that.

BEV: Heck, I'd wreck that home if I could.

Notice that in this interaction Toni tells a story on herself and is labeled by her friends as a "homewrecker." She then offers her justification and excuses ("we've never really done nothing. . . . First time I've
ever done that"), at which time her best friend supports her by saying
that she would behave similarly ("Heck, I'd wreck that home if I
could"). Fine argues that by engaging in these complex exchanges
about morals and social norms, adolescents are attempting to define
the boundaries of what is acceptable, and in the process constructing
and refining their moral stances.

This view of gossip as serving positive developmental functions is
echoed in observations of adolescent friends' conversations by Gottman and Mettetal (1986, pp. 216–217). They suggested that adolescents
gossip as a way of solving problems and establishing their identities, as
shown in the following example:

A: But also, like, we were, remember in the park we were saying how
it's just good to talk about people, because then you can find out
whether you want to be like that . . .

B: Right, right.

A: At least I can think, "Well, boy, I know I do not want to be like that."
And so, . . .

B: Right, that's true . . . I'll listen to people on the bus and they'll be
talking about . . . oh, God, what jerks.

A: Yah, why are they just talking about other people?

B: I hate them.

A: Why don't they just talk about their own lives, you know?

B: Right, right. But then it's true everybody does it, and it is because you learn so much by talking about other people.

A: Yah, plus it's fun just to find out, plus find out what the other person thinks.

B: Really.

A: That's how you get your values too.

In this fascinating conversation, these adolescent friends reveal that they understand both the negative and positive functions of gossip, moving quickly from scorn for gossip to articulating its possible benefits.

If gossip works to fulfill developmental needs to establish an identity, clarify moral issues, and solve problems, then why do many observe or assume that girls engage in it more than do boys? Eckert (1990) argued that because of their less powerful place in society and less direct influence over the worlds of power and work, girls and women must wield more personal influence and evaluate themselves in terms of character rather than accomplishments. Girls examine and develop moral norms by engaging in "girl talk," which Eckert defines as "a typically female speech event including long and detailed personal discussion about people, norms, and beliefs" (p. 91). Eckert proposes that these conversations may include gossip but that they involve much more, because these types of conversations enable girls to understand and perhaps even to modify the social norms that rule their worlds.

Along somewhat similar lines, Merten (1997) argued that meanness toward peers on the part of some popular girls might result from the tension young women feel between hierarchy and equality. Girls pine for popularity, but popularity brings with it the challenges of standing out as different from others and appearing to be "stuck up."

Here it is important to note the distinction between perceived and sociometric popularity (see Parkhurst & Hopmeyer, 1998, for a thoughtful discussion). Perceived popularity refers to being perceived by others as having "glamour, social prestige, and social influence" (Parkhust & Hopmeyer, 1998, p. 126). Sociometric popularity refers either to receiving large numbers of "like most" nominations from peers (Gottman et al., 1975), or to receiving both large numbers of "like most" and few "like least" nominations (Coie, Dodge, & Coppotelli, 1982). Whereas sociometric popularity is associated with peer perceptions of kindness and trustworthiness, perceived popularity is associated with being seen as dominant, aggressive, and "stuck up." As we will see, the type of popularity studied by ethnographers seems to closely correspond to perceived popularity.

A 3-year longitudinal study of junior high school girls in an upper-middle-class U.S. suburban community examined the behaviors of a group of girls who were both mean and popular, dubbed "the dirty dozen" by their teachers (Merten, 1997). These girls engaged in such spiteful, manipulative, backbiting, socially exclusionary behavior that parents complained to the school and widely enjoyed student events were canceled as punishment for their misbehavior.

Nonetheless, these girls were perceived as popular and powerful, such that many girls attempted to join their group and felt rebuffed when rejected, and therefore claimed that the popular girls were "stuck up." In addition, perhaps because these popular girls wielded so much power, they were held to an unachievable standard of niceness, so that failing to anticipate others' needs and desires was construed as deliberate meanness and being snobby.

Merten (1997) proposed that these girls developed their strategies for meanness as a way of being able to enjoy their popularity while intimidating others and discouraging them from conferring on them the dreaded label "stuck up." Although girls expressed that it would be ideal to be popular and nice, being nice was problematic for two reasons: first, being nice interfered with enjoying and demonstrating the higher status of popularity; second, because popular girls were held to unreasonable standards of "superniceness," it was rarely possible to be sufficiently nice and falling short of this resulted in being designated as "stuck up" anyway. By being mean, girls acted out their popularity, frightened others away from trying to compete, and avoided being called "stuck up." Perhaps because of their discomfort with status hierarchies, these girls preferred to be seen as nasty rather than as snobs.

This phenomenon of meanness from the ethnographic work probably comes closest to the behaviors that have been considered to be social or relational aggression in studies using more quantitative methods. These ethnographies offer fine-grained portraits of interactions among a few girls that suggest fascinating hypotheses. However, these studies may suffer from what Thorne (1993) referred to as "Big Man Bias," or in this particular case "Big Girl Bias," overfocusing on the experiences and behaviors of a few highly visible youth. As stimulating as they are, with a few exceptions the ethnographies discussed here depict mostly middle-upper-class white girls who are popular cheerleaders. To understand better the extent to which more typical girls perpetrate and experience social aggression, research is needed with larger samples using more systematic methods.

Quantitative Investigations of Indirect and Relational Aggression

Whereas for middle childhood there is a large body of research on social aggression using large samples and diverse methods, for adolescence only a handful of studies are available, some using peer ratings but most relying on semistructured interviews. Recall from Chapter 6 that some of the early studies of indirect aggression conducted by Bjorkqvist and the Finnish research team included adolescent samples. In a study with 8-, 11-, and 15-year-olds (Bjorkqvist, Lagerspetz, & Kaukiainen, 1992), students rated their classmates for a variety of types of behavior when angry on an instrument called the DIAS (Direct and Indirect Aggression Scale). The results showed that the two older age groups seemed to discriminate clearly between indirect and direct aggression, peers rated girls as higher on indirect aggression than boys, and peer ratings indicated that indirect aggression was most intense in the 11-year-old age group. In another study with 15- and 16-year-olds using this instrument, girls were again rated as higher on indirect aggression than were boys (Salmivalli et al., 2000). In this study, indirect aggression was highly correlated with both physical ($r = .51$) and verbal aggression ($r = .80$). Interestingly, for both genders, engaging in indirect aggression was unrelated to sociometric rejection when physical and verbal aggression were statistically controlled.

Research with adolescents does not consistently show gender differences for indirect aggression. When asked to nominate peers for specific indirectly aggressive behaviors ("Who intrigues behind others' backs?"), a large sample of early, middle, and late adolescents from Finland reported no gender differences for indirect aggression (Pakaslahti & Keltikangas-Jarvinen, 2000). Gender differences also failed to appear in teacher ratings and self-reports (and with $N = 2,002$, there was certainly adequate statistical power to detect even small effects). In another study with a large sample relying entirely on self-report measures, there were no gender differences in relational aggression or victimization (Prinstein, Boergers, & Vernberg, 2001).

In a study that examined gender and developmental differences in indirect aggression across a wider age range, Owens (1996) administered a modified version of the DIAS to Australian children in grades 2, 6, 9, and 11. Rather than asking children to rate specific classmates on individual behaviors, participants were asked to rate how often boys and girls in their grade, in general, engaged in specific types of aggression. Overall the results showed that at all ages girls were rated as less likely to engage in direct and verbal aggression. For the children in the elementary grades there were no gender differences for indirect aggression, but indirect aggression increased with age for girls such that by high school girls were rated by peers as higher on indirect aggression than were boys. In subsequent analysis of this same data set, Russell and Owens (1999) examined boys' and girls' frequency and form of aggression with same- and other-gender partners. In general, the investigators found that other-gender aggression was described as between the quantity and style of boy–boy aggression (which tended to be direct or verbal) and girl–girl aggression (which tended to be indirect). Girls were described as directing more indirect aggression toward other girls than toward boys.

In an effort to analyze the forms, reasons, and functions of indirect aggression among girls, Owens and colleagues (2000a) conducted focus group discussions with 54 middle-class 15-year-old girls at Catholic schools in Australia. They began these group discussions with a vignette describing social exclusion and malicious gossip, asked girls to discuss the specifics of the vignette, then asked, "Does this sort of thing ever happen at this school?" This focus group method has the advantage of not only gathering data from a larger sample but also eliciting more elaborate accounts of girls' experiences (see Owens et al., 2000a, for a thoughtful discussion of the validity and rigor of these procedures). In this study, girls freely discussed several different types of hurtful behaviors: talking badly about others ("bitching," spreading rumors, betraying trust by telling secrets, criticizing others), social exclusion, nonverbal aggression, and physical aggression.

These adolescent girls offered heartbreakingly precise accounts of the effects of indirect aggression ("It hurts a hell of a lot"; Owens, Shute, & Slee, 2000c, p. 351). They reported that right after being the target of indirect aggression, girls were likely to be confused and deny being hurt. Then, girls often experienced anxiety, loss of self-esteem, and depression so severe that it led to a desire to leave school or to commit suicide. Targets of indirect aggression were described as feeling that the harassment would continue without ceasing and as fearing that no one would intervene. Girls said that the agony of victimization may be increased by irrational self-talk ("Everybody hates me and it will never get better"; Owens et al., 2000c, p. 369), which may lead some girls to respond with desperate retaliation. According to girls in this sample, conflicts involving indirect aggression usually ended when one girl sought a resolution by one-on-one communication with another and avoided engaging the entire peer group.

When asked why they engage in indirect aggression, girls cited two main categories of reasons: (1) alleviating boredom/creating excitement and (2) friendship/group processes (attention seeking, group inclusion, belonging to the right group, self-protection, jealousy, and revenge; Owens, Shute, & Slee, 2000b). As we discuss in the latter half of this chapter, others have proposed that indirect aggression is related to properties of girls' peer relationships, but this study provided the first evidence that girls might engage in social or indirect aggression for sheer entertainment value. As diabolical as it sounds for girls to explicitly state that they engage in social aggression for amusement and to protect group standing and friendships, it is fascinating that girls seem aware of the fact that these behaviors are deployed not just to be mean or express anger but also to confirm peer group boundaries and their own sense of belonging and acceptance.

One of the few published studies of social aggression during adolescence also used interview methods to study victimization, but this time with individuals (Paquette & Underwood, 1999). Students in the seventh and eighth grades responded to structured questionnaires assessing self-concept and frequency of experiencing victimization by social and physical aggression. Then, they also responded to a semistructured interview that asked them to recall, in detail, recent experiences of being the victim of social and physical aggression. On the structured questionnaire, there were no gender differences in reported victimization by social aggression and the mean indicated that children experienced social aggression "almost never." Although the overall mean reported frequency was not particularly high, most youth could recall highly salient experiences in which they had been victimized by social aggression.

In response to the interview, the most common type of social aggression reported was being the target of malicious gossip (e.g., "A group of girls spread lies that I was pregnant"; Paquette & Underwood, 1999, p. 253). Although girls and boys reported experiencing social aggression with equal frequency, girls reported being more distressed by particular experiences of victimization than did boys. For girls but not for boys, victimization by social aggression was negatively related to global self-concept, as well as to self-concept in specific domains (athletic competence, physical appearance, romantic appeal, behavioral conduct, and close friendships). Although these data are correlational and therefore the direction of causation cannot be certain, these results add to the growing body of evidence that social aggression may be associated with psychological distress in females.

In another study combining qualitative and quantitative methods, seventh graders provided detailed narratives of peer conflict that were coded as physical aggression, verbal aggression, direct relational aggression, and social aggression (here defined as nonconfrontational behaviors deployed to do interpersonal damage by involving the social community; Xie et al., 2002). These narratives provide vivid portrayals of how aggressive behaviors unfold in children's most salient experiences; they offer clues as to the specific contexts and processes involved in social aggression. More girls than boys were reported to engage in social aggression. Preadolescents reported that social aggression was usually an initiating behavior whereas direct relational aggression more often occurred in response to perceived slights and insults. Most episodes of social aggression involved three or more peers, and engaging in social aggression was related to being a more central member of social networks (defined as being a nuclear member of a social group as determined by detailed social network mapping procedures).

Because these data were collected as part of a larger longitudinal study, it was possible to examine whether particular forms of aggression predicted maladjustment in adolescence (defined as a criminal arrest, a school dropout, and teen parenthood). Engaging in physical aggression predicted all forms of maladjustment, but social and direct relational aggression did not. However, it is important to remember that social aggression here included only nonconfrontational behaviors. Whether it is possible to reliably distinguish between nonconfrontational social aggression and direct relational aggression remains unclear. Also, whether a particular person was mentioned in others' worst peer conflict experiences may not be the most sensitive index of an individual's propensity for social aggression, especially given that by its very nature this behavior often allows perpetrators' identities to be concealed.

In summary, then, research on anger and aggression among adolescent girls' includes a limited number of quantitative studies but a rich body of ethnographic observations. Together, these data paint a picture of girls as suppressing anger, managing conflicts so as to protect the integrity of their social relationships, using physical aggression quite rarely, and engaging in social aggression for a variety of both positive and negative reasons. Ethnographic researchers have arrived at diverse views of gossip among teenage girls as "girl talk" in the service of refining and maybe even changing social standards (Eckert, 1990), as moral negotiation (Fine, 1986), as part of an inevitable cycle of popularity that results when few girls have opportunities for status and visibility (Eder, 1990), and as "meanness" deployed to prevent being labeled as snobs (Merten, 1997). Research with larger samples only partly confirms that girls engage in social aggression more than boys do, but it supports the ethnographic findings that girls engage in these behaviors for a variety of reasons and find victimization painful.

Although few of these studies include age groups from both early and later adolescence, some developmental hypotheses can be formulated on the basis of findings across studies. Perhaps one reason some view social aggression as developmentally normal or even beneficial and some see it as hateful and maladaptive may be that this behavior takes different forms at different ages. Perhaps younger adolescents are more likely to engage in social aggression as a way of protecting the boundaries of groups and their own sense of status, or as a way of alleviating boredom. They may use forms of social aggression that are more crude and immature, for example, bluntly telling someone he or she is not invited to a party or threatening to end the friendship if the person does not comply with a demand. As adolescents mature, maybe some social aggression behaviors, perhaps especially gossip, become transformed into more subtle and sophisticated forms of communication used less for meanness and self-protection and more for problem solving, moral negotiation, and identity development (Gottman & Mettetal, 1986). It also seems highly likely that as youth move through adolescence, social aggression may more often involve manipulating or threatening girls' romantic relationships (Crick et al., 1999).

ORIGINS AND EXPLANATIONS FOR ADOLESCENT GIRLS' ANGER AND AGGRESSION

Why might girls who are becoming socially sophisticated in so many other ways, and who mostly refrain from outward expressions of anger and certainly from physical fighting, sometimes engage in what seem to be such mean-spirited, manipulative behaviors? Why do adolescent girls express anger via social aggression, manipulate relationships for the sake of alleviating boredom, and gossip, whether to harm others or in the service of moral negotiation? Just as for girls in preschool and middle childhood, hard evidence for the causes and explanations of social aggression among female adolescents is sorely lacking. But clues may be found in related literatures on temperament and biological factors, emotion regulation, parental relationships, gender stereotypes, social cognition, and peer and romantic relationships.

Temperament and Biological Factors

Although adolescents are well past the age when personality characteristics can be assumed to be largely inborn, a few studies have examined gender differences in personality dispositions that may be related to temperament. Remember that some studies with younger children found boys to be higher than girls on some forms of difficult temperament (see Brody, 1999, for a review of these findings). However, these gender differences appear less consistently with adolescent samples. When a sample of 82 teenagers (ages 14–18) rated their own temperament on the Dimensions of Temperament Survey–Revised (DOTS-R; Windle & Lerner, 1986), there were no gender differences for difficult temperament. Gender differences were evident for only 2 of the 10 dimensions measured by the DOTS-R; girls reported less flexibility and less regularity of eating than did boys (Kawaguchi, Welsh, Powers, & Rostosky, 1998). In another study in which a much larger sample (N = 975) of 15- to 17-year-olds responded to the DOTS-R, girls were higher than boys on adaptability and positive affect (effect size was .22) whereas boys were higher on rhythmicity (of eating and sleeping; effect size was .27) and on attentional focus (effect size was .28; Windle, 1992). It is important to refrain from making much of small but significant effects from studies with large samples. Still, that teenage girls report higher levels of sociability and positive emotions fits with their tendency to resolve conflicts carefully so as to preserve relationships and, perhaps when furious, to prefer the more indirect forms of aggression.

Although dispositional differences in adolescence are difficult to attribute to biology alone, there is a biological event in adolescence that seems to have powerful effects on girls' relationships—the onset of puberty. Puberty presents girls with considerable challenges (Caspi & Moffitt, 1991). As girls experience hormonal and associated physical changes, they begin to focus more on themselves as sexual beings, be more concerned with their physical appearance and attractiveness to others, and worry more about conforming to stereotyped notions of how women are supposed to behave (Basow & Rubin, 1999). Early maturation may be particularly difficult because it requires girls to meet new developmental expectations when they are not yet psychologically mature (Ge, Conger, & Elder, 1996).

For girls, the onset of menarche seems to be associated with increased negativity in their relationships with their mothers (Holmbeck & Hill, 1991). Seventh-grade girls were observed as they engaged a Structured Family Interaction Task with their mothers and their fathers, which involved discussing preferences for vacations, restaurants, and weekend activities. Shortly after menarche for the daughters, interactions with their mothers were more conflictual and the mothers were observed to be less likely to respond to interruptions and disagreements with positive affect.

The results of this study as well as others suggest that girls maturing early might be at special risk for difficulties. In the study just described, families of girls who matured early seemed more disengaged and less cohesive than other families (Holmbeck & Hill, 1991). In a longitudinal study with families in rural Iowa that compared early-maturing, on-time-maturing, and late-maturing girls on subsequent psychological adjustment, early-maturing girls reported greater psychological distress as adolescents (Ge et al., 1996). Early-maturing girls were more likely than girls in the other two groups to have had prior psychological problems, to affiliate with deviant peers, and to be subject to hostile behavior by their fathers. In a longitudinal study with a more urban sample of youth in New Zealand, early maturation predicted delinquency for girls (Caspi & Moffitt, 1991). In another study of a large community sample of U.S. high school students, early-maturing girls reported more psychopathology than other groups (Graber, Lewinsohn, Seeley, & Brooks-Gunn, 1997).

No published research to date has examined the relation between pubertal maturation and social aggression. However, it seems possible that just as girls' relationships with their mothers may become more turbulent as a result of pubertal changes, so might their relationships with peers. In future studies, it will be important to remember that pubertal development seems to be more of a continuous series of events than a discrete event (there is a great deal of overlap in hormonal levels between pre- and postmenarcheal groups; Dorn et al., 1999). Complex models will be needed to understand the relations between hormones and social behavior during adolescence (Susman, 1997). It would be fascinating to investigate whether pubertal development is associated with more conflict in peer relations and more social aggression, as girls might face increasing demands but also increasing pressure to be nice and ladylike. It also seems possible that early-maturing girls, and possibly late-maturing girls too, might be particularly vulnerable to being victimized by social aggression (Craig, Pepler, Connolly, & Henderson, 2001).

Emotion Regulation

Although theories offer fascinating speculations about emotions and their regulation during adolescence, most of these claims are supported by precious little empirical evidence. The majority of teachers and parents believe that early adolescence is a turbulent, difficult, challenging time of life (Buchanan et al., 1990)—that adolescents are overcome and impelled by strong negative emotions that they have great difficulty regulating. Many seem to believe that these difficulties are linked to hormones and pubertal development, and therefore are universal and inevitable. It is not uncommon to go to parent orientations for middle or junior high schools and hear warnings such as "teenagers are walking hormones" and "hang onto your hats—adolescence is a wild ride." A pioneering psychologist, G. S. Hall (1904), proposed long ago that adolescence is a period characterized by "storm and stress," a point of view that seems to have been widely adopted for the better part of the last century.

In a thoughtful examination of the empirical evidence for adolescence as stormy and stressful, Arnett (1999) points out that the argument that adolescence is difficult is based on three primary problem areas: conflict with parents, emotional dysregulation (mood disruptions), and reckless, norm-breaking behavior. In none of these domains do the research findings suggest that storm and stress is universal, nor is it linked directly to biological factors such as the onset of puberty. Arnett offered instead a modified storm and stress theory that "not all adolescents experience storm and stress, but storm and stress is more likely during adolescence than at other ages" (p. 317). Arnett noted that there is considerable individual and cultural variation in the extent to which teenagers experience storm and stress; difficulty seems greatest for Western cultures that encourage teenagers to develop independence. Arnett also pointed out that several positive emotional features are hallmarks of this developmental period, including exuberance and passionate idealism.

Another balanced view of adolescents' emotional development was offered by Gottman and Mettetal (1986), who proposed that adolescence is characterized by "the fusion of emotion and reason" (p. 202). Adolescents use their increasingly sophisticated cognitive skills as they try to understand the complex worlds of emotions and social relationships and to explore their identity in relation to others. Adolescents appreciate that they and others can have both positive and negative features and that it is possible to dislike a particular characteristic of something or someone but still appreciate the whole. Gottman and Mettetal proposed that the primary goal of conversation for this age group is to understand the self in relation to others and that key processes are sometimes brutal honesty between friends, making oneself vulnerable by self-disclosure, helping others explore the meaning of their disclosures, and working with friends to solve problems even if it requires confrontation. Gottman and Mettetal (p. 203) even refer to their theory of emotional development as the *Star Trek* theory, where early childhood is predominated by raw emotion (the human side of Mr. Spock and the kindness of Dr. Leonard "Bones" McCoy), middle childhood is characterized as extreme rationality and an emphasis on controlling emotions at all costs (the Vulcan side of Mr. Spock), whereas adolescence represents the balanced persona of Captain James T. Kirk.

Whether adolescents are beset by storm and stress or are indeed more balanced characters remains in large part to be determined because very little empirical research has focused specifically on emotional development in this age range (Zahn-Waxler, Klimes-Dougan, & Kendziora, 1998). Emotion researchers seem to have been reluctant to study teenagers, perhaps because many of these scholars come from the ranks of infancy or early-childhood researchers. Another possible reason might be that adolescents are perceived as especially challenging to study because they may be so capable of dissemblance, so busy with other activities, or even disagreeable enough so as to be noncompliant. In addition, researchers might have difficulty getting access to high school samples because teachers are all the more reluctant to relinquish precious instructional time. Others might hesitate to study emotion regulation with adolescents because teenagers may be more vulnerable to particular types of harm from research participation in their capacity to experience pain from social comparison (Thompson, 1990). However, some cleverly conceived methods have provided extremely useful descriptive information about adolescents' emotional lives, for example, Larson's *experience sampling method* (see R. Larson & Richards, 1994). Adolescents have proven to be cooperative research participants, even when they are required to wear pagers and to fill out forms in response to intermittent beeps; thus more research on their emotion regulation seems entirely possible and is important for understanding their anger and aggression. Findings from these studies are discussed in later subsections.

Additional research on adolescents' emotional regulation may be especially important for understanding girls' social aggression. Evidence suggests that girls experience greater interpersonal stress during adolescence, and this may contribute to their greater risk for depression and for some forms of anxiety disorders (Rudolph, 2002; Zahn-Waxler et al., 1998). In one study, fifth through eighth graders reported how stressed they would feel in response to particular types of peer experiences; girls reported more stress than boys did in response to friendship disruptions, whereas boys reported greater stress than girls did in response to difficulties in the larger peer group (Rudolph, 2002). Girls' abilities to cope with the stresses of friendship problems may well be related to individual differences in social aggression.

Parental Relationships

Another fertile ground in which to search for developmental origins of social aggression among girls may be their relationships with parents. During this developmental period, adolescents' relationships with parents undergo processes of disengagement and transformation (R.

Larson, Richards, Moneta, Holmbeck, & Duckett, 1996). Adolescents present their parents with myriad dramatic changes in every aspect of their being, push their parents to alter their parenting practices to accommodate their strong desire for autonomy, while at the same time they rely on their parents for support and value their responsiveness (Holmbeck, Paikoff, & Brooks-Gunn, 1995).

With increasing age, adolescents seem to spend less time with family members. According to experience-sampling data, overall time with family members decreased from 35% of waking time in the fifth grade to 14% of waking time in the 12th grade (R. Larson et al., 1996). However, time spent talking alone with parents stayed stable throughout this period. Especially for girls, time spent talking with family about interpersonal issues increased with age.

Because girls continue to rely on parental support and talk with their parents about relationship issues, features of parental relationships may well be related to girls' social aggression during adolescence. A detailed account of the wealth of research on parenting of adolescents is beyond the scope of this chapter (see Holmbeck et al., 1995, for a comprehensive review). The discussion in the following subsections focuses on three aspects of parent–child relationships that may relate to social aggression among adolescent girls: attachment, differential socialization of girls and boys, and exposure to marital conflict.

Attachment

As discussed in Chapter 6, the extent to which youth have secure relationships with sensitive, responsive parents may foster developing positive working models that influence their later relationships (Bowlby, 1969). Although no published research to date has examined the relation between parental attachment and social aggression, it seems reasonable to hypothesize that children with insecure parental attachment might be more vulnerable to feeling threatened in their peer relations and therefore might be more likely to engage in social aggression.

Research using various methods suggests that there may be a small-to-moderate relationship between some dimensions of parental attachment and qualities of peer relations. In one longitudinal study conducted in Germany, infants participated in "strange situation" assessments with mothers and fathers, then when they were 16 years old responded to the Adult Attachment Interview (AAI; Main, 1991) and participated in a peer social problem-solving task (a complex computer simulation involving ecological conditions in a Third World country; Zimmerman, Maier, Winter, & Grossman, 2001). The results showed that adolescents who appeared insecurely attached to their fathers as infants showed less adept emotion regulation with their peers at age 16. Also, teenagers who were classified as insecurely attached on the AAI were more disruptive when emotions were intense in the peer problem-solving task.

Investigations using questionnaire methods also show modest relationships between parental attachment and peer relations. Armsden and Greenberg (1987) developed a self-report measure of three dimensions of attachment to parents and to peers: trust, alienation, and communication (the Inventory of Peer and Parent Attachment, IPPA). The correlations between parent and peer attachment, within and across domains, were all in the expected directions and in the range of .24 to .47. In a study with a fairly small sample of 10th graders, Schneider and Younger (1996) examined the relation between adolescents' responses to the IPPA and their self-reports of interpersonal competence. The results showed that parental alienation, especially with fathers, was related to poor social competence, but that positive dimensions of attachment were not related to positive social adjustment. In a study with 16-year-olds in Germany, secure attachment as assessed by the AAI was related to adaptive responding to vignettes describing social rejection (Zimmerman, 1999).

Other research suggests that parent–child attachment is related to adolescents' overall psychological adjustment, and it seems reasonable that this finding might extend to children's peer relationships. In one study, 13- to 19-year-olds who were rated as securely attached on the AAI had fewer psychological symptoms and higher self-concept than insecure groups (although they were not the lowest on risky behaviors; Cooper, Shaver, & Collins, 1998). In another study that did not specifically invoke the label of attachment but that measured relevant dimensions, parents with high warmth, low hostility, and good management skills had children who were less likely to have externalizing problems and less likely to show increases of problems over time (Scaramella, Conger, & Simons, 1999). Other research and theory suggests that insecure parental attachment may contribute to children being sensitive to social rejection (Downey, Lebolt, Rincon, & Freitas, 1998), which, as discussed in a later subsection on marital conflict, may also be related to social aggression. All of these findings together suggest at least the possibility that parental attachment may relate to ways that girls express anger and behave aggressively.

Differential Socialization of Girls and Boys

Another feature of parent–child relationships that may well relate to girls' preference for social over physical aggression is the extent to which parents relate differently to girls and to boys. Few investigations to date have examined gender differences in the relation between parental attachment and children's peer relations. However, some evidence indicates that girls describe their relationships with their mothers as deeper than do boys (Kawaguchi et al., 1998). Given the closeness of girls' relationships with their mothers and the disruption in these that occurs around menarche (Holmbeck & Hill, 1991), and given that with age girls increasingly talk with their families about relationship issues, the possible link between mother–daughter attachment and girls' social aggression may well merit further exploration.

Moving beyond the realm of attachment, how else might mothers and fathers treat adolescent girls and boys differently? In their review, Holmbeck and colleagues (1995) note that as compared to fathers of adolescents, mothers spend more time with their sons and daughters and are slightly more likely to be involved in caregiving. Relationships between mothers and adolescents are more disrupted by the onset of puberty than father relationships, but mothers continue to be perceived as a more important source of support than fathers: mother–daughter relationships seem to be especially close; daughters and mothers report relying on one another more than do all other parent–child pairs; and mother–daughter relationships are more mutual than father–daughter relationships. All of these findings suggest that girls' relationships with their mothers might be related to their social aggression with peers. It seems especially important to begin exploring the extent to which girls observe their mothers engaging in these behaviors, and how mothers respond to girls' experiences as victims and perpetrators of social aggression.

Exposure to marital conflict

Another important way in which parent–child relationships may relate to social aggression among girls is exposure to parents' marital conflict. As discussed in Chapter 6, marital conflict may relate to children's social aggression because it threatens their emotional security and therefore increases their risk for behavioral problems more generally. Also, by observing parents in conflict, children may learn to hurt others by harming their social relationships.

Although no published research to date has examined the influence of exposure to marital conflict on adolescents' social aggression, marital conflict seems to relate to psychological problems more generally. In a longitudinal study beginning with seventh graders and their families in rural Iowa, children's perceptions of parents' marital conflict predicted later internalizing and externalizing problems for boys but not for girls (Harold & Conger, 1997). However, another study with middle adolescents showed that girls were more vulnerable to family discord then were boys; family discord mediated the relation between maternal depression and girls' depression and conduct disorder (but did not mediate this relation for boys; Davies & Windle, 1997). Other research showed that marital conflict that occurs in front of young adolescents adds to the prediction of teenagers' psychological problems, above and beyond general family conflict (David, Steele, Forehand, & Armistead, 1996).

Although such speculations await empirical tests, it seems reasonable to imagine that if adolescents observe parents attempting to hurt each other by triangulating others in conflicts or by threatening to withdraw from the relationship, these adolescents might be more likely to engage in these behaviors with peers. And children might learn these behaviors from observing other family members. Research suggests that adolescent girls may learn control tactics from their brothers that they import to their friendships with others girls (Updegraff, Moltale, & Crouter, 2000), so it may not be so farfetched to expect that girls may learn at least some elements of social aggression from their relationships with sisters and brothers.

Gender Stereotypes

Another important influence on adolescent girls' anger and aggression may be gender stereotypes. Girls' adherence to stereotypes and others' expectations that they conform to these may be strengthened around the time of the onset of puberty. According to the gender intensification hypothesis, perhaps as a result of puberty and its associated changes, girls experience an "acceleration of gender differential socialization during adolescence" (Hill & Lynch, 1983, p. 201). As girls mature physically and also move to bigger schools and begin dating, the theory suggests that parents become less permissive with girls and hold them to higher standards of achievement and behavior than they do boys. Girls may respond to all of these changes by conforming more strictly to gender stereotypes, perhaps especially in early adolescence. As possible support for this theory, Hill and Lynch (1983) outlined several broad types of gender differences: girls are more likely than boys to be anxious, have low self-esteem, and engage in less aggression. However, none of these are sufficient evidence for the gender intensification hypothesis. Few studies have examined age differences in differential socialization by parents or the relation between pubertal onset and magnification of gender differences, and those studies that have examined these issues found only mixed support for gender intensification (Galambos, Almeida, & Petersen, 1990).

Research on adolescents' adherence to gender stereotypes confirms that overall adolescence is a time of decreasing flexibility but that these changes seem not to be related to the onset of puberty. In a study that used a combination of cross-sectional and longitudinal methods, Alfieri, Ruble, and Higgins (1996) examined the flexibility of gender stereotypes for children in grades 4–11. In this study, flexibility was operationally defined as the number of times that participants responded "both" when asked whether a particular personality characteristic was associated with men, women, or both. The results showed that flexibility increased immediately after the transition to junior high school, regardless of whether this transition occurred at seventh or eighth grade, perhaps as a result of children being exposed to a large group of new peers and different routines. After this transition, gender beliefs became less flexible across the middle and high school years. There was no increase in gender flexibility upon entry to high school, which the authors speculated might have been due to the fact that this transition involved less novelty. Overall, these results suggest that flexibility of gender stereotypes may be influenced by changes in social ecology.

In a longitudinal study that examined the gender intensification hypothesis more directly, children completed measures of masculinity, femininity, and beliefs about gender roles in the sixth, seventh, and eighth grades (Galambos et al., 1990). The results indicated that, with age, gender differences in masculinity and sex role attitudes increased but there were not developmental changes for gender differences in femininity. None of these changes were strongly associated with pubertal timing. Galambos and colleagues (1990) interpreted these results as providing some support for gender intensification in early adolescence, but not for puberty as a strong causal factor. They speculated that the lack of developmental increases in femininity might be due to young adolescents' perceptions that femininity is less desirable than masculinity.

Moral Development

Almost no research to date has examined the relation between moral development and social or relational aggression (but see Goldstein et al., 2002, for one study with preschoolers). Still, existing research on moral development more broadly suggests that social aggression may well be related to moral development, perhaps especially for girls and in particular during the adolescent years.

First, several experts have suggested that youth consider their interpersonal difficulties in moral terms. When asked to describe their own real-life moral dilemmas, youth in grades 7, 9, and 12 told stories about interpersonal difficulties 24–38% of the time (Yussen, 1977). Remember from earlier in this chapter that theorists have conceived of girls' gossip as moral negotiation (Fine, 1986; Gottman & Mettetal, 1986).

Second, adolescents' moral reasoning becomes increasingly sophisticated in ways that make morality all the more likely to be related to social aggression. Kolhberg (1976) proposed that most adolescents are in the process of moving from conventional moral reasoning (what is moral is determined by others' rules and standards) to post-conventional moral reasoning (morality is internally determined). Gilligan (1982) countered that for girls moral reasoning focuses less on justice and rules and more on care and relationships, and that girls' moral development involves their learning to balance their own needs with care for others. Both theories suggest that adolescents may be prone to wrestling with the moral implications of interpersonal behavior in a way that may relate to social aggression. All of the basic components of moral development (Rest, 1995) may be related to social aggression: moral sensitivity (awareness of how behaviors affect others), moral judgment (deciding what is right and wrong), moral motivation (choosing to prioritize moral over personal principles), and moral character (persisting in moral behavior in the face of challenges).

A third reason to examine how moral development relates to social aggression is that previous research has shown that moral cognition relates to physical aggression and other antisocial behavior. Even when people believe in moral ideals, these can become disengaged from their actual behavior. As described by Bandura (1999), moral disengagement involves four primary mechanisms: cognitive restructuring to make behavior morally justifiable, denying one's own agency by diffusing or displacing responsibility, minimizing the harmful effects of one's behaviors, and blaming or dehumanizing victims. Studies with children and adolescents have found that self-reported disengagement is related to a variety of types of antisocial, transgressive behavior for both genders (Bandura, Barbaranelli, Caprara, & Pastorelli, 1996; Bandura, Caprara, Barbaranelli, Pastorelli, & Regalia, 2001). One survey with 14- and 16-year-olds found that endorsement of attitudes related to moral disengagement predicted 38% of the variance in self-reported bullying (Hymel, Bonanno, Henderson, & McCreith, 2002).

Fourth and last, further examining moral development may be especially important for understanding social aggression among girls. Girls' care and concern for relationships (Gilligan, 1982) may be related to their greater distress when friendships are disrupted (Rudolph, 2002). Investigating the relation between moral reasoning and social aggression may illuminate why some girls engage in social aggression and some do not.

Social Cognition

In addition to gender stereotypes, other features of social cognition may be related to adolescent girls' anger and aggression: social information processing, preoccupation with others' perceptions ("the imaginary audience"; Elkind, 1967), rumination, and rejection sensitivity. No published research to date has examined how social information processing may be related to social aggression in adolescent girls, but it seems reasonable to expect that these behaviors may be related to particular types of interpretations of social cues, social goals, and outcome expectations.

One feature of adolescents' thinking that may be related to social or indirect aggression is their seeming preoccupation with what Elkind and Bowen (1979) called "the imaginary audience." Because young adolescents are moving away from parents and still in the process of developing supportive peer relationships and clear identities, they "enhance, maintain, and defend self-esteem in relation to the audience" (Elkind, 1983, p. 435). Early research using questionnaires to assess children's views about the imaginary audience showed that young adolescents were especially reluctant to reveal their true selves to others and that girls were less willing to reveal themselves than were boys (Elkind & Bowen, 1979–although subsequent studies showed that gender and developmental differences may be less clear; see Gossens, 1984; Peterson & Roscoe, 1991). Because adolescents seem so preoccupied with others' perceptions of everything they do, they may engage in strategic interactions specifically designed to manipulate audience perceptions, "interpersonal interactions that have as their aim the acquisition, concealment, or revelation of information *through indirect means*" (Elkind, 1990, p. 434; emphasis added). Elkind (1990) hypothesized that these strategic interactions may include staying on the telephone so others get a busy signal, cutting a conversation short in case others are trying to get through, and snubbing someone in front of higher-status others. Some of these strategic interactions resemble social aggression.

Another feature of adolescent cognition that might enhance the likelihood of perpetrating and feeling the pain of social aggression is rumination, thinking obsessively about one's problems and their consequences. A large body of research has demonstrated that, in response to depression, women are more likely to ruminate on their symptoms than are men and that rumination contributes to longer-lasting depressive symptoms (Nolen-Hoeksema, Morrow, & Fredrickson, 1993). Adolescent girls are more likely to ruminate than are adolescent boys (Nolen-Hoeksema, 1994). It seems quite possible that ruminating about interpersonal problems could lead girls to engage in social aggression, as well as to make them feel worse when they are victims. Ruminating could lead girls to magnify the important of relationship problems, and even to be oversensitive to social exclusion. When girls describe victimization experiences, they report thinking more about feeling hurt than boys do (Paquette & Underwood, 1999). Remember also that in the study with focus groups of teenage girls, Owens and colleagues (2001a) found that girls reported that thinking obsessively about victimization by indirect aggression was a common response by victims and that such thinking made girls feel helpless.

Girls also have been shown to be more likely than boys to engage in corumination with friends, defined as "excessively discussing personal problems within a dyadic relationship" (A. J. Rose, 2001, p. 2). Corumination might provide girls with opportunities for social aggression, especially for maligning others.

The last type of social cognition that may relate to social aggression for girls is rejection sensitivity. Rejection sensitivity is "the disposition to defensively (i.e., anxiously or angrily) expect, readily perceive, or overreact to social rejection" (Downey et al., 1998, p. 1074). Rejection sensitivity might lead children to engage in social aggression as a defensive tactic or even as a preemptive strike when they feel that friendships or social status are threatened.

Most research on the effects of rejection sensitivity on relationships has focused on romantic relations in adolescence (Downey, Bonica, & Rincon, 1999; Purdie & Downey, 2000) and adulthood (Ayduk, Downey, Testa, Yen, & Shoda, 1999; Downey & Feldman, 1996). This body of work demonstrates that rejection-sensitive people overattribute rejection when their partners behave insensitively. Rejection-sensitive people feel chronically threatened and behave in ways so as to undermine the quality of the relationship (Downey et al., 1999). Specifically, adult women who are rejection sensitive engage in more conflict with partners and make more hostile, spiteful remarks during conflicts, which results in decreases in partners' satisfaction with and commitment to the relationship (Downey & Feldman, 1996). A model of rejection sensitivity proposes that reactions of rejection-sensitive people to perceived slights lead them to experience even more social rejection and to become increasingly rejection-sensitive (Levy, Ayduk, & Downey, 2001).

Research on children's rejection sensitivity is only beginning. Recently, Downey and colleagues (1998) developed a measure of rejection sensitivity for children's expectations of and responses to peers and teachers, and found that for a sample of fifth through seventh graders rejection sensitivity predicted self-reported and teacher-rated aggression 1 year later (the measure of aggression included items to assess physical and verbal—but not social—aggression). Because one important function of social aggression may be to protect one's own social standing and reputation (Paquette & Underwood, 1999; Xie et al., in press-a), it seems possible that rejection-sensitive children will be more likely to perceive social slights and more likely to respond by harming others by social exclusion, relationship manipulation, and spreading rumors.

Peer Relations

As so much of the evidence reviewed thus far suggests, girls' expressions of anger and aggression are embedded in the culture of their peer relationships. What features of adolescent girls' friendships, networks, and romances may be related to their preference for social aggression, to their capacity for breaking each other's hearts? Here again, a comprehensive review of gender differences in adolescent peer relations is beyond the scope of this chapter (and this is an area begging for a thoroughgoing meta-analytic review). The discussion in the following subsections highlights the most recent studies and emphasizes those that include measures other than self-report questionnaires.

Friendships

As youth move through adolescence, they confide more in friends, friendships become more focused on conversation and less on play, and friends engage in self-exploration together and offer each other social support while continuing to need to work through conflicts (Buhrmester, 1996). Overall, girls report having higher-quality friendships than boys do (Jones & Coston, 1995), but also that they are more vulnerable than boys are to interpersonal difficulties (Leadbeater, Kuperminc, Blatt, & Hertzog, 1999).

In many studies, girls report on questionnaires that their same-gender friendships involve more intimacy and self-disclosure than boys do (Blyth & Foster-Clark, 1987; Buhrmester, 1996; Papini, Farmer, Clark, Micha, & Barnett, 1990). However, a study that examined effect sizes of gender differences in disclosure to best and good friends of the same and other gender found that many of the gender differences in self-disclosure were small in magnitude (Dolgin & Kim, 1994). Still, girls reported disclosing more to girls than to boys; girls reported hearing more disclosures of moderately or highly intimate topics, whereas boys reported more disclosures related to low-intimacy issues; and the discrepancy between self-disclosure to best and close friends was greater for girls than for boys.

Observational studies as least partly confirm that girls' friendships may feature more intimacy and self-disclosure than those of boys do, but also suggest that gender differences may depend on how intimacy is defined. In one study mentioned earlier, 15-year-old same-gender best friends completed a questionnaire assessing friendship quality, then were observed as they discussed what each does that angers the other and as they discussed other peers (Brendgen et al., 2001). The results showed that girls reported higher friendship quality on the questionnaire than boys did. In the observed interaction, as compared to boys, girls were more responsive, self-disclosing, showed less negative emotion, were less critical, and engaged in less conflict. For both girls and boys, questionnaire ratings of friendship quality corresponded moderately to observed behaviors.

In another observational study, intimacy was defined as the sharing of emotional experiences (McNelles & Connolly, 1999). In this longitudinal study of youth in grades 9, 10, and 11, best friends participated in a semistructured task that required them to make complex decisions jointly. These interactions were rated on global scales that assessed shared affective involvement, activity-centered intimacy, and personal disclosure. From grades 9 and 10 for both genders there was an increase in intimate conversation and disclosure, and from grades 10 and 11 sustained shared affect increased. Girls were higher than boys on intimacy in their discussion and self-disclosures, but boys were higher than girls on intimacy in shared activities. Overall, these results suggest that girls may be higher than boys on the forms of intimacy typically assessed but that to understand intimacy among boys we may need to observe them in activity contexts.

Although girls' greater propensity for intimate, self-disclosing conversations may sound extremely positive, it is not difficult to imagine that it is exactly these features of girls' friendships that might make them vulnerable to engaging in and experiencing social aggression. If girls' friendships are particularly close and intimate, then threats to their exclusivity could feel all the more threatening. Girls may also use their intimate knowledge of friends to hurt and betray them when they are angry; girls may be vulnerable to social aggression exactly because they disclose so much to their friends.

Although many of these speculations have yet to be tested directly, recent research offers hints of some negative features of adolescent girls' friendships. For example, although children and adolescents view girlfriends as more likely to know personal information about each other and would be more likely to enjoy sitting and talking than boys would, they also report that girls are less likely to be friends with each other if they are each friends with a third target child (Markovits, Benenson, & Dolensky, 2001). In response to hypothetical vignettes describing situations in which a close friend succeeded and they did not, young adolescent girls reported that they would be more bothered than boys about a friends' greater success in the domains of close friendships, romance, popularity, and attractiveness (Benenson & Benarroch, 1998). In another questionnaire study, although girls and boys in grades 7–11 reported similar levels of social stress and social support, for girls but not for boys social stress was related to depression and lower self-esteem (Moran & Eckenrode, 1991). For boys but not for girls social support was related to lower depression and to higher self-esteem. Together, the findings from all of these studies suggest that girls may pay higher costs than boys do for the intimacy of their friendships, in resenting possible interlopers and friends' success, and in being more distressed by social difficulties (see also Leadbeater et al., 1999). Feeling more resentful of friends' other friends and friends' successes may well contribute to the urge to hurt someone else by manipulating his or her relationships, and having intimate knowledge of friends may supply the ammunition.

As intuitively appealing as these hypotheses may be, it is important to take care in generalizing these ideas to all types of friendships. Most friendship research has focused on same-gender friends; we know very little about other-gender friendships that are not romantic (Sippola, 1999). Most research on friendship has been conducted with mostly white middle-class and upper-middle-class samples from Canada and the United States. On the basis of a large-scale interview study with a more diverse sample, Giordano, Cernkovich, and DeMaris (1993) concluded that African American youth remain closer to their families during adolescence than European American youth do and have less intense friendships. In a thoughtful review, Brown, Way, and Duff (1999) pointed out that most of what we know about the intricate processes of adolescent girls' friendships comes from research with samples of white girls from the upper Midwest. Very different friendship processes may emerge when other groups are studied. For example, urban ethnic minority girls report being extremely outspoken with friends, which they view as one way of expressing care in the relationship (Way, 1995). If these girls are more assertive in pursuing their social goals, perhaps they are less likely to engage in social aggression. We need much more research on how girls of different ethnicities and social classes negotiate the tensions between individual success and solidarity with peers.

Networks

Girls fulfill their communal needs not only within the context of dyadic friendships but also in larger groups and peer networks. Social networks have proven challenging to measure for at least two reasons. First, adolescents' social networks operate at many levels: interactions occur in dyadic relationships, which are in turn embedded in specific social groups within global networks (Furman & Simon, 1998). Second, social networks have been defined and measured in various ways, including self-reports, sociometric status, and complex social-cognitive mapping procedures in which several members of the peer group report who among them hang around together (Cairns, Leung, & Cairns, 1995).

Although girls' social networks are often characterized as smaller than boys' networks are (Maccoby, 1998), most recent studies do not find differences in network size although some suggest that girls may be more connected to and concerned with their social networks than are boys. In a rare observational study, Pellegrini (1994) followed a small sample of children during their first 2 years of middle school and found no gender or grade differences in the size of children's social networks as observed during free play. In a large study with children in grades 6–12 in three different school systems, boys and girls reported their close friends, best friends, friendship groups, and social crowds, and complex statistical procedures were used to map networks (Urberg, Degirmencioglu, Tolson, & Halliday-Scher, 1995). Girls' and boys' social networks did not differ in size, but girls were more embedded than boys in social networks in that they made and received more network choices, had more mutual nominations, and were more likely to have a best friend and to be a clique member. In another study by this same research group, there were few gender differences in the stability of friendship networks across a single school year for middle and high school students, although girls were more likely to stay affiliated with any network (but not necessarily the same one) from the fall to the spring (Degirmencioglu, Urberg, Tolson, & Richard, 1998).

In addition to being more connected with their social networks than boys are, girls may be more concerned than boys about the inner workings of their social groups. In a questionnaire study with early, middle, and late adolescents, girls reported more positive group interactions, but also more distress about negative interactions within the groups and more permeable group boundaries (Gavin & Furman, 1989).

As adolescence progresses, social networks may become more permeable and expand to include other-gender peers. As compared to younger teens, older adolescents report less concern with being in the popular group, less conformity and leadership within their networks, and fewer difficult and more positive interactions among group members (Gavin & Furman, 1989). A large-scale sociometric study with children in grades 3–12 found that after sixth grade the percentage of youth who are group members decreases and more youth become liaisons, individuals who have weak ties to multiple groups and less integrated networks of friends (Shrum & Cheek, 1987). However, in this study, groups were measured only by friendship nominations. In other research that assessed network structure more directly by asking children to report who they "hang around with," evidence for this degrouping process has not been found (Urberg et al., 1995).

Romance

Regardless of whether degrouping occurs, it is clear that as adolescence progresses groups expand to include other gender peers, and this process may set the stage for romantic involvement. From middle school onward, adolescents' preference for same-gender friends seems to decrease (Shrum, Cheek, & Hunter, 1988). During grades 6 and 7, girls and boys begin to interact more on the playground (Pellegrini, 1994). Boys increasingly direct rough-and-tumble play and teasing toward girls (Pellegrini, 2001), which appears to serve as a playful and perhaps safe way to begin to initiate potentially risky other-gender interactions (sometimes referred to as "pushing and poking" courtship; Maccoby, 1998, p. 70). Links develop between girls' and boys' social clusters, and mixed-gender networks form (Cairns et al., 1995). In a longitudinal study of Canadian adolescents in grades 9–11, small groups of close friends were found to expand to become other-gender networks, and participating in these was related to the beginning of romantic involvement (Connolly, Furman, & Konarski, 2000). The quality of same-gender friendships was related to the quality of early romantic relationships, confirming theories suggesting that peer friendship groups and networks facilitate the emergence of romance (Dunphy, 1963). This facilitation may occur for good or for ill; adolescents who report they bully peers also report that they are more coercive and aggressive in their romantic relationships than nonbullies are (Connolly, Pepler, Craig, & Taradash, 2000).

By the eleventh grade, more girls (52%) than boys (33%) reported being involved in a romantic relationship (Connolly, Furman, & Konarski, 2000). For many girls across ethnic and social class groups, some

degree of romantic involvement begins in adolescence, and preliminary evidence suggests that as girls mature their social aggression begins to involve others' romantic partners (Werner & Crick, 1999).
Research on adolescent romance is just beginning, and theoretical
frameworks are still being formulated and refined. Note that the following discussion will focus on girls who are heterosexual; more research on gay and lesbian youth is desperately needed (Savin-Williams,
2001).

Even early adolescents share adult conceptions of romance, and
many are involved in romantic relationships, however fleeting. When
asked to respond to questionnaires about qualities of romantic relationships and other-gender friendships, even 9- to 14-year-olds with little actual experience described romance as featuring passion and commitment, and other-gender friendships as featuring affiliation (no
gender differences emerged; Connolly, Craig, Goldberg, & Pepler,
1999). When asked to describe their romantic involvement, 88% of 15-
year-olds reported having dated, the average duration of dating someone was 12 weeks, and there were no gender differences for romantic
involvement (Feiring, 1996). When asked to describe the positive features of romantic relationships, girls mentioned intimacy more than
did boys, and boys mentioned physical attractiveness more than did
girls.

Older adolescents report more romantic involvement than do
younger adolescents, and older girls are also more likely than older
boys to report greater attachment and care in their romantic relationships (Shulman & Scharf, 2000). In this interview and questionnaire
study with teenagers in Israel, the affective intensity of the youths'
same-gender friendships, but not parental relationships, was related to
the affective intensity of their romantic partnerships. This result confirms the findings of Connolly, Furman, and Konarski (2000) that romantic involvement increases across the high school years and that
qualities of same-gender friendships may relate to qualities of early romances.

How does the development of romantic involvement relate to social aggression? Remember that the experience-sampling research
shows that for adolescent girls most of the developmental increase in
negative emotions is due to increasing anger, hurt, and worry about op-
posite-gender peers. For girls, developing relationships with boys may
generate exuberance, passion, and love, but also emotional pain. As
some of the examples in the first portion of this chapter indicate all too
clearly, one way that girls may harm each other is by manipulating their
romantic relationships as well as their other friendships. Perhaps because girls report valuing attachment and care in their romantic rela-

tionships more than do boys, stealing someone's boyfriend or otherwise engineering a romantic betrayal might become a particularly lethal form of social aggression for adolescent females.

SUMMARY

Both ethnographic and more qualitative studies have provided a rich and interesting portrait of girls' social aggression in adolescence. In the service of organizing the overwhelming amount of information here, I return to the primary questions that organize this book:

• *What does research evidence suggest about how adolescent girls express anger and behave aggressively?* Here again, it is important to remember that although it is not clear that girls engage in social aggression more than do boys during adolescence, the evidence does suggest that girls prefer to express anger and pursue social goals in ways that may prominently feature social aggression, certainly much more than physical aggression and other overt anger expressions. For girls, relationships with peers may be significant sources of angry feelings, but girls seem to prefer to avoid open expressions of anger, especially with close friends. Girls tend to prefer to deal with conflicts by using mitigating strategies such as negotiation and compromise, but they also often respond with what appears to be submission and disengagement, at least in the immediate sense (whether these sometimes then lead to more covert retaliation remains unknown). Very few girls fight physically. However, given that girls value relationships so intensely and that social and physical aggression are often highly correlated, the rare episodes in which girls do fight likely also involve social aggression. We need to know more about how and why social aggression leads to physical aggression for some few girls.

Various types of evidence converge to suggest that social aggression is fairly widespread among adolescent girls and that they engage in it for diverse reasons. Girls may engage in social aggression to express anger, seek revenge, or to assert social dominance. However, research suggests that other reasons for social aggression are to confirm girls' own sense of belongingness and acceptance by excluding others, to negotiate norms and moral standards by using gossip to test the boundaries of acceptable behavior, and even to relieve boredom. As youth move into later adolescence, social aggression increasingly involves girls' threatening and even manipulating each others' romantic relationships.

• *How does social aggression unfold among adolescent girls, and how does this differ from that among boys?* Very few studies have examined carefully how social aggression might proceed differently among teenage girls and boys. The quantitative studies have relied mostly on peer rating and nomination methods, which are poorly suited for revealing gender differences in group processes. And they have yielded mixed evidence for gender differences. Most of the ethnographic studies of social aggression have focused specifically on social aggression among girls and have not carefully observed boys (e.g., Eder, 1985, 1990; Fine, 1986; Merten, 1997). One exception is the ethnographic account of social exclusion among preadolescents by Adler and Adler (1995), who concluded that both genders engage in social aggression, but for different reasons: for girls to be emotionally vindictive and for boys to assert dominance in hierarchies. It could be fruitful to examine these intriguing hypotheses in more systematic quantitative research.

A few studies using structured interviews suggest that social aggression is firmly embedded in children' social groups and may take different forms for girls and boys. For both boys and girls, social aggression typically involves three or more peers, and engaging in social aggression is related to being a more central member of a social network. Girls are more likely than boys to describe social aggression when asked to recall peer conflicts or victimization experiences. Girls report thinking about and being more distressed about social aggression than boys do.

Much additional research is needed to understand whether there are indeed gender differences in how social aggression unfolds in girls' and boys' groups. As compared to that of boys, is girls' social aggression longer lasting, more intense, more worrisome to all involved, and (perhaps most importantly) more likely to be deployed among friends rather than directed toward outsiders? For girls in particular, is social aggression related to being perceived by peers as popular? As the ethnographic investigations suggest, is social aggression a way for girls, but not for boys, to demonstrate and even protect their popularity? Do girls more than boys engage in malicious gossip as a way of negotiating and confirming boundaries for acceptable behavior?

• *Are there developmental differences in the forms and functions of social aggression?* Because few studies include different age groups and longitudinal evidence has yet to become available, developmental differences in social aggression remain somewhat unclear. Some evidence suggests that social aggression increases in junior high school, but other studies do not find developmental differences. Research to date offers some clues as to developmental differences in the functions served by social aggression. Younger adolescents' social aggression may seem more mean and exclusive because it might be used more in the service of protecting the boundaries of social groups and for confirming and perhaps even enjoying high peer status. However, as girls move through adolescence, another arena in which to be mean opens up and that is romantic relationships. As romance becomes more prominent in girls' lives, a particular powerful way of seeking revenge and pursuing social goals may be to threaten a peer's relationship with a man. For older adolescents, social aggression, gossip in particular, may be used less for self-protection and more in the service of self-understanding, identity development, and moral negotiation.

Adolescents' gossip in the service of self-understanding may presage adult behaviors that might seem like social aggression but also serve other important functions. Although we adults can certainly gossip to hurt and exclude others, sometimes we talk about other people for the purpose of enhancing our understanding of a difficult interpersonal situation or generating strategies for how best to respond. To choose an example close to home, one academic may consult another about challenging matters such as political struggles within a department, difficulties involved in reviewing research for Institutional Review Boards, or how best to help an ill colleague who is unable to meet professional obligations. Discreet individuals might take pains to contain the harm done by these conversations by discussing the problem with someone not centrally involved, or by concealing the identities of the people about whom negative information is being conveyed. By being less careful about whom to talk with or what details to reveal, less prosocial individuals might strategically use these very same types of conversations to inflict serious social harm. Acknowledging these potential complexities could inform our understanding of the development of social aggression and its possible functions in younger age groups.

• *What are the developmental antecedents of girls' anger and aggression? How and why might girls come to express anger and aggression in this particular way?* Although little quantitative evidence exists for the possible origins of social aggression among teenage girls, the research presented in this chapter suggests some fascinating hypotheses. Perhaps girls engage in social aggression because they tend to be temperamentally sociable individuals who face disruptions in relationships around puberty but also increasing pressure to conform to standards of womanhood, including not fighting. Girls report close supportive relationships with their mothers, which might make them more vulnerable to feeling threatened by relationship difficulties with their moms, or might make them more likely to learn some forms of social aggression by observing their mothers talking about friends and husbands. Girls may be particularly vulnerable to interpersonal difficulties, perhaps in part because

they are self-conscious about how others view them and likely to ruminate over interpersonal problems, even to coruminate with friends.
These cognitive vulnerabilities might make girls especially sensitive to
social rejection, which might lead them to engage in social aggression
as a preemptive strike to protect relationships, and might also make
them feel greater pain from victimization. For girls, social aggression
may be even more possible because their friendships are intimate and
involve high levels of self-disclosure, which means that they may have
ample opportunities to betray friends and may feel especially pained by
disloyalty. Given that girls value care and attachment in their romantic
relationships, an especially nasty new avenue for social aggression may
be disrupting emerging romances of others.

• *What are the developmental consequences of girls' anger and aggression?* As is discussed at length next in Chapter 8, the longer-term developmental outcomes of perpetrating and being victimized by social
aggression remain largely unknown. Research on the shorter-term consequences for adolescents suggests that victimization results in distress,
perhaps especially for girls. Frequently being the target of social aggression is related more strongly to poor self-concept for young adolescent
girls than for boys. When girls describe victimization experiences, they
report being more upset and thinking and talking about the victimization more than do boys.

Less clear is whether perpetrating social aggression is related to
maladjustment. Using peer narratives to identify those who frequently
perpetrate social aggression, one study found that social aggression in
seventh grade was not related to later maladjustment (delinquency,
dropping out of school, and adolescent pregnancy). These findings fit
with the suggestions of some of the ethnographic studies that for girls
social aggression may serve a variety of positive and negative developmental functions. However, as discussed next in Chapter 8, another
study with late adolescent college women found that those nominated
as high on relational aggression by sorority sisters were more likely to
report borderline personality features and symptoms of bulimia (Werner & Crick, 1999). These discrepant findings could be due in part to
the different forms of social aggression (nonconfrontational vs. direct
relational) and different types of maladjustment studied. Additional research is badly needed to clarify which specific forms of social aggression may predict particular forms of maladjustment, and it will be important to focus on psychopathology symptoms that may be more
common for women: depression, eating disorders, and some types of
personality disorder.

• *What does research on the processes involved in social aggression suggest for intervention?* Because research with this age group has used qual-

itative and well as quantitative methods to elucidate specific processes involved in social aggression, some interesting possibilities for intervention emerge.

First, if social aggression indeed does serve positive developmental functions such as confirming belongingness and negotiating identity, interventionists should proceed carefully in seeking to eradicate social aggression and consider developing alternative frameworks in which these needs might be met. For example, educators, parents, and policy makers might consider offering more and more varied school activities so that more youth would have opportunities to feel a sense of acceptance and status. Girls could be encouraged to conceive of broad possibilities for their future plans and goals, perhaps helping them focus their identities on more than their perceived popularity at any given moment.

Second, if girls are indeed engaging in social aggression to alleviate boredom and for the sheer entertainment value of manipulating others' relationships, we may want to take a serious look at how girls are spending their time. As argued convincingly by R. W. Larson and Verma (1999), time can be considered a developmental resource that can be invested in meeting developmental goals. As compared to youth in other cultures, North American teenagers spend more time in leisure activities—in particular, consuming diverse forms of media entertainment and hanging around with friends. R. W. Larson and Verma's comprehensive analysis suggests that girls spend more time talking with peers than do boys, that adolescents in Western industrialized nations spend an average of 2.5 hours per day in conversation, and that all of this conversation time "might exceed the necessary time for youth to gain the benefits of this developmental niche" (R. W. Larson & Verma, 1999, p. 721). Although such use of time has not been examined specifically in relation to adolescent social aggression, it is not hard to imagine that all of this discretionary time for hanging around and talking might contribute to boredom that girls say they alleviate by social aggression. If we want to reduce social aggression, it might be worthwhile to consider encouraging girls to be involved in other types of activities: increased academic work, organized sports or clubs, or volunteer work or community service. Recent evidence suggests that U.S. youth of both genders are spending increasing proportions of their leisure time in structured, organized activities (R. Larson, 2001). Could we capitalize on this trend to reduce social aggression among girls if we chose and structured the activities carefully?

A third possibility for intervention comes from the few studies of conversational processes involved in social aggression. One close analysis of gossip episodes showed that if an initial negative evaluation of a peer was immediately challenged, the gossip halted immediately (Eder & Enke, 1991). However, if the initial negative evaluation was met with even one or two confirming comments from peers, the bout of gossip was likely to continue and to become sharply negative in tone. Perhaps girls could be taught to offer these immediate challenges when peers malign others. And perhaps intervention could focus on girls most likely to be involved in social aggression, those central in social networks (Xie et al., 2002), not only because they are likely perpetrators but also because their high status would make their challenges likely to be successful. Chapter 9 discusses in detail these and other possibilities for intervention.

FUTURE RESEARCH

Just as for the earlier developmental periods, almost all of the questions raised here have yet to be tested empirically. For adolescent girls, the following questions seem most pressing:

- Just how frequent and typical is social aggression among adolescents, and does social aggression increase or decrease with age?
- How does social aggression unfold differently in girls' and boys' groups? Is social aggression among girls more likely to be directed at friends than outsiders, is it more intense, does it last longer, and does it threaten girls more severely?
- Are there disruptions in girls' peer relationships around menarche such that social aggression may increase?
- How are girls' relationships with mothers related to their social aggression? Are girls with close maternal relationships more likely to engage in social aggression because they may be more exposed to this behavior by their moms, or are they less likely to be socially aggressive because they are securely attached and less likely to feel threatened?
- Are cognitive styles such as preoccupation with others' perceptions, rumination, and rejection sensitivity related to individual differences in social aggression?
- Are adolescents with particularly close friendships or those who are more embedded in social networks more or less vulnerable to engaging in or being victimized by social aggression?
- Are girls involved in romantic relationships more likely or less likely to engage in social aggression with both friends and romantic partners?
- Which particular forms of social aggression relate to specific

types of maladjustment for girls and women? Is nonconfrontational social aggression less predictive of risk than direct relational aggression?

Clearly, some women continue to engage in social aggression into
adulthood. The next chapter considers the consequences—concurrent
and future, developmental and clinical—of perpetrating social aggression.

PART III

CLINICAL IMPLICATIONS

Chapter 8

Developmental and Psychosocial Consequences of Girls' Aggression

Why is there so little known about girls' own experiences of hostility, resentment, and anger (and about the clinical implications of these negative emotions for females)?

—Zahn-Waxler (1993, p. 84)

Females carry children for nine months then care for them. . . . Females also care for the elderly and the sick. Consequently, the overall damage to the society due to the criminality and/or antisocial behavior of females may be greater than the prevalence rates of offending or antisocial behavior among females would lead us to believe.

—Kratzer and Hodgins (1999, p. 69)

Events of unexplained aggression and loss mark some girls forever. The worry that there is always a hidden layer of truth beneath a façade of "niceness" can leave girls permanently unsure about what they can trust in others and in themselves.

—Simmons (2002, p. 269)

Aggressive, nasty "bad girls" often capture our imaginations. A recent late-evening newscast featured three lead stories, two of which were tragic. First, a woman in a nearby small town had shot and killed her three young children, then shot and attempted to kill her husband before killing herself. Second, a nurse at a small rural hospital was accused of murdering 20 patients by injecting them with poison. Third, the newly crowned Miss Teen Texas had been accused of underage drinking. The news anchors (successful professionals in a large media

181

market) could barely conceal their fascinated glee at such a trio of stories about women gone wrong.

When friends and colleagues heard I was writing a book on anger and aggression in girls, many instantly assumed that my primary focus was going to be girl murderers or female gang members. After all, the goal of writing a book would be to sell as many copies as possible, and what could be more compelling than the baddest of the bad girls? (Little did many of us then realize that in the year or so during which this book was written there would be an explosion of public interest in more subtle forms of aggression in girls; see the popular books by Simmons, 2002; Wiseman, 2002; and others.)

So far, this book has addressed forms of anger and aggression that are common among typical girls, though the milder forms of social and physical aggression may well be related to extreme violence. The last few chapters have described the development of anger and aggression mostly for normal samples, but now it is time to discuss the developmental and clinical consequences of extreme levels of angry, aggressive, and even antisocial behavior.

This chapter focuses not only on developmental correlates and outcomes associated with girls' social aggression but also on girls' physical aggression because these outcomes provide a framework for beginning to understand risks for girls. Although it is important to understand developmental outcomes linked to other forms of girls' anger and aggression (e.g., anger regulation, conflict behavior, and verbal aggression), research on the long-term consequences of these is scarce. Fortunately, recent research has provided a large and growing database on the developmental consequences of girls' physical aggression in childhood. What about social aggression?

When a girl spreads a malicious rumor out of anger or contempt for a peer, is she engaging in normative though nonetheless hurtful behavior, inviting rejection from her peers or earning their respect, putting herself at risk for later negative outcomes, or learning valuable lessons about the subtleties of adult interactions? Experts disagree as to whether social aggression is fairly frequent and even developmentally normative or whether these behaviors are rare and deviant and maladaptive for girls (Underwood et al., 2001b). Because social or relational aggression among girls has been likened to physical aggression among boys (Crick et al., 1999), it is tempting to assume that social and physical aggression are similarly maladaptive. However, preliminary evidence suggests that this may not be so. This chapter examines whether girls' physical and social aggression relate to concurrent problems and to later outcomes. Then, I discuss several fascinating controversies that have arisen as investigators have begun to focus more systematically on physical aggression among girls and its consequences, because these same conceptual debates may inform future progress in understanding social aggression. In keeping with a developmental psychopathology approach, this chapter next considers the possibility that social aggression may also serve some important developmental functions for children. Last, I consider the possible consequences of continuing to engage in social aggression into adulthood.

Before beginning, it is important to acknowledge that some of the same forces that compel our fascination with bad girls may also cloud our attempts to understand them. In part, our fascination has to be related to the fact that girls' bad behavior (be it violence or social aggression) severely violates our stereotypes of girls as nice, compliant, and prosocial. That such behavior undermines our deepest-held assumptions about what it means to be female might tempt us to pathologize all forms of girls' aggression rather than to seek to understand why girls might engage in them. To speak in the most extreme terms possible, pathologizing girls' ways of asserting their social goals might be one more way of keeping women in their place. As Chesney-Lind (1986) argued in relation to serious antisocial behavior, "Clearly, harsh public punishment of a few 'fallen' women as witches and whores has always been integral to enforcement of the boundaries of the 'good' woman's place in patriarchal society" (p. 78). In considering the research evidence for outcomes associated with girls' aggression, it seems important to be mindful of the historical and cultural context in which we are trying to understand these behaviors.

CONCURRENT PROBLEMS ASSOCIATED WITH AGGRESSION IN GIRLS

Researchers have investigated several types of concurrent problems associated with perpetrating physical and social aggression: peer rejection, academic maladjustment, and internalizing problems. Many older studies were conducted with samples of boys or included too few girls to examine gender differences in current adjustment problems related to aggression, but more recent research has explored correlates for girls and for boys. This section first reviews research on the psychosocial correlates associated with physical aggression in girls, then addresses concurrent difficulties associated with social aggression.

Physical Aggression

Research conducted mostly with North American boys indicates that physical aggression is associated with peer rejection, poor school achievement, and possibly also internalizing disorders (for reviews, see the Conduct Problems Prevention Group, 1992; Parker & Asher, 1987). Few of the older studies included aggressive girls in sizable enough numbers to examine gender differences in concurrent problems associated with physical aggression, but recent studies have suggested that the strength of some of these relationships may differ for girls.

For example, for girls, physical aggression seems to be even more strongly related to peer rejection than for boys (Coie, Belding, & Underwood, 1988; Coie & Dodge, 1998; Underwood et al., 2001b). In the Carolina Longitudinal Study, physically aggressive girls were more stable in their aggression than were boys and differed more from their nonaggressive peers (Cairns & Cairns, 1984). When examined as continuous variables, in another study, aggression was more strongly correlated with peer rejection for girls ($r = .73$) than for boys ($r = .37$) (Lancelotta & Vaughn, 1989). For a sample of 9- and 10-year-olds in Canada, playground observations of aggression were negatively related to peer acceptance for girls but not for boys (Serbin, Marchessault, McAffer, Peters, & Schwartzman, 1993). For girls aggressiveness is related to peer rejection regardless of the level of aggression in the classroom group, whereas for boys physical aggression is less strongly related to peer rejection in the context of highly aggressive classrooms (Stormshak et al., 1999).

Remember also that the relation between aggressive behavior and peer status may vary with development. According to Moffitt's (1993) theory of adolescent onset antisocial behavior, many teenagers respond to perceiving the gap between their biological maturity and the few adult privileges available to them by engaging in antisocial behavior. If these negative behaviors are more normative during adolescence, then engaging in them may be less strongly related to peer rejection during this developmental period and may even be related to peer acceptance. In a longitudinal study investigating exactly this claim with a Canadian sample followed from the end of elementary school through the beginning of middle school, attraction to physically aggressive peers was found to increase with age (Bukowski, Sippola, & Newcomb, 2000). However, note also that at each age of assessment girls were not attracted to aggressive female peers, whereas with age they did become more attracted to aggressive boys.

Recent evidence suggests that adolescent girls who fight may be more likely to be aggressive in their concurrent romantic relationships. One investigation by Connolly, Pepler, Craig, and Taradash (2000) found that early-adolescent girls (and boys) who report engaging in bullying are likely to date earlier, are more likely to have a current boyfriend, are more advanced in their romantic involvement, and are likely to report perpetrating physical and social aggression with their romantic partners. These findings suggest that "young adolescents whose peer relationships are characterized by bullying may be at risk for continued difficulties when they begin to initiate romantic relationships" (p. 305). Another study with a high-risk sample of couples in which the men were 18–20 years old found that 36% of women and 31% of men reported being physically aggressive toward their dating partners (the men in these couples were part of the Oregon Youth Study in which the sample was selected to be at high risk for delinquency; Capaldi & Crosby, 1997). In a 36-minute sequence of laboratory interaction tasks including discussing problems and marriage issues, 16% of women engaged in nonplayful forms of physical aggression (as compared to 6% of men). Whereas men's partner aggression was related to antisocial behavior, women's partner aggression was related more to poor self-esteem and symptoms of depression.

As discussed in detail later in this chapter, some of these results support the theory of the "gender paradox" for physical aggression in girls, namely, that physically aggressive girls may be more severely disturbed than are aggressive boys. However, before we can reach this conclusion, additional research is needed about whether physical aggression is more strongly associated with other difficulties for girls, such as academic failure and internalizing problems. We know that childhood physical aggression is associated with academic difficulties, for normal samples in longitudinal studies in North America (see the Conduct Problems Prevention Group, 1992, for a discussion) and in China (Chen, Rubin, & Li, 1995, 1997). However, it is not clear whether girls' physical aggression is more strongly associated with academic problems than is boys' aggression. Research with clinical samples suggests that girls referred to treatment foster care have more concurrent adjustment problems than do boys, including associating with deviant peers, engaging in health-risk-taking behavior, teen pregnancy, running away, and attempting suicide (Chamberlain & Moore, 2000; Leve & Chamberlain, in press). However, almost no research has examined whether, for normal samples, physical aggression in girls is more strongly related to other difficulties (anxiety, depression) than is aggression in boys.

Social Aggression

As discussed in previous chapters, research on the relation between social aggression and psychosocial adjustment is only beginning. Early evidence suggests that for girls social aggression may be related to at least some of the same difficulties as physical aggression.

Previous research suggests contradictory hypotheses as to the relation between social aggression and peer status. Some studies indicate that engaging in relational aggression is related to peer rejection (Crick & Grotpeter, 1995), but other research indicates that social aggression may also relate to high peer regard. The sociometric group highest on relational aggression is the controversial group (Crick & Grotpeter, 1995)—children who are both intensely liked and disliked. Engaging in social aggression has also been found to relate to being a central member of a social network (Xie et al., 2002).

Together, these findings suggest that the relation between social aggression and peer status may be complex. In the studies of Crick's research team, peer nomination data are used to select the most extremely relationally aggressive children, who may engage in this behavior so frequently and so crudely that they are indeed intensely disliked. However, manipulating others' friendships requires having at least some connection to and influence on the peer group, and some average or well-liked children may at times engage in social aggression, perhaps in less intense or even more suave and sophisticated ways.

No published research to date has examined whether social aggression is related to poor school achievement. On the one hand, it seems reasonable to expect that the mental energy required to manipulate and exclude others might detract from focusing on academics. Educators have begun to recognize that social aggression may impair academic performance for at least some students and are calling for assessment and intervention strategies for low-achieving, socially aggressive girls (Talbott, 1997). On the other hand, it may also be that social aggression requires high intelligence because it is such a subtle and complex behavior, and thus some socially aggressive children may still succeed academically despite distractions. Remember that for adolescents indirect aggression has been shown to be correlated with social intelligence (Kaukiainen et al., 1999), which may also in turn help socially aggressive children to survive academically.

Both perpetrators and victims of social aggression have been shown to have internalizing difficulties, perhaps especially girls. For a sample of third through sixth graders, children high on peer nominations for relational aggression reported higher levels of loneliness, depression, and social isolation than did their nonaggressive peers (Crick & Grotpeter, 1995). Children's self-reports of victimization by relational aggression were related to self-reported depression and loneliness (Crick & Grotpeter, 1996). In another study, self-reports of victimization by social aggression were related to poor self-concept, especially for girls (Paquette & Underwood, 1999).

Overall, the evidence to date suggests that for girls extreme levels of both engaging in and being victimized by social aggression seem related to concurrent adjustment problems. What are the longer-term developmental and clinical consequences of these behaviors?

CLINICAL OUTCOMES ASSOCIATED WITH GIRLS' AGGRESSION

In searching for clinical outcomes related to engaging in social aggression, researchers have explored three types of disorders (Crick et al., 1999): syndromes related to physical aggression (i.e., externalizing disorders), disorders with symptoms that resemble social aggression (e.g., borderline personality disorders), and disorders with higher base rates in females (depression, anxiety, and eating disorders). A sizable number of studies have examined clinical outcomes associated with physical aggression in childhood. Published research exploring these outcomes for social aggression remains scarce, though reviews and book chapters cite promising though unpublished evidence.

Outcomes Associated with Physical Aggression in Girls

One reasonable way to begin the search for later outcomes associated with girls' social aggression in childhood is to examine outcomes related to girls' physical aggression. This seems sensible because social and physical aggression share key features (intent to harm, perceived harm), and because social and physical aggression are highly correlated (Crick et al., 1999). Several longitudinal studies have demonstrated that girls who fight as children are at risk for a fairly broad range of negative developmental outcomes: dropping out of school (Cairns, Cairns, & Neckerman, 1989; Kupersmidt & Coie, 1990; Serbin et al., 1998); adolescent pregnancy, gynecological problems, and sexually transmitted diseases (Serbin et al., 1998); teenage motherhood (Miller-Johnson et al., 1999; Serbin et al., 1998; Underwood et al., 1996); obstetrical complications, close spacing of births, and multiparity (Serbin et al., 1998); and unresponsive parenting and having children who are slow to develop language and cognitive skills (Serbin et al., 1998).

If we examine outcomes associated with broader syndromes including other antisocial behaviors besides aggression, the developmental picture looks even worse (see Pajer, 1998, for a review). In examining the predictive utility of retrospective reports of conduct problems, a broader set of behavior problems than aggression alone, Robins (1986) concluded "an increased rate of almost every disorder was found in women with a history of conduct problems" (p. 399), including externalizing problems, internalizing problems, and personality disorders. The personality traits of aggression and alienation at age 18 predicted several high-risk behaviors at age 21: alcoholism, violent crime, unsafe sex, and dangerous driving (Caspi et al., 1997). According to data from the National Youth Survey (Elliott, 1994), equal proportions of women (18%) and men (22%) who were violent offenders as adolescents continue to commit serious violence offenses into adulthood (including assault, robbery, and rape).

Evidence is converging to suggest that for young women (and young men too) engaging in antisocial behavior as a teenager predicts perpetrating physical aggression in romantic relationships as a young adult. In research in New Zealand with a community sample (again, as in Chapter 7, from the Dunedin longitudinal study, i.e., formally called the Dunedin Multidisciplinary Health and Development Study), girls' problem behavior and delinquency at age 15 predicted perpetrating aggression toward romantic partners at age 21 (Magdol, Moffitt, Caspi, & Silva, 1998). Another study with a U.S. community sample found that adolescent girls' delinquency predicted women's self-reported partner violence 10 years later (Giordano, Mulhollen, Cernkovich, Pugh, & Rudolph, 1999). In research with a high-risk sample of couples (the young men had been involved in the Oregon Youth Study), antisocial behavior at age 17 predicted aggression between dating and married couples at age 23 for both girls and boys (Andrews, Foster, Capaldi, & Hops, 2000). Assortative mating seems to occur whereby antisocial women are likely to end up with antisocial male partners (Capaldi & Crosby, 1997; Krueger, Moffitt, Caspi, Bleske, & Silva, 1998), and much of young adults' partner violence seems to be bidirectional (Capaldi & Owen, 2001). Regardless, women generally experience more serious injuries from partner violence than do men (Cantos, Neidig, & O'Leary, 1994).

This predictive relation between girls' physical aggression and antisocial behavior in childhood and later negative outcomes is so robust that it persists despite methodological variation. Aggressive girls are demonstrated to be at risk in prospective longitudinal studies (e.g., Serbin et al., 1998), follow-back studies (Robins, 1986), and studies that select highly aggressive girls within gender (Serbin et al., 1998) or across gender (Underwood et al., 1996).

Why might girls' physical aggression in childhood be related to so many diverse negative outcomes? Longitudinal studies that assess youth at particular points in time and assess outcomes by using court or medical records may be limited in their ability to illuminate what may be complex developmental processes. For example, the sequence of events that leads a physically aggressive girl to become a teenage mother is not immediately obvious. However, hypotheses about developmental processes are beginning to emerge. First, for girls, fighting in childhood may be a marker for some earlier or perhaps broader risk factors, such as a difficult temperament, impulsivity, or cognitive deficits that might contribute to diverse negative outcomes (Caspi et al., 1997). A second possible explanation may be that childhood aggression increases the likelihood of associating with deviant peers, which in turn contributes to the development of diverse problem behaviors. In the Carolina Longitudinal Study, belonging to an aggressive peer clique in seventh grade predicted dropping out of school, which in turn predicted adolescent motherhood (Cairns, Cairns, Neckerman, Gest, & Gariepy, 1988). Aggressive girls have as many friends and belong to social networks as frequently as do nonaggressive girls, but they tend to socialize with other aggressive girls (Cairns, Cairns, Neckerman, et al., 1988). These girls may form groups in which antisocial behavior and risk taking are the norm. Childhood aggression and adolescent motherhood can also be viewed through the lens of *behavior problem theory*, which argues that various types of problem behaviors cluster together (Jessor & Jessor, 1977). Following this logic, some of these predictive relations simply become instances of persistence forecasting, where problem behavior today (childhood aggression) predicts problem behavior tomorrow and into the future (early unprotected sex leading to adolescent motherhood; Underwood et al., 1996).

Outcomes Associated with Social Aggression in Girls

To what extent is social aggression related to some of these outcomes for girls? Very little published research is currently available, but preliminary evidence suggests that social aggression may relate similarly to other problem behaviors. A comprehensive review of research to date on relational aggression cited some still unpublished evidence that relationally aggressive youth were higher than their nonrelationally aggressive peers on some forms of delinquent behavior (C. D. MacDonald & O'Laughlin, 1997, as cited in Crick et al., 1999). In a study of adolescent girls and boys referred for assessment as a result of adjudication for delinquent behavior, self-reports of relational aggression were correlated with having committed physical assault ($r = .47$; Moretti, Holland, & McKay, 2001). Antisocial girls referred to Treatment Foster Care in Oregon reported extremely high rates of relational aggression (72% reported engaging in relational aggression in a single 24-hour period; Chamberlain & Moore, 2000). A study with young high-risk couples found that engaging in verbal aggression in a discussion task with parents at age 17 predicted perpetrating physical aggression with romantic partners 6 years later (Andrews et al., 2000). Because these studies of clinical samples may well overestimate the extent to which social aggression relates to and predicts other externalizing problems, longitudinal research with normal samples is needed.

Clinical Outcomes with Symptoms Resembling Social Aggression

Another approach to exploring clinical outcomes related to social aggression has been to examine disorders for which symptoms resemble social or relational aggression (Crick et al., 1999). In the *Diagnostic and Statistical Manual of Mental Disorders*, 4th ed. (DSM-IV), no childhood disorder perfectly matches social aggression, but social aggression appears related to at least some symptoms of the adult category of borderline personality disorder. Borderline personality disorder is characterized as "a pervasive pattern of instability of interpersonal relationships, self-image, and affects, and marked impulsivity" and includes at least two symptoms that may result from or contribute to social aggression: "frantic efforts to avoid real or imagined abandonment" and "a pattern of unstable and intense interpersonal relationships characterized by alternating between extremes of idealization and devaluation" (American Psychiatric Association, 1994, p. 654). In addition to these stated criteria, many clinicians have the strong impression that people with borderline personality disorder are socially manipulative and engage in "emotional hypocrisies" (Zanarini & Gunderson, 1997). Some features of borderline personality disorder may stem from an underlying difficulty with overly close relationships (Geiger & Crick, 2001).

Very few studies have examined the relation between social aggression and borderline personality disorder, but the initial results are intriguing. Unpublished evidence suggests that third graders high on relational aggression report more borderline personality features than do nonrelationally aggressive children (Crick, Werner, & Rockhill, 1997, as cited in Crick et al., 1999). In a study with college students, relational aggression was assessed with peer nominations by fraternity brothers and sorority sisters (Werner & Crick, 1999). Relational aggression was correlated ($r = .20$) with self-reports of borderline personality features. In hierarchical regression analyses examining the prediction of specific symptoms, relational aggression predicted 5% of the variance in affective instability, 7% of the variance in negative relationships, and 4% of the variance in self-harm. Additional research is needed to examine the strengths of these relationships in more diverse samples.

Clinical Outcomes with Higher Base Rates in Females

Given that some experts believe that social or relational aggression is more common among girls, a third approach to investigating outcomes has been to explore the links between social aggression and disorders that have higher base rates in females, such as eating disorders and depression (Crick et al., 1999). Almost no published work to date has examined whether childhood social aggression predicts either of these outcomes. Here again, unpublished evidence indicates that a clinical sample of girls with eating disorders was higher on relational aggression but not physical aggression as compared with other children (Crick, Casas, & Werner, 1997, cited in Crick et al., 1999). And, in the Werner and Crick (1999) study described above, for women only, relational aggression was related to self-reported symptoms of bulimia ($r = .20$; when entered in hierarchical regressions after age and gender, the interaction between relational aggression and gender explained 3% of the variance in bulimic symptoms).

Although these preliminary studies suggest that relational aggression may relate to borderline personality features and eating disorders, longitudinal research is needed to determine whether childhood or adolescent social aggression indeed predicts later borderline, eating, and internalizing symptoms. In conducting these studies, it will be important to use measures appropriate for detecting subclinical levels of symptoms in normal samples, but also to remember that findings related to borderline features or bulimia symptoms do not necessarily mean that social aggression is related to the full-blown clinical disorders. Exploring the relationships between behaviors and outcomes that are all so subtle and complex will be challenging indeed, and will require all of the methodological sophistication that researchers can muster.

CONTROVERSIES SURROUNDING RESEARCH ON AGGRESSION IN GIRLS

Now that I have outlined what we know to date about developmental correlates and clinical outcomes associated with girls' aggression, it seems important to discuss in detail some conceptual and methodological challenges. Until recently, our understanding of physical aggression among girls was limited by the slim research evidence available. Because so few girls fight physically, much less empirical research had explored the processes, development, and outcomes associated with girls' physical aggression. Some girls do fight, and just as the paucity of research on women and heart disease is a grave problem, so is the lack of research on physical aggression in girls (Cairns & Cairns, 1994).

Compounding matters further, as mentioned earlier in the chapter, the extent to which violent, antisocial behavior violates our gender stereotypes for girls and women may have interfered with careful, impartial examination of what physical aggression really means for girls.

Behaviors considered deviant for girls seem to have changed over historical time (Schlossman & Cairns, 1994). Decades ago, girls became involved in the juvenile justice system most often due to allegations of sexual precocity or promiscuity. Even if girls' misbehavior was not always related to their sexuality, they may have been sexualized in some ways within the juvenile justice system. In one study of case files from the 1960s, male intake workers at youth detention facilities made comments about delinquent girls' physical attractiveness in 63% of cases, and this was all the more likely if girls' behavior problems were characterized as involving immorality (Rosenbaum & Chesney-Lind, 1994). In modern times, caseworkers less often document girls' attractiveness. Research in the 1980s and early 1990s indicated that girls are most often arrested for nonserious status offenses (such as truancy or running away; see Chesney-Lind, 1988; Shelden & Chesney-Lind, 1993). More recent evidence suggests that girls are more likely to exhibit clusters of more serious problem behaviors, and in recent years these problem behaviors increasingly include physical aggression (H. N. Snyder & Sickmund, 1999).

As researchers have begun to focus more systematically on physical aggression in girls, controversies have emerged as to how to best understand and measure these behaviors. These challenges have arisen as a direct result of the increasing quantity and richness of the research literature on girls' physical aggression; they are testimony to the rapidly advancing state of the art in this research area. Although most of these challenges pertain to research on physical aggression, we would be wise to attend to some of these same issues as research on social aggression advances.

Are Physically Aggressive Girls More Deviant Than Physically Aggressive Boys?

That girls who fight are somehow more deviant and disturbed than aggressive boys fits with our gender stereotypes, and is also supported by some of the empirical evidence. Investigators have observed a phenomenon called the "gender paradox"—that the members of the gender group least frequently afflicted by a disorder are often the most severely disturbed (Eme, 1992; Keenan, Loeber, & Green, 1999). The logic of the gender paradox seems to be that to develop a highly gender-atypical disorder, individuals must have several strong risk factors that could contribute to other types of problems. In support of the gender paradox for criminal property offenses, female offenders may be more genetically predisposed to criminal behavior than male offenders. In a large Danish adoption cohort, female offenders had more biological relatives who were also offenders than did males, suggested a stronger genetic component to the women's criminality (Baker, Mack, Moffitt, & Mednick, 1989). In a study of adolescents referred to residential treatment for a variety of types of antisocial behavior, girls had more disturbed families and chaotic backgrounds than did boys (Chamberlain & Moore, 2000).

Other support for the gender paradox comes from research on physical aggression. Fewer girls fight physically, but those who do seem to have more problems than do physically aggressive boys. As discussed earlier, for girls, physical aggression is more strongly related to peer rejection than for boys. In another study, teachers rated physically aggressive girls as higher on both internalizing and externalizing problems than both relationally aggressive and nonaggressive girls (Crick, 1997). Sisters of delinquent boys who were rated by their mothers as high on conduct disorder symptoms were more likely to have other problems (relational aggression, impulsivity) than were brothers who were so rated (Tiet et al., 2001). Unfortunately, research on the gender paradox has rarely been conducted with normal samples, nor has it specifically examined aggressive behavior, and evidence available so far is conflicting (see Keenan et al., 1999, for a review).

What are the implications of the gender paradox for understanding outcomes associated with social aggression? If it is indeed the case that the gender group least frequently affected is more seriously disturbed and that boys are typically lower on relational aggression than are girls, then relationally or socially aggressive boys might be more maladjusted than socially aggressive girls. This speculation was confirmed by a study that found that children who engage in gender-nonnormative forms of aggression may be most at risk, namely, physically aggressive girls and relationally aggressive boys (Crick, 1997). In this study, peers provided nominations for relational and physical aggression, and teachers reported problem behaviors on the Teacher Report Form of the Child Behavior Checklist (CBCL). The results indicated that teachers perceived relationally aggressive boys and physically aggressive girls to be higher than all other groups on adjustment problems (internalizing and externalizing symptoms combined). Additional research on the gender paradox for social aggression is badly needed, and this research may be all the more challenging because research on behavior problems with boys tends to focus either on physical aggression or on clinical syndromes such as conduct disorder.

Are We Best Served by Focusing on Aggressive Behavior or More Broad Clinical Syndromes?

A serious challenge for integrating the few available studies on girls' aggression and violence is that investigators have focused on overlapping but not identical categories of behavior. Some research has examined outcomes related specifically to girls' physical aggression in childhood (e.g., Serbin et al., 1998; Underwood et al., 1996), whereas other studies have focused on outcomes relating to conduct disorder (e.g., Cote, Zoccolillo, Tremblay, Nagin, & Vitaro, 2001; Zoccolillo, Tremblay, & Vitaro, 1996) or antisocial behavior more broadly (e.g., Bardone, Moffitt, Caspi, Dickson, & Silva, 1996; Moffitt & Caspi, 2001). Conduct disorder is the DSM-IV diagnosis of childhood that includes symptoms for many different kinds of behavior problems, including aggression but also damaging property, stealing or lying, and violating rules (American Psychiatric Association, 1994). Focusing on conduct disorder has the advantage that this clinical diagnosis can be detected from medical records and includes a range of problem behaviors that sometimes occur together. Investigators studying antisocial behavior in adolescents tend to rely on self-reports or police records of delinquent behaviors, which again include aggression but also property and status offenses. Both of these strategies have the disadvantage of sometimes obscuring the correlates or outcomes related specifically to aggression, and samples identified as antisocial frequently include large numbers of children who are not aggressive. In fact, in the aforementioned large, well-designed Dunedin longitudinal study in New Zealand (i.e., the Dunedin Multidisciplinary Health and Development Study), none of the girls met criteria for aggressive conduct disorder as children (Bardone et al., 1996). For all of these reasons, it is important to be cautious in generalizing findings from studies of antisocial girls to aggressive girls.

Here it seems important to note that there is currently no childhood DSM-IV diagnosis that corresponds perfectly to relational or social aggression. If relational aggression is as maladaptive as some have argued and centrally important for understanding girls' psychopathology, perhaps it would be sensible to formulate a diagnostic category that would be practically useful in helping these children get treatment but also in identifying girls at risk for later serious problems. However, it also seems important to be cautious in generating labels that would further stigmatize girls or discourage them from expressing their anger (Zahn-Waxler, 1993). Additional research is needed to clarify whether social aggression is always maladaptive and linked to negative outcomes, which will require also understanding the normative development of these behaviors for both genders.

Do Developmental Trajectories Differ for Girls and Boys?

As the results of well-designed longitudinal studies have become available, researchers have proposed that antisocial behavior may develop along two distinct trajectories, referred to in the research literature as (1) the early-onset, life-course-persistent trajectory and (2) the adolescent-onset or adolescent-limited trajectory (Moffitt, 1993; Moffitt & Caspi, 2001). The early-onset, life-course-persistent (LCP) trajectory is described as beginning when a child inherits or acquires from the early environment neuropsychological problems, a difficult temperament, and hyperactivity, and as a result, becomes noncompliant. These noncompliant, difficult behaviors may be exacerbated by inadequate parenting and poverty. As the child begins school, aggressive, noncompliant behaviors might result in poor school performance and rejection by peers, which subsequently could lead to affiliating with deviant peers in adolescence and the development of antisocial behavior that persists into adulthood. The adolescent-limited (AL) trajectory begins near the time of puberty, when it is hypothesized that some youths perceive a gap between their biological maturity and the social privileges and responsibilities available to them. Youths on this trajectory may engage in particular forms of antisocial behavior (such as drinking, smoking, or violating curfews) as one way of demonstrating their maturity, autonomy from parental demands, and connectedness with older peers. Youths who follow this trajectory tend to cease most antisocial behavior when they are able to assume more adult roles and responsibilities. Several longitudinal studies have demonstrated the distinctiveness and the validity of these two developmental trajectories (Mazerolle, Brame, Paternoster, Piquero, & Dean, 2000; Moffitt & Caspi, 2001; Patterson, Forgatch, Yoerger, & Stoolmiller, 1998).

However, experts disagree as to whether these two developmental trajectories describe the antisocial behavior of girls as well as boys. In a thoughtful and detailed review of studies with both clinical and community samples, Silverthorn and Frick (1999) proposed that the LCP/AL typology does not fit well for girls, because so few girls fit the childhood-onset LCP pattern, and those who began antisocial behavior in adolescence have more negative, distressed childhood histories that are more similar to those of LCP boys. They argued that a third developmental trajectory is needed to characterize the development of antisocial behavior in girls, the delayed-onset pathway, in which girls share many of the same risks as LCP boys but do not begin antisocial behavior until they are faced with the biological and social challenges of puberty. In confirmation of some aspects of the delayed-onset pathway, a large, prospective, longitudinal study of a Danish sample found that girls who fit the AL trajectory (according to criminal records) shared some of the same childhood risk factors as the early-onset boys (Kratzer & Hodgins, 1999).

On the basis of data from the Dunedin longitudinal study, however, Moffitt and Caspi (2001) argued that the LCP/AL model fits equally well for girls and for boys and that no gender-specific trajectory is required. Moffitt's (1994) original formulation of the LCP/AL trajectories predicted that because girls are lower than boys on most of the risk factors, many fewer females than males would follow the LCP trajectory. On the other hand, girls have more "equal access" to the AL trajectory because they face the same maturity gap as do boys; therefore, the gender ratio for the AL trajectory should be more even. This theory was confirmed by the data; the ratio of males to females for the LCP group was 10:1, whereas for the AL group it was only 1.5:1. For the Dunedin sample, girls in the AL group did not share the risk factors of the LCP group, as had been suggested by Silverthorne and Frick (1999). Moffitt and Caspi suggested that these conflicting conclusions may be because Silverthorne and Frick included data from clinical rather than community samples in which the AL girls would have appeared more deviant. Another reason for inconsistent results may be different methods for assessing antisocial behavior; Moffitt and Caspi relied on self-reports, whereas Kratzer and Hodgins (1999) consulted court records. What these approaches share, however, is the recognition that for most girls, problem behaviors first appear later than for boys. Would this be equally true if childhood diagnostic criteria were modified to include forms of aggression more typical for girls?

Before I address the specific issue of diagnostic criteria, it is important to recognize that experts in criminology and sociology have also been calling for gender-specific models for understanding delinquency and antisocial behavior for different but perhaps related reasons. Chesney-Lind (1989) argued that juvenile justice systems operate with an androcentric bias, in insisting on viewing girls' problem behaviors as related to their sexuality and arresting girls for behaviors that might constitute strategies for resisting abuse (e.g., hitting parents and running away). Chesney-Lind (1989) proposed that scholars and policy makers work together toward a *feminist theory of delinquency*, which would acknowledge that girls' behavior problems may relate to their being forced to exist within patriarchal systems. What this theory would look like in positive terms remains unclear, but some of its goals might be served by studying carefully the developmental trajectories of aggression in both genders and perhaps by defining clinical conduct problems differently for girls and for boys.

Should Diagnostic Criteria Be Adjusted for Girls?

In recognition of the fact that existing definitions and criteria seem to detect girls' problem behaviors either less frequently or at a later developmental point than those of boys, some have suggested that criteria for childhood conduct disorder should be altered to be more sensitive to and inclusive of girls with early behavioral difficulties (Zoccolillo, 1993). If girls and boys do indeed grow up in separate and different peer cultures, then it should not be surprising that girls and boys manifest conduct disorder in different ways—girls with fewer aggressive and more somatization symptoms than boys. Zoccolillo (1993) suggested that the thresholds for the number of symptoms required should be lower for females and that the criteria should be altered to include symptoms more common in girls. In an empirical investigation of the sensitivity and specificity of DSM-III-R criteria for conduct disorder in girls as predictors of later antisocial behavior (American Psychiatric Association, 1987), of girls who went on to develop persistent and pervasive antisocial behavior, only 3% met DSM-III-R criteria for conduct disorder in childhood (Zoccolillo et al., 1996). Altering criteria for girls by requiring two rather than three symptoms and adding rule violation as a symptom resulted in 35% of antisocial girls meeting criteria for childhood conduct disorder. If the goal of diagnosing children with conduct disorder is to predict later antisocial behavior, these researchers have argued that gender-specific criteria may be needed (Zoccolillo, 1993; Zoccolillo et al., 1996).

Other experts have argued that altering diagnostic criteria so that equal numbers of girls and boys are labeled with conduct disorder would be seriously misguided. Zahn-Waxler (1993) questioned the wisdom of deemphasizing aggression as an important criterion of conduct disorder and of adopting gender-specific criteria, because this would serve to obscure real gender differences in important behaviors such as physical aggression and possibly stigmatize girls. Zahn-Waxler wrote, "There is reason to question any approach that potentially serves to discourage females from expressing anger and aggression and reminds them of their subordinate positions in society" (p. 81). Zahn-Waxler acknowledged that diagnostic criteria or even categories may need to be added in order to understand and include the externalizing behaviors of women and men, but that author urged caution in relying overmuch on diagnostic categories whose criteria are not always useful for identifying the earliest forms of antisocial behavior. Zahn-Waxler advocated a developmental psychopathology approach. As opposed to beginning with diagnostic categories and working backward to understand their origins, the developmental psychopathology approach involves prospective longitudinal studies. These investigations focus on specific early behaviors (such as physical aggression) that might predict later negative outcomes. Later in this chapter, we return to other important implications of the developmental psychopathology approach.

What about Girls in Gangs?

To date, research on girls in gangs has suffered from the lack of integration of the work of criminologists on gangs with research by developmental psychologists on friendships and social networks (Cairns, Cadwallader, Estell, & Neckerman, 1997). The research base for understanding girls' gangs is especially limited, perhaps because girls' groups may be less prone to antisocial behavior than boys' groups are (Cairns et al., 1997). In describing research to date on girls who participate in gangs, Joe and Chesney-Lind (1995) concluded, "girls' involvement in gangs has been neglected, sexualized, and oversimplified" (p. 412). Estimates of the percentage of gang members who are female vary from 3.6% (Curry, Fox, Ball, & Stone, 1992) to just under 10% (W. B. Miller, 1980) to about one-third in an ethnographic study conducted in Los Angeles (J. Moore, 1991). Female gang members have been characterized as the property, "little sisters," and girlfriends of male gang members (see Chesney-Lind, 2001, for an extremely thoughtful review of research to date on girls in gangs). Researchers are only beginning to move beyond the focus on violent behavior more common among boys in gangs to begin to focus on the wider range of functions that gangs might serve for girls.

How can research on physical and social aggression among girls help us understand the phenomenon of girls who participate in gangs? Experts disagree as to the extent to which girls in gangs engage in extremely violent behavior. Female gang members typically do not seek opportunities to engage in aggressive, violent behavior, and recent increases in girls' arrests for violent offenses may be due to girls who commit status offenses instead being charged with violent offenses (e.g., a girl who has run away might be arrested for hitting her mother—criminologists call this practice "bootstrapping"; Chesney-Lind, 2001). However, in one study of female gang members adjudicated by the California Youth Authority in 1990, 94% had been arrested for a violent crime and most were described by themselves and by authorities as extremely angry and hostile (Rosenbaum, 1996).

No published research to date has examined the extent to which girls in gangs are involved in social aggression. However, a small but growing body of research suggests that girls may join gangs for some of the same reasons that girls engage in social aggression—to alleviate boredom (Owens et al., 2000b) and to confirm their own sense of belonging and acceptance (Paquette & Underwood, 1999). One interview study with ethnic gang members in Hawaii found that although there was not any one type of gang girl, many girls were drawn to join gangs for protection from abusive families and peers, for relief from boredom, and for social outlets and support (Joe & Chesney-Lind, 1995). In the aforementioned study of female gang members adjudicated by the California Youth Authority, 30% said they joined gangs to help meet their needs for family support, and 26% said they joined gangs out of loyalty to friends because those friends gave them what they needed (Rosenbaum, 1996). In a study that compared gang members and girls not in gangs among a sample of female arrestees, gang members were younger, were more often from dysfunctional families, and were attracted to gangs by close friends who were already members (Chang, 1996).

Clearly, the few girls who join gangs do so for complex reasons, only some involving physical and social aggression, and most beyond the scope of this book. Readers who seek detailed descriptions and analyses of groups like the Nasty Fly Ladies, Vice Queens, and Just Every Mother's Angel will need to turn to other sources (see Sikes, 1997; Chesney-Lind, 2001; and Joe & Chesney-Lind, 1995, respectively). For particularly vivid portrayals of female gang members in New York, Los Angeles, and Milwaukee, I especially recommend Eight Ball Chicks (Sikes, 1997). As researchers continue to examine more carefully girls' involvement in gangs and to acknowledge that gangs may serve different functions for girls and for boys, it will be important to recognize that for some girls in especially bleak or disadvantaged circumstances, gang participation may serve some of the same developmental needs felt by more typical girls—to feel a sense of belonging and acceptance, to feel safe and okay and part of a group.

Could There Be Positive Developmental Functions of Social Aggression?

> Nearly all of the great systematizers in psychology, psychiatry, and psychoanalysis have argued that we can learn more about the normal functioning of an organism by studying its psychopathology, and likewise, more about its psychopathology by studying its normal condition. (Cicchetti & Olsen, 1990, p. 263)

In this chapter and really throughout the entire book, I have attempted to adopt this developmental psychopathology approach. I have focused on specific forms of aggression rather than on clinical syndromes, included studies of normal as well as clinical samples, highlighted prospective longitudinal studies, and attempted to acknowledge that behaviors may take different forms and serve different functions at different points in development. One step remains, though, which is to consider the possibility that social aggression may have both positive and negative correlates, and serve both positive and negative developmental functions.

The best understanding of social aggression will be informed by research with both normal and clinical samples and will be guided by developmental theory. Most of the research to date on the relation between social aggression and psychological adjustment has utilized peer nomination methods, which by definition identify those relatively few youths who engage in these behaviors most frequently and intensely. Because relational aggression has been hypothesized to function similarly in the developmental psychopathology of girls as physical aggression does for boys (Crick et al., 1999), many researchers seem to assume that social and physical aggression may be similarly maladaptive.

However, there are at least two reasons to question this claim (Underwood et al., 2001b). First, several studies have shown that even physical aggression is sometimes related to social competence. Among fourth through sixth-grade boys in one study, two subgroups of popular boys emerged (Rodkin, Farmer, Pearl, & Van Acker, 2000). Popular-prosocial (model) boys were perceived by peers to be cool, studious, good leaders, well behaved, and nonaggressive. Popular-antisocial (tough) boys were described as cool, athletically talented, and antisocial. Several other studies suggest that, at least in particular developmental periods in some contexts, physical aggression may be related to social competence (Hawley, 2001; Prinstein & Cohen, 2001; Vaughn, Bost, & Vollenweider, 2001). If physical aggression can be related to some types of social competence, then it seems reasonable to examine whether social aggression might be also. Second, specific features of social aggression suggest that it might not always be maladaptive. Many children as well as adults may at times resort to social aggression. In older age groups, most children do not fight physically (Cairns & Cairns, 1994; Coie & Dodge, 1998). One reason may be that when children develop verbal skills, they instead use them to harm others because the risk of punishment is so much less than for physical aggression (Bjorkqvist, 1994). Remember also that the derivation of the word "gossip"—"god" plus "sibb" (meaning "kinsman")—suggests that gossip need not always be malicious (Gottman & Mettetal, 1986). Gossip may indeed be one way of maligning someone else or seeking to harm his or her friendships or social standing, but it may also be used to serve more positive purposes, such as informing others of someone's need for help and support. The boundaries between these negative and positive types of gossip may at times become unclear.

Developmental theory also suggests that gossip may not always be harmful. During middle childhood, children strongly value feeling accepted and included by their same-gender peer groups, and negative evaluation gossip may be one way that children join with each other and test the boundaries of important social norms (Fine, 1986; Gottman & Mettetal, 1986). For youths who may be desperate to fit in, one way to maintain their own sense of belongingness may be to exclude others (Paquette & Underwood, 1999). Social aggression may also be important in helping children and adolescents to protect the integrity of their social groups (Eder, 1985; Leckie, 1999). Remember also that peer ratings of indirect aggression are positively correlated with social intelligence, defined as accurately perceiving other people, flexibility in social contexts, success in accomplishing social goals, and engaging in desired behaviors (Kaukiainen et al., 1999). Additional research with normal samples will be important for learning more about the possible positive functions of gossip, and perhaps also other forms of social aggression.

It is also important to recognize that not all longitudinal research has demonstrated that social aggression is linked to later negative outcomes. For the data from the Carolina Longitudinal Study, social aggression for cohorts of fourth and seventh graders was measured by determining the number of times that individual girls were mentioned in others' accounts of peer difficulties involving social manipulation and peer ostracism (Xie et al., 2002). The results indicated that girls high on social aggression were more likely to be central than peripheral members of their social networks. Whereas physical aggression predicted low academic competence, dropping out of school, and criminal behavior, childhood social aggression was related to none of the later negative outcomes examined (nor was direct relational aggression; Xie et al., 2002). In another longitudinal study conducted in Finland, facial and verbal aggression as assessed by peer nominations in childhood predicted adult women having higher grade point averages (GPAs) and longer educational careers than their nonaggressive counterparts (Pulkkinen, 1992). These findings await replication with other samples and different measures of the constructs of indirect, relational, and social aggression, but they do suggest that social aggression may not always bode ill for girls.

As important as it has been to acknowledge that social aggression may be harmful for both perpetrators and victims, it also seems important to recognize that these behaviors may not always predict negative developmental outcomes, may occur for developmental reasons, and may even be related to some types of social skills. None of this is to suggest that "girls will be girls," that social aggression cannot be hurtful and harmful, but simply to urge that the fullest understanding of this fascinating set of behaviors will require that we consider both its positive and negative features and outcomes. Considering all of the possible functions of social aggression demands that we examine whether and how these behaviors may persist into adulthood.

SOCIAL AGGRESSION INTO ADULTHOOD

A member of a large Protestant church sent an anonymous electronic mail message to members of governing bodies of the congregation as well as to numerous other parishioners, stating dissatisfaction with the head minister for general reasons of his not being sufficiently spiritual. This led to a great deal of negative gossip about why various families had recently left the church, and to widespread speculation that the minister would not stay in his job.

When adults hear descriptions of the phenomenon of social aggression, they often say, "how interesting–but of course adults do that all the time." Research has only begun to explore social aggression among adults. What does social aggression look like in the adult years, and how does it relate to psychological adjustment?

Research on Indirect and Relational Aggression among Adults

Several different research groups have investigated the specific phenomenon of indirect/relational/social aggression among adults, and the items used on their questionnaires paint a rich and detailed portrait of possible elements of social aggression in adult life. Here again, that different research groups described many of the same features of social aggression suggests that this phenomenon continues to be robust into adulthood. However, that such a wide array of behaviors has been included under the rubrics of indirect and relational aggression suggests that additional research is needed to refine what these constructs mean for adults.

Preliminary evidence suggests that gender differences are unclear and that some forms of social aggression may be more harmful than others. In one study, adults were asked to report on their own direct and indirect aggressive behavior in response to the Richardson Conflict Response Scale (Green, Richardson, & Lago, 1996). Indirect aggression items included the following: "made up stories to get them in trouble"; "made negative comments about their appearance to someone else"; "spread vicious rumors"; "gossiped behind their back"; "told others not to associate with them"; "told others about the matter"; and "gathered other friends to my side" (Green et al., 1996, p. 83). The results showed that although adult males reported engaging in more direct aggression than females did, there were no gender differences for indirect aggression.

However, indirect aggression may take more or less subtle forms in adulthood; gender differences may well depend on the specific type of behavior. Among adults, indirect aggression may include both rational-appearing aggression and more overt social manipulation (Bjorkqvist, Osterman, & Lagerspetz, 1994). Rational-appearing aggression includes deliberately trying to hurt others by reducing their opportunities for self-expression, interrupting, judging their work in an unfair manner, criticizing, and questioning their judgment. Social manipulation was defined as follows: "insulting comments about one's private life"; "insinuative negative glances"; "backbiting"; "spreading of false rumors"; "insinuations without direct accusation"; "not being spoken to"; and "do-not-speak-to-me behavior" (Bjorkqvist, Osterman, & Lagerspetz, 1994, p. 30). In a study with university staff members in Finland, males were rated as higher on rational-appearing aggression than were females, whereas females were reported to engage in more social manipulation than were males (Bjorkqvist, Osterman, & Lagerspetz, 1994). These results support the intuition that some forms of social aggression might be subtle enough that the perpetrators and victims may not be aware of them until the negative consequences are all too clear.

Very little research has examined the relation between social aggression and psychological adjustment for adults, but the available studies are intriguing. In a study with university students, fraternity and sorority members provided peer nominations for prosocial behavior and for relational aggression (items included the following: "When angry, gives others the silent treatment"; "When mad, tries to damage others' reputations by passing on negative information"; "When mad, retaliates by excluding others from activities"; "Intentionally ignores others until they agree to do something for him/her"; "Makes it clear to his/her friends that he/she will think less of them unless they do what he/she wants"; "Threatens to share private information with others in order to get them to comply with his/her wishes"; and "When angry with same-sex peer, tries to steal that person's dating partner" [Werner & Crick, 1999, p. 618]). Because the peer nomination data were standardized within gender groups, gender differences could not be examined. The results showed that peer nominations for relational aggression explained proportions of the variance in several types of psychological problems: peer rejection (12%); self-reports of antisocial personality features (5% for stimulus seeking and 9% for eccentricity); borderline personality features (5%); and for women, symptoms of bulimia (3%).

Although ethnographic and more quantitative studies together suggest that social aggression among older adolescents and adults may occur concerning and within romantic relationships, this possibility has only begun to be examined. One study investigated the use of indirect aggression among women of Buenos Aires, Argentina, using a combination of survey and ethnographic methods (Hines & Fry, 1994). Participants were some university students, but also older adult women who were acquainted with the investigators. Adults were asked to judge the likelihood of men and women engaging in indirect and direct aggression. Items that loaded on the indirect factor included "judge," "lie," "exclude," "gossip," and "interrupt." Participants of both genders reported that women more often engage in indirect aggression than do men and that men are more physically aggressive than are women. The ethnographic observations suggested that although the "marianismo role" for women prohibits direct, physical aggression, Argentine women are quite competitive with one another and engage in multiple forms of rough but still somewhat indirect behavior (pushing on buses but never making eye contact, expressing annoyance by providing customers extremely poor service, and the like). Businesses are described as avoiding hiring female workers because of the high conflict level among them: "If many women are together, they fight. . . . Therefore, we say sometimes amongst us men, that it is impossible for women to have friendships because there is always one woman who tells a secret to the other and then the other divulges it, and the feud begins between them" (quoted in Hines & Fry, 1994, p. 20). Women were described as often competing for men and engaging in indirect aggression toward their rivals. Nonverbal behaviors seemed to be important forms of social aggression among women competing for a man: "[T]he tendency is not to talk with each other at all, but rather to exchange nasty looks. They don't say anything . . . but look aggressively at each other" (Hines & Fry, 1994, p. 19).

Although research on this issue is just beginning, social aggression may also take place between romantic partners. In a study with a midwestern U.S. university sample, men and women completed self-report measures of relational aggression and victimization within romantic relationships, and measures of romantic, peer, and parent relationship quality (Linder, Crick, & Collins, 2002). Items assessing romantic relational aggression included the following: "I have threatened to break up with my romantic partner in order to get him/her to do what I wanted"; "I try to make my romantic partner jealous when I am mad at him/her"; "I have cheated on my romantic partner because I am angry with him/her"; " I give my romantic partner the silent treatment when [he/she] hurts my feelings in some way"; and "If my romantic partner makes me mad, I will flirt with another person in front of him/her" (Linder et al., 2002, p. 86). On this self-report measure, there were no gender differences for engaging in romantic relational aggression, but men reported higher levels of relational victimization than did women. Not surprisingly, reported romantic relational aggression and victimization both related to negative qualities of romantic relationships (frustration, ambivalence, lack of trust, jealousy, and anxious clinging; all correlations ranged from .4 to .58). Romantic relational aggression was related to reports of feeling alienated from mothers and having poor communication with fathers. Both romantic relational aggression and victimization were related to feeling alienated from peers. This study provides some of the first evidence that relational aggression disrupts young adult romantic relationships, and it will be important in future work to validate self-reports of romantic relational aggression and perhaps observe couples talking together to understand more about the processes involved.

One observational study of a related form of aggression, *psychological aggression* (sometimes referred to as *emotional abuse*), confirms that such behavior is frequent in young adult couples and may be related to serious relationship problems (Capaldi & Crosby, 1997). In this investigation, 18- to 20-year-old men who had been part of the Oregon Youth Study participated with their romantic partners in an observational and questionnaire study assessing physical and psychological aggression between dating partners. Psychological aggression includes threats of violence, ridicule, jealousy, threats to terminate the relationship, restriction, property damage, and abrupt withdrawal from the interaction (Follingstad, Rutledge, Berg, Hause, & Poleck, 1990; Kessler, 1990). When observed in the lab, women engaged in higher rates of psychological and physical aggression toward their partners than did men. Psychological aggression within the relationship was strongly related to physical aggression between partners ($r = .55$ for women and $r = .6$ for men), and psychological (but not physical) aggression was negatively related to relationship satisfaction.

Together, these studies suggest that social aggression occurs both among adult women and between women and men, and is viewed by different groups of investigators as taking similar forms, whether studies are conducted at upper-midwestern U.S. universities or in Argentina. In future research, it will be important to understand the extent to which social aggression occurs in community samples of adults beyond college age and relates to a person's capacity for meeting the challenges of adulthood. How does engaging in extreme levels of social aggression affect one's ability to get along with coworkers and to form and maintain close friendships and romantic relationships? Does intense involvement in social aggression interfere with being a sensitive or responsive parent? Is resorting to social aggression occasionally a normal part of adult life, and perhaps even adaptive as a way of maintaining superficially smooth social relations while addressing difficulties more covertly?

SUMMARY AND CONCLUSIONS

> Man, it is so hard to live down that sugar-and-spice rep. We women try, Lord do we try, and still people are shocked—shocked!—when we are mean to each other, humiliate our partners, scream at our children, spread nasty rumors, lie on our résumés, embezzle from our employers, demean our employees, give slower drivers the finger, have extramarital affairs, commit murder, enter the military, join the Aryan Nation or the Islamic Jihad, and fail to send Christmas cards to the family. How dare women behave like . . . like . . . people? (Tavris, 2002, p. B7)

This chapter has wrestled with the complex issue of the developmental and clinical outcomes associated with girls' social aggression. Considering these outcomes at this particular time requires some struggle and no small measure of patience, for several reasons. First, objective consideration of all forms of aggression among girls is difficult because mean behavior violates our strongly held stereotypes about how girls should behave, stereotypes that influence how we design research and interpret results in ways that may be beyond our ken. Second, because research on social aggression is fairly new, a natural way to begin has been to liken social aggression to physical aggression and to assume that their outcomes may be similarly negative. This approach has been fruitful in many ways, but it also has its limits, and many of the same controversies that have dogged those attempting to understand physical aggression may plague us as we seek to understand social aggression. Third, little truly developmental research has investigated social aggression, so developmental trajectories remain unclear and we know little about what this behavior means in adulthood. Fourth and perhaps most important, consider the possibility that social aggression may serve some developmental functions conflicts with the prevailing cultural Zeitgeist about social aggression—that these behaviors are nothing but harmful and heartbreaking—and to contemplate other possibilities is dismissed as "girls will be girls" thinking. These beliefs about girls' meanness have grown so fervent so rapidly that we seem to have gone quickly from modest substantive knowledge about girls' aggression to the backlash, an insistence that all girls are not mean and that those who are mean become that way because they are human (see Tavris, 2002, quoted above).

Researchers have made tremendous progress in understanding what social aggression means for girls, and the importance of acknowledging that social aggression can hurt cannot be underestimated. Still, much remains to be known about the negative and positive consequences of these behaviors. In future investigations, a developmental psychopathology approach might well be helpful in conducting prospective longitudinal studies that examine multiple and specific forms of social aggression, outcomes important for both genders, and whether social aggression might serve both positive and negative developmental functions. Further understanding of the multiple functions of social aggression and its adult manifestations will guide our understanding of developmental trajectories and outcomes, and it might also inform our decisions about whether, when, and how to intervene.

Prevention and Intervention
Harnessing the Power of Sisterhood

Turning sixty, I am more aware of the voices of exclusion in the classroom. "You can't play" suddenly seems too overbearing and harsh, sounding like a slap from wall to wall. How casually one child determines the fate of another. . . . Must it be so? This year I am compelled to find out. Posting a sign that reads YOU CAN'T SAY YOU CAN'T PLAY, I announce the new social order and, from the start, it is greeted by disbelief.
                    —PALEY (1992, p. 4)

In order for patterns to change, systems must lose stability so they may be sensitive to perturbations. To maximize the potential for change, change should be introduced in multiple systems simultaneously. An isolated effort for change at one level will be thwarted by the other systems that remain stable and draw the target system back into line. For example, within interventions to reduce bullying, dynamic systems theory suggests that it is futile to intervene with the bully or victim alone. Not only does each of their behaviors depend on the others, but they are embedded in the larger frames of the peer group, classroom, and school. There may also be supporting interactional systems at home, suggesting that parents may also need to be involved.
                    —PEPLER, CRAIG, AND O'CONNELL (1999, pp. 449–450)

Our smiles and glances,
the ways we walk, sit, laugh, the games we must play
with men and even oh my Ancient Mother God the games
we must play among ourselves—these are the ways we pass
unnoticed, by the Conquerors.
They're always watching,
invisibly electroded into our brains,
to be certain we implode our rage against each other,
and not explode it against them. . . .
                    —From "Letter to a Sister Underground"
                    (Morgan, 1970, p. xii)

208

What greater gift can we give girls than the ability to speak their truths and honor the truths of their peers? In a world prepared to value all of girls' feelings and not just some, girls will enjoy the exhilarating freedom of honesty in relationship. They will live without the crippling fear of abandonment. It is my hope that as they, and any woman who has ever been the odd girl out, collect their thoughts to speak their minds, they will whisper to themselves, "What I most regretted were my silences. Of what had I ever been afraid?"
—SIMMONS (2002, p. 270)

Social aggression hurts children, perhaps especially girls, and this fact has quite naturally led to calls for developing prevention and intervention programs to reduce these behaviors (Owens et al., 2001). Some have argued that considering relational or social aggression is critically important in identifying girls who are aggressive (Crick et al., 1999; Henington et al., 1998). If socially aggressive girls are indeed at risk for concurrent and subsequent psychological maladjustment, then it is only logical that prevention and intervention programs be developed to reduce these behaviors.

However, intervening to reduce social aggression is not without controversy. As discussed in Chapter 8, experts disagree as to whether these behaviors are necessarily maladaptive, and some have suggested that social aggression may even serve some developmental functions that are not entirely negative. Because much of the research on indirect/relational/social aggression has been conducted so recently, most of this knowledge has yet to be incorporated into existing interventions to improve children's social relations. To date, the scientific literature includes no prevention or intervention programs that have been developed specifically for the purpose of reducing social aggression and whose effectiveness has been empirically demonstrated.

This chapter reviews how research might inform efforts to prevent or reduce social aggression. First, I consider reasons for and against intervention programs addressing social aggression. Second, the chapter reviews possible approaches to intervention: parents as interveners, the wisdom of adapting intervention programs for physical aggression and bullying, and school-based approaches to reducing bullying (whole-school policies, intervening via the curriculum, working with individual children involved, and efforts to change the overall school climate). Next, I consider how research to date might guide specific clinical practices to reduce social aggression. Last, the chapter discusses special challenges likely to make reducing social aggression particularly difficult, but also how girls' strengths and distinctive characteristics might be harnessed in intervention efforts.

WHY INTERVENE TO REDUCE
OR PREVENT SOCIAL AGGRESSION?

The first and foremost reason cited for intervening to reduce social aggression is that it harms both its victims and its perpetrators. Frequent
victimization by social aggression is related to increased loneliness and
depression (Crick & Grotpeter, 1996) and to low self-concept, especially for girls (Paquette & Underwood, 1999). Perpetrating social aggression is related to peer rejection, loneliness, depression, and social
isolation (Crick & Grotpeter, 1995). Engaging in relational or social aggression may also be related to eating disorder symptoms and to borderline personality features in young adult samples (Werner & Crick,
1999).

A second reason for developing programs to reduce social aggression is that it may create a negative climate in school classrooms, disrupt learning, and annoy teachers. In fact, educators are beginning to
call for assessment and intervention tools to help them recognize and
decrease social aggression among their students (Talbott, 1997).

A third argument for intervening to reduce social aggression is
that it may lead some children to become physically aggressive. Of the
conflicts that girls (kindergarten through grade 5) brought to peer mediators in one study, 29% involved physical aggression and 71% involved verbal or relational aggression (Cunningham et al., 1998). In
one observational study of 11-year-olds on the playground, 25.9% of
physical fights started as aggressive retaliations to teasing (Boulton,
1993). Although teasing is more typically considered to be verbal aggression, the definition used in this study was sufficiently broad that
some of what was coded as teasing may have been social exclusion or
taunting related to relationships. According to one large school survey,
12% of girls in grades 7, 9, and 11 reported having engaged in a physical fight during the last 30 days (these data were screened carefully and
invalid responders eliminated; Cornell & Loper, 1998). Although no research to date has examined the role of social aggression in physical
conflicts among girls, it seems reasonable to expect that social relationships may be involved. Remember that for a sample of adjudicated girls
referred for antisocial behavior, relational aggression and physical assault were highly correlated (Moretti et al., 2001).

As discussed in detail in Chapter 8, girls' physical aggression is related to a long list of later negative outcomes, including delinquency,
dropping out of school, substance abuse, internalizing disorders, and
adolescent motherhood. In addition, engaging in bullying has been
linked to suicidal ideation (Rigby & Slee, 1999), and severe aggression
in adolescence has been linked to suicidal behavior for both boys and

girls (Cairns, Peterson, & Neckerman, 1988). Intervening to reduce social aggression may be a fruitful avenue for reducing physical violence among girls, which in turn might help prevent a wide array of negative outcomes.

A fourth argument for addressing social aggression in intervention programs is that these behaviors may pose special challenges for the treatment of antisocial girls. In one study of the effectiveness of Treatment Foster Care in Oregon, foster parents reported that during the first month of the program, girls had fewer behavior problems than boys did (Chamberlain & Reid, 1994). However, after 6 months of treatment, whereas boys' behavior had improved dramatically, girls' behavior problems had increased to the 1-month levels of boys' symptoms. Foster parents reported feeling extremely frustrated by girls' relationship difficulties and poor response to treatment. In a later study of a sample of girls in Treatment Foster Care in this same community, 72% of the girls reported engaging in at least one act of relational aggression in a single 24-hour period (Chamberlain & Moore, 2000). In a thoughtful review of clinical interventions for antisocial girls, Leve and Chamberlain (in press) concluded that programs for girls would be enhanced by efforts to reduce the chaotic, conflictual nature of the antisocial girls' peer relationships and to help them to develop positive relationships with other young women.

Fifth and last, for all girls, intervening to reduce social aggression might help girls become more assertive and straightforward in resolving their interpersonal difficulties, and might even help them resist the pressures of gender stereotypes as they enter adolescence. As discussed in previous chapters, girls may engage in social aggression because they have few other options for acting on their anger, contempt, or desire for dominance. Feminists have long suggested that women engage in indirect aggression with each other in part due to men's unwillingness to tolerate women's anger (the poem from the opening of this chapter comes from an introduction to an anthology of writings from the Women's Liberation Movement called *Sisterhood is Powerful*; Morgan, 1970). Pressures to mask straightforward expressions of anger might become especially intense in early adolescence. Developmental psychologists have proposed the gender intensification hypothesis (Hill & Lynch, 1983)—that pressures on girls to be feminine increase as they go through puberty and enter adolescence. However, in a qualitative study of conversations among girls from the working class, middle class, and upper class in Maine, preadolescent girls attempted to resist social pressures to be ladylike by encouraging each other to speak up, show their strength, and resist abuse and discrimination (Brown, 1998). Working with girls to reduce social aggression may be one way to build on their own efforts to defy gender stereotypes that discourage anger expression, to encourage them to assert themselves and speak their minds, and to "educate the resistance" (Brown, 1998). I return to this idea later in this chapter.

WHY NOT INTERVENE?

Although many hold high hopes for the potential benefits of intervening to reduce social aggression, there are also several reasons to proceed cautiously.

First, some have argued that it would be unwise to work to reduce social aggression because these behaviors serve some positive goals: fostering and maintaining group allegiance (Adler & Adler, 1995), moral negotiation (Fine, 1986), identity development (Gottman & Mettetal, 1986), protecting the integrity of social groups (Leckie, 1999), and confirming one's own sense of belonging and acceptance (Paquette & Underwood, 1999). Acknowledging that social aggression may serve some positive goals need not require denying that these behaviors may also have some negative consequences; both may well be possible.

Further understanding possible positive developmental functions of social aggression is important for two reasons. (1) Failing to consider them may result in intervention programs unwittingly doing harm, having iatrogenic effects that might make the social environment worse rather than better. Remember that in the focus group study with 10th-grade girls in Australia, girls were extremely skeptical about the effectiveness of adult intervention to reduce indirect aggression and often asserted that the efforts of well-intentioned adults resulted in even worse peer scorn for victims (Owens et al., 2000a). (2) The fact that these behaviors serve some positive functions may make them resistant to intervention efforts and require that those creating prevention programs consider creative means for how these needs might otherwise be met.

A second argument for why some seem reluctant to intervene to reduce social aggression is that resources are scarce and therefore intervention efforts should concentrate on physical violence because its immediate effects are so much more dangerous. Recently I spoke on social aggression at a junior high school Parent–Teacher Association (PTA) meeting, and a father present (also a faculty colleague of mine) offered the opinion that social aggression is good compared to physical aggression and that we should be teaching our children to be socially aggressive instead of fighting and using guns so "no one ends up bleeding on the sidewalk." Before I could answer, he said, "But, then there's

Columbine," referring to the sad sequence of events in which two boys shot several classmates at their Colorado high school and left a video-tape claiming that they had suffered taunting and social exclusion. Re-searchers should further examine the extent to which social aggression leads to physical aggression, so at the very least programs to prevent physical violence might address social aggression as a possible causal factor.

A third argument against intervening to reduce social aggression is that intervention efforts should be based on empirically derived devel-opmental models of how problematic behaviors develop and that the knowledge base for social aggression may still be too small. An excel-lent example of a comprehensive intervention based on a vast body of developmental research and theory is the Fast Track Intervention Pro-gram for the Prevention of Conduct Disorder (Conduct Problems Pre-vention Research Group, 1992). In the absence of detailed knowledge about the developmental origins and outcomes of social aggression, some might argue that we simply do not know enough to intervene yet and that resources should instead be focused on additional basic re-search.

As compelling as this argument may be, it seems important to note two points here. (1) An inadequate knowledge base has certainly not prevented efforts to ameliorate other psychological problems. Scan-ning the DSM-IV (American Psychiatric Association, 1994) makes clear that, although great progress has been made, the research evidence for many established disorders and their treatment is quite weak though clinicians have been diagnosing and treating some of these disorders for decades. Sometimes human suffering cannot wait for science to catch up, and the consequences of social aggression may be worrisome enough that developing interventions while basic research proceeds may be the best course. (2) The recent increased attention to social ag-gression has resulted in a growing knowledge base that may well al-ready provide some important clues for intervention and prevention programs (Owens et al., 2001). What does research to date suggest about how we might intervene?

HOW TO INTERVENE?

What might actually be done to reduce social aggression among chil-dren? Programs need not be invented out of whole cloth. The creation of intervention and prevention programs might be guided by at least two existing bodies of research evidence. First, it could be fruitful to consider intervention programs that already exist to reduce or prevent physical aggression and/or bullying, and to examine whether these programs already have components that address social aggression or could be adapted to do so. Second, some research on specific features of social and relational aggression suggests possible strategies for intervention.

ADAPTING OTHER APPROACHES

Because social aggression among girls has been likened to physical aggression among boys (Crick et al., 1999), it might be tempting to assume that interventions to address antisocial behavior and physical fighting might well work for social aggression too. However, this may not be the case because social and physical aggression may be so different in form and function. For example, many programs to reduce physical aggression include "Stop and think" components to reduce impulsivity and help children consider social choices more carefully; children high on social aggression may have no difficulty inhibiting immediate reactions and may be all too capable of deliberation and social planning. Still, other more broad features of intervention programs for physical aggression might also work to reduce social aggression, such as training in positive play, appropriate conversational skills, interpersonal sensitivity, and empathy. In considering how intervention programs might be adapted to address social aggression, we first consider parent interventions, then school interventions to reduce bullying.

What Parents Might Do

When I give public presentations about social aggression, parents plead with me for suggestions as to what they might be able to do to help their children refrain from perpetrating social aggression and to help them cope with victimization. Although parent training and parent intervention have been used to reduce antisocial behavior in young children to excellent effect (Patterson, 1982), no published parent-training programs address what parents can do about social aggression.

However, research suggests several promising ways in which parents might help children have positive peer relations overall, and perhaps some of these strategies could be useful in helping children to resist social aggression. On the basis of others' research and their own investigations in China, Russia, and the United States, Hart and colleagues (2001) outlined two broad categories of parenting practices that foster positive peer relations: managerial practices and educational practices. Managerial practices include the roles of designer (choosing children's schools and activities and selecting social opportunities for peer contact) and mediator (initiating play dates and friendships). Educational practices include supervision and advice/consulting. Parents can supervise their children's peer activities by interactive interventions (being actively present and involved when children play with peers to help them engage in activities and resolve conflicts—more common with younger children), directive interventions (staying nearby when children are playing together to intervene or redirect if needed—more likely with older children), and monitoring (being continually aware of children's activities, companions, and whereabouts when the child and the parent are apart, which seems particularly important for adolescents). Parents serve in the advising/consulting role when they discuss with their children peer encounters after the fact or outside of the social context in which they are occurring. (For other important scholarship on how parents may promote positive peer relations, see also Ladd & Pettit, 2002; Parke & O'Neil, 1999; Putallaz, Klein, Costanzo, & Hedges, 1994.)

How might parents use some of these practices to help their children refrain from social aggression and respond optimally to victimization? The supervision and advice/consulting roles seem to be especially promising avenues for parent intervention. Parents could play with younger children and point out the hurtfulness of statements like "I won't be your friend if you don't play my way" and quickly redirect conversations and activities when these episodes occur. Parents could make the most of opportunities to overhear older children's conversations (e.g., when parents are driving carpools) to intervene by interrupting or challenging malicious gossip, and parents could attempt to monitor the levels of social aggression in girls' groups by engaging in discussions about whom their daughter socializes with and invites to various events. Parents may assume the advice/consulting role when helping their children cope with victimization. Not all children may go to parents with their victimization experiences, but some will, and adults can use these opportunities to help children respond optimally. At a recent parent presentation, a mother (also a clinical psychologist) told me that she struggled with what to suggest to her 8-year-old son who was being teased at school. She was having trouble convincing him of the power of ignoring teasers until she thought of a more concrete metaphor she could use (she encouraged him to think of himself as wearing a "word raincoat," a protective covering to keep hurtful statements from bothering him).

To explore the possibility of parents as interveners, it might well be useful to investigate parents' perceptions of their children's social aggression, whether they attempt to socialize children to refrain from these behaviors or not, and how they talk with their children about victimization. Teaching parents to help children refrain from social aggression may be challenging, because some parents might not perceive these behaviors to be serious problems or be aware that their children are engaging in them. Or parents themselves might engage in social aggression with their friends and colleagues and be modeling the behaviors for their children, thus requiring intervention on several levels.

School-Based Approaches

Because not all parents are willing or able to be involved in intervention efforts and because the school is such a critically important setting for children, many programs to reduce physical aggression and bullying have been implemented in the school setting (Coie et al., 1988; Lochman, Coie, Underwood, & Terry, 1993). Several of these programs might serve as models for efforts to reduce social aggression, and some include components that already address these behaviors. A comprehensive review of these programs is beyond the scope of this chapter (for reviews of interventions to reduce aggression, see the Conduct Problems Prevention Research Group, 1992; Kazdin, 1987; for bullying, see Smith & Sharp, 1994; Smith et al., 1998).

Because the goal here is to describe how we might intervene to reduce social aggression among girls and how existing programs might be adapted, the following discussion highlights details of one existing comprehensive school-based program, the Sheffield Anti-Bullying Project (described in detail by Smith & Sharp, 1994). An intervention program to reduce bullying was chosen rather than a program to reduce conduct disorder or physical aggression because bullying programs as a group tend to view the behaviors as a group phenomenon rather than an individual problem, and bullying is often defined broadly enough (see Olweus, 1996) that, as we discuss below, some of these programs already address social aggression. This discussion focuses on the Sheffield Anti-Bullying Project in particular because it is an excellent model of how school interventions might operate on several levels: whole-school policies, curricular interventions, targeting individual bullies and victims, and otherwise altering classroom and playground environments.

Whole-School Policies

Experts intervening to reduce bullying have long recognized that an essential step is establishing clear school policies that support the program (Sharp & Thompson, 1994). Such policies may take the form of policy statements formulated by staff or even by students themselves. However, these policies need to go beyond general statements so as to provide guidelines at several levels: (1) delineating what behavior is acceptable at school; (2) specifying strategies that teachers and students should implement when bullying is suspected; and (3) setting up focused programs that target individual bullies and victims (Sharp & Thompson, 1994). Establishing an effective whole-school policy is a process that requires identifying the need, developing the specific guidelines, implementing the new policy, and evaluating its effectiveness (Sharp & Thompson, 1994).

Challenges in implementing whole-school antibullying policies include finding the right people to whom leadership responsibilities can be assigned, making changes in school personnel, overcoming reluctance to involve all groups in the school community, coping with a lack of trained staff, and dealing with concern as to public reactions (Sharp & Thompson, 1994). Implementing whole-school policies to discourage social aggression may be all the more challenging because the behaviors are subtle and varied, less widely recognized as problematic, and less often subject to discipline of any kind. Whole-school policies to reduce social aggression might be more effective if they were stated in positive terms, such as building a community and including everyone, rather than more specific prohibitions of particular behaviors. Whether policies are stated in terms of desired behaviors or community attributes or in terms of prohibitions, it is important to recognize that these policies only set the stage for more focused intervention efforts.

Curricular Interventions

Given that all school children are taught according to an academic curriculum, a promising avenue for prevention of social aggression is adapting the form and content of the curriculum in ways that might serve to decrease the likelihood of bullying episodes. Intervening via the curriculum might include instituting cooperative learning practices that foster a climate of belonging and acceptance, or even studying literature or films whose content specifically addresses the issue of social aggression (Cowie & Sharp, 1994).

Cooperative learning programs have long been recognized as a means for helping students achieve academically and for creating a more positive social climate. Several different cooperative learning approaches have been studied empirically (e.g., the jigsaw method; see Aronson, Blaney, Stephin, Sikes, & Snapp, 1978; Aronson & Patnoe,

1997), and others have been marketed commercially (thousands of schools every year purchase and implement the TRIBES program; Gibbs, 2001). All cooperative learning programs share the goals of helping children feel responsible for creating a learning community, helping them understand and tolerate that individuals can have diverse perspectives on the same problem, and marshaling the power of the group for both academic accomplishments and positive social behavior.

In the Sheffield Anti-Bullying Project, a cooperative learning technique popular in industry called the Quality Circles Method was adopted for the classroom. Quality Circles are groups of five or six students who meet regularly to solve various kinds of problems through a process of brainstorming, doing research to investigate the causes of the challenging situation, hypothesizing causes, proposing solutions, presenting the causes and solutions to "management" (in this case, teachers and school staff), and assessing the outcome of the implemented solutions (Cowie & Sharp, 1994).

Quality Circles might be an effective technique for helping students to generate solutions to the problem of social aggression. In the Sheffield Anti-Bullying Project, ideas implemented at the suggestion of Quality Circles included the following (Cowie & Sharp, 1994, p. 92):

• A lunchtime games tournament to reduce boredom
• A survey of bullying in the whole school
• A booklet on bullying written by the Quality Circles and disseminated to other classes
• A play on bullying devised by pupils and performed for other pupils
• Teaching younger children cooperative games
• Special discussion groups with a particularly high-bullying class
• Gardening teams to improve the school playground

In addition to Quality Circles developing creative and concrete solutions to problems concerning social aggression, of course these kinds of cooperative techniques might also work to reduce social aggression by helping everyone to feel included.

Another strategy for intervening to reduce social aggression via the curriculum may be to have students read literature or view films depicting social aggression. In the Sheffield Anti-Bullying Project, classrooms discussed a story about racism in India called the "The Heartstone Odyssey," which was highly effective in generating discussions concerning racism and diverse forms of harassment including social exclusion (Cowie & Sharp, 1994).

Targeting Individual Aggressors and Victims

School-based intervention programs typically include strategies for helping teachers and peers to intervene with individual bullies and victims. The Sheffield Anti-Bullying Project included several techniques designed to help empower students to stop bullying: collaborative conflict resolution, peer counseling, and assertiveness training for victims (Sharp & Cowie, 1994).

In perhaps the only published work to date to address specific possibilities for intervening to reduce indirect aggression, Owens and colleagues (2001) offered thoughtful suggestions for how these and other existing techniques could be adapted to address the more subtle forms of hurtful behavior. These techniques include the *no blame approach* (Maines & Robinson, 1992), the *method of shared concern* (Pikas, 1989), *peer counseling* (Cowie & Sharp, 1996), and *peer mediation*. Other techniques have been developed to assist victims, such as the *circle of friends* (Taylor, 1996) and *assertiveness training* (Sharp & Cowie, 1994). Although all of these programs seem potentially useful, none is designed specifically to reduce social aggression and their effectiveness has not yet been supported by research evidence.

Other Strategies for Changing the School Climate

Still other strategies may be helpful in altering the overall school atmosphere in subtle but important ways. Some experts have suggested that bullying may be less likely in schools with a less competitive ethos (Besag, 1989). Although reducing the competitiveness of a school culture is easier said than done, it is not difficult to imagine experimenting with strategies such as reducing the emphasis on winning and social comparison and offering a variety of ways for youth to excel and to feel a sense of belonging and acceptance.

Another means of changing the school environment may be training teachers and other staff to sensitize them to the prevalence and potential hurtfulness of social aggression. Observational studies of bullying show that although teachers claim that they are aware of and seek to reduce bullying, they intervene in only one-sixth of bullying episodes on the playground and one-fifth of such episodes in the classroom (Craig, Pepler, & Atlas, 2000). As part of the Sheffield Anti-Bullying Project, playground supervisors were trained to recognize bullying, intervene when it occurred, encourage positive play on the playground, enhance the quality of play, and improve the quality of activities offered on rainy days (Boulton, 1994). In schools in which lunchtime supervisors completed the training program, several forms of bullying decreased, including those in which someone was "threatened," "teased," the "target of nasty stories," and "deliberately excluded" (Boulton, 1994, p. 158). This intervention for playground attendants may have been effective because they were trained to recognize and intervene to stop these behaviors, but it may also have been effective because activities were enhanced and children were likely more happily occupied. Remember that girls in focus groups cited alleviating boredom as a primary reason why they engage in indirect aggression (Owens et al., 2000c).

In summary, school-based programs to prevent or reduce bullying offer excellent examples of frameworks for intervention and prevention programs for social aggression. However, some of the empirical evidence suggests that these programs may be more effective in reducing bullying by boys. For example, in a follow-up study of the effectiveness of the Sheffield Anti-Bullying Project conducted 1 year after the formal evaluation was concluded, the intervention had led to reduced levels of bullying by boys but to an increase in bullying by girls in three of the four schools assessed (Eslea & Smith, 1998). The authors interpreted this discouraging result as suggesting that the intervention program had been more focused on the needs and behaviors of boys, and that girls' bullying takes indirect forms that are extremely difficult to address. They proposed that "efforts must be made to ensure that anti-bullying work is not skewed by a male stereotype of bullying behavior, and that it properly reflects and addresses the problems experienced by girls, and especially the nature of indirect bullying" (Eslea & Smith, 1998, p. 217).

TECHNIQUES FOR DECREASING SOCIAL AGGRESSION: CLUES FROM EMPIRICAL RESEARCH

Programs to prevent or reduce social aggression will likely need to include techniques specifically designed to prevent or interrupt social aggression. Devising these techniques will require more research on the social contexts in which social aggression occurs and the specific social processes by which social aggression unfolds. What does the research to date suggest for strategies that might be especially effective in reducing these behaviors? The following discussion is highly speculative because no published research has examined intervention strategies, but the literature points to some fascinating practical suggestions. Although the focus here is primarily social aggression among girls, suggestions are offered in terms of both genders when strategies follow directly from research results pertaining to both boys and girls.

Measuring Social Aggression

First, to intervene to reduce social aggression, it will be important to assess the behavior using reliable, accurate methods. Research to date on relational aggression suggests that teacher questionnaires may be the most valid method for preschool children (Crick, Casas, & Mosher, 1997). Peer nominations may be especially useful for children in middle childhood (Crick & Grotpeter, 1995), although teacher reports may still have some validity (Crick, 1996). Although few assessment tools have been developed to measure social aggression in adolescence, research with college students suggests that peer nominations from fellow members of organized groups may be useful (see Werner & Crick, 1999, for a study in which sorority and fraternity members report on each other's relational aggression). An important first step for gender-sensitive interventions is assessment tools that tap important behaviors for both genders (Kavanaugh & Hops, 1994), and researchers are making great progress in developing these measures for social and relational aggression.

Once we are able to measure who is socially aggressive or even overall levels of social aggression in a school or a community, the question remains: What can be done to reduce these behaviors? The suggestions given in the subsections below are strategies that follow directly from empirical research to date on the processes and contexts of social aggression. They are organized developmentally, because different strategies may be needed for children at different developmental levels.

Teaching Preschool Children That Social Aggression Is Hurtful and Wrong

For preschool children, the available evidence suggests that several strategies could be fruitful in reducing social aggression. One possibility may be for adults to be more explicit in communicating to children that social aggression is unacceptable. In one of the very few studies to assess children's moral judgments of different forms of aggression, preschoolers rated relational aggression as more acceptable than verbal or physical aggression (Goldstein et al., 2001). It may be important for teachers (and parents) to tell young children explicitly that social aggression hurts others' feelings, that it is harmful and wrong to exclude others (see Paley, 1992, for a fascinating discussion of what occurred when she told her kindergarten students, "You can't say you can't play.")

Encouraging Preschool Children to Seek Adult Assistance When Victimized

Explicit teaching about the harmfulness of social aggression might have another helpful effect; it might make children more likely to seek adult assistance when they are victimized. Remember that preschool children sought adult aid only 4% of the time when they were socially rejected by peers (Fabes & Eisenberg, 1992). If children knew that adults view social aggression as hurtful and wrong, they might be more willing to seek their help and, in so doing, might help teachers become even more aware of social aggression in their preschool classrooms.

Helping Children Respond Optimally to Physically Aggressive Peers

Because social and physical aggression are often highly correlated (Crick et al., 1999) and likely closely linked in time (Arnold et al., 1998), one way to reduce classroom levels of social aggression might be to teach children more optimal responses to peers who are physically aggressive. Remember that for preschool girls and boys, when a child is physically aggressive, it is highly likely that he or she will immediately be the target of socially rejecting behaviors (Arnold et al., 1998). Social aggression could be reduced by teaching children to respond to peers who hit in other ways—with verbal assertiveness, by seeking adult aid, or perhaps even by ignoring the physical aggressor, depending on the situation. Children could be helped to understand that as wrong as it is for one child to hit, it is also problematic to respond to physical aggression with social aggression.

Sensitizing Parents to How Children May Learn Social Aggression by Observing Marital Difficulties

For children in preschool and beyond, one strategy for reducing social aggression may be to educate parents about the harmfulness of this behavior and the possibility that children can learn it from observing particular types of marital conflicts. Remember that in families where parents are divorcing, girls' relational aggression has been shown to be linked to their triangulation in parents' marital conflicts (Kerig et al., 2001). All parents could be counseled that children may learn social aggression by observing their parents resolve conflicts in ways that harm relationships: giving one another the silent treatment when angry, enlisting other family members or friends to support their point of view in an argument, threatening to end the relationship, withdrawing love or affection, and in particular, involving the child in arguments or conflicts.

Social-Cognitive Interventions

Another way to intervene to reduce social aggression might be to interrupt particular types of social cognition that may relate to social aggression. Perhaps as a result of family experiences, some children are prone to making particular types of errors in processing social information that may be related to engaging in physical aggression (Crick & Dodge, 1994) and perhaps social aggression as well. For example, girls high on relational aggression tend to overattribute hostility in relationally provoking situations (Crick, 1995; Crick et al., 2002). This suggests that one way to intervene might be to teach children to make more benign attributions in ambiguous social situations. School-age children might be sophisticated enough to benefit from techniques borrowed from cognitive therapy, such as learning to entertain alternative interpretations and recognizing automatic, overly negative thinking.

Assertiveness Training

If social aggression in middle childhood is related to girls' struggling between feeling furious but wanting to be nice and to dissemble negative emotions, one strategy for reducing social aggression might be assertiveness training. Girls could be taught to express their needs and desires more directly and to accept that conflict is a natural part of relationships. Moreover, girls could be taught to express their negative feelings calmly and in the least threatening manner possible, and could practice these skills in role plays with friends or in groups. Feminist scholarship confirms that assertiveness training can be helpful for girls. In their broad review of gender and treatment, Kavanaugh and Hops (1994) argued that "more emphasis needs to be given to arming both genders with the skills and the abilities that are normally built into the other's repertoire" (p. 72). This might not require teaching girls to fight physically, but instead to feel more comfortable directly voicing their concerns and asserting their social goals.

Harnessing Girls' Distaste for Social Aggression

Because research suggests that girls in both the United States and Indonesia dislike those who engage in social aggression (French et al.,

2002), girls' distaste for social aggression in others could be harnessed to encourage them to refrain from the behavior themselves and to stop others from excluding and manipulating peers. Parents, teachers, and counselors might discuss with girls how social aggression hurts, reflects badly on the perpetrator, and undermines everyone's trust in the peer group. Discussions might also focus on how social aggression may be a way to meet immediate needs or exact revenge in the short term but the longer-term consequences could be social rejection and reputational harm.

Focusing on Girls Who Spend Time Alone

Another important suggestion for intervention comes from research showing that for 8- or 9-year-old girls on the playground, time alone was related to peer victimization and, in fact, low levels of time alone predicted the greatest increase in peer social preference 5 months later (Boulton, 1999). For girls, time alone may be a marker or perhaps even a cause of their vulnerability to victimization, whereas time engaged with peers seems related to becoming better liked. If prevention programs seek to identify those who may be at risk for victimization by social aggression, it might be important to attend to girls who spend a great deal of time by themselves. Part of the intervention strategy may include trying to integrate these girls into the peer group by seeking to increase their interest in interacting with others, teaching them appropriate social skills, or strategically assigning them to classroom groups or activities with peers.

Providing Multiple Opportunities for Girls to Belong

If girls in middle childhood and early adolescence indeed engage in social aggression as a way of affirming their own sense of belongingness (Adler & Adler, 1995), one way to reduce social aggression might be to offer multiple frameworks within which youths can feel accepted. Developmental theory suggests that preadolescent girls desperately want to fit in, to feel part of a same-gender peer group (Gottman & Mettetal, 1986). Too often in late elementary or junior high school, girls can feel as if there is only one possible group and a person is either in or out. Some girls in this age range may have limited access to activities in their schools—sometimes only athletics, a few clubs, and cheerleading are available. If girls were able to engage in a broader array of activities at earlier ages, such as drama, choral singing, service organizations, and academic interest groups, there might be more diverse opportunities for girls to feel accepted within at least one group.

Engaging Girls in More Structured Activities

Because research indicates that a primary reason that girls engage in social aggression may be to alleviate boredom (Owens et al., 2000b), another strategy for reducing overall levels of social aggression might be to encourage girls to participate more in structured activities. Studies of adolescents' time use across cultures suggest that teens in the United States spend enormous amounts of discretionary time hanging around with friends and talking—up to 18% of their waking time, approximately 2.5 hours per day in conversation with peers (R. W. Larson & Verma, 1999). In one study with European American girls ages 10–15, the proportion of waking time spent talking with peers increased from 9 to 18% (Raffaelli & Duckett, 1989). Some developmental consequences of spending leisure time in this way may be negative (R. Larson, 2001), including increased opportunities to engage in relational aggression (R. W. Larson, Wilson, Brown, Furstenberg, & Verma, 2002). Recent evidence suggests that U.S. youth are spending increasing amounts of their discretionary time in structured, voluntary activities (including sports, drama, music, service organizations, and other clubs (R. Larson, 2001). These activities may foster various types of competence and growth; they also may reduce boredom that may lead girls to manipulate relationships for sheer entertainment.

Helping Girls to Become More Comfortable with Appropriate Competition

Another positive consequence of engaging girls in more structured activities might be helping them to become more comfortable with competition, which could further enhance their skills in assertiveness and help them to engage in less social aggression. One reason why girls may be more prone to indirect aggression is that they have less experience in competing in organized games (Lever, 1976) and experience negative emotions in competitive situations (Benenson et al., 2002). In this cleverly designed study, kindergarten and fourth-grade girls and boys were observed in two laboratory experiments. In Study 1, same-gender groups of four friends were observed as they chose a group leader. Although girls and boys did not differ on their levels of involvement in this task or their negotiation time, girls were observed to exhibit greater discomfort in this context than were boys (discomfort was coded for nonverbal behaviors such as tightly crossed arms, refusing to make eye contact, frowning, or looking around anxiously). In Study 2, same-gender dyads played games while separated by a barrier, then the barrier was removed while they awaited the results of the competition.

Girls and boys did not differ in observed discomfort when separated by the barrier, but when the barrier was removed girls showed more discomfort than did boys.

If girls had more experience in competitive organized activities, they might become more comfortable with competing within the contexts of games, sports, and even other activities (e.g., musicians engage in keen regular competition for chair placements in orchestras). If girls could become more comfortable competing within particular contexts without taking competitive behavior personally (Lever, 1976), they might be better prepared to resolve friendship conflicts more assertively. One promising context in which these skills could be taught is games: "Game situations may provide a productive and safe context for helping children with the emotional side of their lives with peers" (Asher & Rose, 1997, p. 216).

Teaching Specific Peers to Actively Defend Victims

Another promising avenue may be to mobilize particular children to interrupt or discourage social aggression. Recent research on bullying has found that in addition to the roles of bully and victim, children assume other participant roles in bullying situations: assistant, reinforcer, defender, and outsider (Salmivalli, Lagerspetz, Bjorkqvist, Osterman, & Kaukiainen, 1996). With a sample of sixth graders in Finland, these investigators found moderate agreement between self- and peer-reports of children's participant roles. In this study, girls who were bullies were high on both social rejection and social acceptance. Perhaps girls' bullying does not always lead to social rejection precisely because it is covert and tolerated more (Salmivalli, Kaukiainen, & Lagerspetz, 2001). Girls more often assumed the roles of defender and outsider in bullying situations, whereas boys were more likely to be bullies, reinforcers, or assistants (Salmivalli et al., 1996). Children who served as defenders were low on rejection by peers and high on peer acceptance, and 43% had popular peer status. These results suggest that some children quite naturally assume the defender role. In intervention programs, some of these defenders, maybe especially the ones with high peer status, might be taught specific strategies to interrupt social aggression in situations in which they witness it occurring, contexts in which adults are often far out of earshot.

Teaching Girls to Interrupt Malicious Gossip

If peers are to be trained to intervene to halt or discourage social aggression, what exactly should they be urged to do? One practical suggestion comes from Eder and Enke's (1991) careful analysis of gossip among young adolescents at junior high school lunch tables. Although the structure of these interactions encouraged the tone becoming increasingly negative, this structure was also flexible in important ways. Gossip usually began with one person offering an initial negative evaluation. The first immediate response to the initial evaluative comment influenced the nature of all remarks to follow. If the first response was supportive of the initial negative remark, then all remarks following were likely to reinforce the negative evaluation. However, if the initial response to the negative evaluation was a challenge, regardless of whether the challenge was offered by a high- or a low-status peer, then subsequent comments were also likely to be more positive and less negative. Challenges to negative gossip were only effective if they were offered immediately following the first negative evaluative comment.

The power of peers' immediately resisting negative evaluations of others suggests that intervention programs could teach girls strategies for quickly challenging malicious gossip, and perhaps also social exclusion. Because girls are prone to being agreeable, it would likely be important to teach them very specific statements and to practice these in role plays to help them become more comfortable and effective in voicing disagreements. Although challenges could be effective from high- and low-status youth (Eder & Enke, 1991), it might be especially effective to teach these skills to high-status girls who are already prone to assuming the defender role and likely to have the greatest impact on their peers.

These preliminary suggestions are only the beginning elements of the techniques that will be needed to interrupt social aggression. As researchers continue to study how these behaviors occur in particular social contexts and begin to understand more about their developmental origins, psychologists will be much better prepared to design effective intervention and prevention programs.

CHALLENGES FOR INTERVENING TO REDUCE OR PREVENT SOCIAL AGGRESSION

Although there is reason to believe that intervention to reduce social aggression is possible, it is important to acknowledge that by their very nature these behaviors may be very difficult to change for several reasons. First, social aggression is subtle, rarely visible, and may not respond to global interventions to reduce aggression or bullying (Eslea & Smith, 1998). Second, given that social aggression involves dissemblance and talking behind others' backs, girls high on these behaviors

may sabotage intervention efforts by conveying to adults that they support the goals of the program while continuing to surreptitiously exclude others, gossip, and manipulate friendships. Third, girls who are
highly socially aggressive may frustrate and alienate adults: teachers
(Talbott, 1997), Treatment Foster Parents (Chamberlain & Reid, 1994),
and perhaps counselors or therapists or even parents may simply give
up. Fourth, children who bully seem to see themselves as strong and accepted (Salmivalli, 1998); therefore, some children who are socially aggressive may not wish to change because they perceive no problems
with their peer relations and may not even be aware of the impact of
their social aggression.

Another formidable challenge for intervention programs is that
children may face few peer consequences for social aggression (Salmivalli et al., 2001). Victims of social aggression may be afraid to speak
up for fear of even worse reprisals, and those who have not been victimized may not be aware of which individuals are perpetrators. Even
when peers are present in physical bullying situations, observational research suggests that they support the bully 75% of the time (O'Connell,
Pepler, & Craig, 1999) and this may be similarly true for social aggression. Even though some youth do seem to assume the role of defending the victim, children with similar participant roles tend to hang
around together (Salmivalli et al., 2001); thus some naturally occurring
groups may have bullies and victims but no defenders.

The last feature of social aggression that will need to be addressed
in intervention programs is that the intimacy and self-disclosure that
makes girls such wonderful friends may make them formidable ene-
mies to one another. To hurt someone else via social aggression, it is
necessary to understand a great deal about the social desires and fears
of that person: the nature of her other friendships, social groups she
may wish to join, romantic interests or friendships she may wish to pursue, and other personal information to use in the service of malicious
gossip. Social aggression may be most effective when one person un-
derstands what makes the other feel most threatened and vulnerable.
Because girls share so much of this information with one another,
many may never lack ammunition for social aggression.

To make matters even more complicated, because girls are accus-
tomed to sharing so much personal information, the withholding of
such information might actually constitute a form of social aggression.
For example, if adolescent girls are close friends, one would be deeply
insulted if the other failed to tell her about a new romantic interest.
Even among adults, withholding of information can be a way to manipulate and exclude. In work contexts, colleagues can hurt and exclude
one another by withholding valuable information, for example, neglect-

ing to tell a colleague of a higher position becoming open or failing to share insights about a supervisor's less than clearly stated goals. Intervening to reduce hurtful withholding will be challenging because all of us keep some information private for the sake of discretion or simply due to limited time and energy for sharing. Still, it might be productive to discuss with girls the hurtful power of withholding information that could potentially help another.

STRENGTHS OF GIRLS TO HARNESS FOR INTERVENTION

Although reducing social aggression poses daunting challenges and qualities of girls' friendships may contribute to these, girls also have important interpersonal strengths that could be mobilized in intervention programs. Girls expect more intimacy, loyalty, and dependence in their peer relations than do boys (Salmivalli et al., 2001); therefore it is not surprising that they are more supportive of interventions to reduce peer harassment (Rigby, 2001). Many girls have strong verbal skills and high social intelligence, which would likely help them think through complex scenarios and be quick students of skills and strategies for interrupting social aggression. As compared to boys, girls are more prone to feeling shame and guilt for bullying, more distressed by victimization, and more likely to tell someone when they are victimized (Rigby, 2001). Even preschool girls view relational aggression as more wrong than do preschool boys (Goldstein et al., 2002). In bullying situations, girls are more likely than boys are to assume defender or outsider roles (Salmivalli et al., 1996), and observational evidence indicates that girls are more likely to intervene in bullying on the playground (O'Connell et al., 1999). The most effective intervention programs will carefully and creatively capitalize on girls' verbal skills, social intelligence, and some individuals' proclivities for peer intervention.

SUMMARY AND CONCLUSIONS

Although discussions of prevention and intervention to reduce social aggression are just beginning, the potential for innovative, effective programs seems great. Researchers have made substantial progress in developing methods for assessing social and relational aggression, and in understanding both its negative consequences and possible positive developmental functions. Already existing intervention programs provide excellent frameworks that may be adapted to address social aggression; the best and most likely effective interventions will follow from research on the specific processes involved in these subtle, complex behaviors. Research to date offers some precise, practical, promising strategies. As we learn more about the forms and functions of social aggression in particular social contexts and its developmental origins, we will be all the more able to design creative means of reducing these behaviors while supporting children's developmental needs.

In further developing intervention programs, two goals seem most pressing. First, as noted by many experts on aggression and bullying, reducing these behaviors will require intervening on multiple levels (Smith & Sharp, 1994), systems thinking (Owens et al., 2001), and perhaps even adopting a dynamic systems perspective (Pepler et al., 1999). Next, in Chapter 10, I consider different models for understanding the developmental origins, social contexts and processes, and outcomes associated with social aggression. Second, efforts to reduce social aggression among girls will be most effective if they are designed to build on girls' relationship strengths and perhaps even their own efforts to resist gender stereotypes (Brown, 1998). Helping girls learn to refrain from social aggression with one another could be an important way of reinforcing their assertiveness, self-worth, and sense of opportunities unbound by conventional femininity. Helping girls recognize their strengths as relationship partners could lead them to appreciate the importance of not undermining one another. Some girls have friendships that are so intense, intimate, and even turbulent that they seem much like sisters, and girlfriends and women friends sometimes refer to each other as "Sister" or even "Sisterfriend." The greatest hope and the worst fear for interventions to reduce social aggression is that, for good or for ill, sisterhood is powerful.

Chapter 10

New Models of Social Aggression
For Its Own Sake

Some say the world will end in fire,
Some say in ice.
From what I've tasted of desire,
I hold with those who favor fire.
But if it had to perish twice,
I think I know enough of hate
To say that for destruction ice
Is also great
And would suffice.
—From "Fire and Ice" (Frost, 1923/1949, p. 268)

As Robert Frost so eloquently argued, hateful behavior may take forms that may be likened to fire, with its flashy, overt, immediately and intensely painful qualities, or to ice, with its cooler, subtle, more slow but no less lethal pain and destruction. Physical aggression may be more fiery and social aggression may be more icy, but (as we discuss below) it may not be so simple.

Note that in his poem Frost seems to liken the icy forms of hate to the fiery ones, saying that both suffice for destruction. Similarly, researchers studying relational and social aggression have attempted to justify the importance of these behaviors by demonstrating their similarity to physical aggression (Crick et al., 1999; Galen & Underwood, 1997). We have argued that social aggression matters because social aggression hurts, just as much if not more than physical aggression, perhaps especially for girls (Galen & Underwood, 1997; Paquette & Underwood, 1999). Likening social to physical aggression may also make sense because they are highly correlated; children who aggress likely do so in multiple ways. Finally, although more systematic research is needed on this point, it seems quite likely that the rare episodes in which girls behave violently may have been preceded by social aggression.

In this final chapter I propose that, though much has been learned by applying theories, methods, and constructs from research on physical aggression to our understanding of social aggression, new models and approaches may well also be needed. First, I summarize the considerable advances that have been made by comparing social aggression to physical aggression, but I also consider the dangers of relying only on this approach. Next, I point out some of the important differences between these two forms of behavior that may require new models. On the basis of research to date, possible new models are presented for defining and classifying aggressive behavior; understanding the forms, processes, and functions of social aggression in particular social contexts; and developmental precursors and outcomes of social aggression. The chapter ends with a discussion of 10 important future directions.

WHAT HAVE WE LEARNED FROM LIKENING
SOCIAL TO PHYSICAL AGGRESSION?

Most research to date has considered behaviors such as social exclusion, friendship manipulation, and malicious gossip to be forms of aggression. Using the term "aggression" has likely helped scholars take behaviors such as friendship manipulation very seriously. Who would dispute that aggression is bad and worthy of research and intervention? Conceiving of these behaviors as aggression has been extraordinarily helpful also because as a result of decades worth of research on physical aggression, sophisticated models, constructs, and methods were already available that could be rapidly and profitably applied to understanding social aggression.

What have we learned by studying social aggression within these frameworks? From studies using peer nomination questionnaires, we know that relational aggression is associated with peer rejection in a manner not dissimilar to physical aggression (Crick & Grotpeter, 1995). Studies asking children to respond to hypothetical vignettes have shown that some of the same social information-processing biases seem associated with both relational aggression and overt aggression (Crick, 1995; Crick et al., 2002). Studies relying on self-reports have shown that relational/social victimization hurts children as much as physical victimization does (Crick & Grotpeter, 1996; Paquette &

Underwood, 1999). Peer nomination data indicate that both relational and physical aggression are relatively stable over short periods of time (a span of 6 months within the same school year) and predict negative consequences (here again, 6 months later; Crick, 1996). Theories and constructs from research on physical aggression will continue to be useful as guides to understanding further the developmental origins and outcomes of social and relational aggression.

However, likening social to physical aggression may also have limitations. First, this choice may lead to an excessive focus on gender differences. Second, this approach may obscure important differences between social and physical aggression. These two issues are discussed at length below.

ARE GIRLS AND BOYS EQUALLY AGGRESSIVE, AND DOES THIS QUESTION REALLY MATTER?

Designating social exclusion, friendship manipulation, and malicious gossip as forms of aggression has generated great excitement because it has done much to "counter the stereotype of the 'sugary, nonaggressive female' " (Crick et al., 1999, p. 98). Calling these behaviors aggression has highlighted that girls too can be mean and hurt one another, and has forced skeptics to take these behaviors seriously.

However, some have gone one step further and argued that girls and boys are equally aggressive but their mean behaviors take different forms:

> Taken together, the previously described studies provide strong evidence that gender differences in aggression are minimal (or nonexistent) when both physical and relational forms of aggression are considered. (Crick et al., 1999, p. 99)

This claim seems problematic for several reasons. First, do we really wish to argue, without overwhelming, compelling evidence, that girls are as aggressive as boys are? Is this really an honor that anyone would want to claim for girls? To embrace the proposition that girls are just as aggressive as boys, in the absence of well-replicated findings, seems a sort of odd perversion of "honorary maleness" (a phenomenon where women succeed by adopting characteristics of the male gender stereotype, sometimes to extreme degrees). Second, the argument that girls and boys are equally aggressive is a difficult claim to support, and focuses efforts squarely on gender differences rather than understanding the meaning of these behaviors for each gender group. Third, the intriguing claim that girls are just as aggressive as boys falls apart in light of the empirical evidence reviewed in Chapters 4–7. Given that boys are clearly higher than girls on physical aggression, if girls are to be "as aggressive" they need to be dramatically and consistently higher than boys on social aggression. Although some studies find that girls are higher on relational aggression than boys are (Crick & Grotpeter, 1995; Lagerspetz et al., 1988), the gender difference is smaller than that for physical aggression and many other studies find no gender differences (e.g., Rys & Bear, 1997) or even that boys are higher on relational aggression than are girls (e.g., Henington et al., 1998; Tomada & Schneider, 1997). The final problem with the claim that girls are just as aggressive as boys is that it is difficult to understand what this means, given that these behaviors are so very different in form.

For all of these reasons, it seems premature to argue that girls and boys are equally aggressive. I concur with Bjorkqvist (1994), who argued that "there are good reasons to doubt whether it is meaningful at all to debate whether one sex is more or less aggressive than the other" (p. 178). Of course, it will be important to continue to measure gender differences in social aggression and seek to understand them as evidence accumulates, but it seems much more interesting to focus on other questions, such as the meaning of these behaviors for girls and for boys, how they might relate differently to girls' and boys' social functioning, and their developmental origins and outcomes. Our efforts to begin to explain social aggression will likely be more fruitful if we acknowledge that social and physical aggression differ in important ways.

DIFFERENCES BETWEEN SOCIAL AND PHYSICAL AGGRESSION THAT MAY REQUIRE NEW MODELS AND METHODS

Although both social and physical aggression hurt victims and create social difficulties for perpetrators, these behaviors differ on some other very basic dimensions. Punching someone in the face is plainly and simply a very different act than, say, not inviting someone to a party, trying to turn a person's friends against her, or spreading a malicious rumor about her. These differences may require that we use alternative constructs and methods for understanding social and physical aggression.

First, physical fighting must occur face-to-face, whereas social aggression may be well underway before the victims are aware that they are targets. Victims of physical aggression usually know exactly who has hurt them and when the specific act of aggression has ceased, but victims of social aggression may not know who the perpetrator is or when the aggression will end, and they must cope with the fear that everyone, even close friends, may be working against them surreptitiously. These features of social aggression require that researchers use creative methods for capturing subtle and extended sequences: remote audiovisual recording using wireless microphones (Asher et al., 2001; Pepler & Craig, 1995), diary or experience-sampling methods (R. Larson & Richards, 1994), or even examining exchanges over the telephone or the Internet (see Warren & Tate, 1992, for a study of younger children's telephone exchanges from a cognitive developmental perspective).

Second, whereas a single act of physical aggression occurs within a brief time frame, one episode of social aggression may play out over hours, days, or even weeks. Researchers who wish to observe physical aggression may be able to learn much by observing free play or asking children to report on others' specific behaviors, but those seeking to understand social aggression may need to observe events over longer periods of time. Here again remote audiovisual recording technology could be helpful, as could more qualitative methods such as interviews or diaries to capture the more extended sequences of hurtful, exclusionary behavior.

Third, whereas physical aggression causes immediate physical pain (and perhaps also hurt feelings and disrupted relationships), social aggression usually causes emotional and psychological harm that may develop over time—and possibly may linger. Here again, studies of victimization by social aggression may need to assess more subtle long-term effects and examine the extent to which youth ruminate on these behaviors.

Fourth, whereas it is possible for physical aggression to occur between only two children, much social aggression by definition often involves groups, either invoking the group by threatening a person with exclusion or directly involving at least a third if not fourth of fifth parties to spread gossip or exclude someone. Researchers who seek to understand social aggression need to consider that these behaviors may be properties of groups, that youth who engage in these behaviors may form social networks in which social aggression is normative or even encouraged, or that networks may socialize their members to engage in these behaviors. In a manner similar to research on bullying by Salmivalli and colleagues (1996), investigators will need to examine different roles played by peers in social aggression, not just perpetrators and victims but also assistants, reinforcers, and defenders.

Fifth, because social aggression is so much more subtle than physical aggression, it may take place in very different settings, maybe in private, but perhaps also under the watchful eyes of parents and teachers, and certainly via many different types of communication such as telephone conversations, e-mail, voice mail, and Instant Messenger interactions. Researchers who seek to witness social aggression may need to move beyond playground observations and watch children in settings such as classrooms or lunchrooms, as well as study how peers may engage in social aggression via the telephone and the Internet.

POSSIBILITIES FOR NEW MODELS

All of these differences between social aggression and physical aggression and the methods needed to measure them suggest that new theories and models might well be needed to understand social aggression in addition to those that have been usefully borrowed from research on physical aggression. The following subsections present possible models for defining and classifying aggression, processes of social aggression, developmental origins of social aggression, and developmental outcomes of social aggression. Many are highly speculative and thus will be presented here as brief outlines to generate empirical research.

Alternative Approaches to Defining and Classifying Types of Aggression

As discussed in detail in Chapter 2 on definitions and subtypes, how we define social aggression will greatly influence our theories, methods, results, and interpretations. As presented in Figure 2.1 on page 30, most current systems for classifying subtypes of aggression, including social aggression, are categorical. Most researchers who try to discriminate between indirect/relational/social aggression and physical aggression work on the assumption that these are discrete categories with firm boundaries and that any one behavior can be placed in one subtype or the other. Categorical systems are enormously helpful because they organize information in a clear, concrete way that translates well to researchers' needs for operational definitions, particular questionnaire items, and discrete observational codes.

However, categorical systems can also be problematic. First, most aggressive behaviors cause more than one type of harm; for example, physical aggression sometimes also causes damage to the victim's social standing or relationships. If one child hits or kicks another, certainly physical pain results but relationships might suffer as well. Damage would be done to the relationship between the victim and the perpetrator, but perhaps also to the victim's social standing with present observers or peers who may subsequently hear accounts of the victimization (depending of course on how peers perceived the perpetrator's and the victim's behaviors). Second, although the social/physical aggression dichotomy is based on the "vehicle of harm" (Lagerspetz et al., 1988, p. 405), other distinctions are just as important. Social aggression may be direct or indirect, proactive or reactive, deliberate or impulsive, and further dividing categories into more and more subcategories leads to a sort of infinite regress in which the units become so small as to be less meaningful. What are some alternatives to the present categorical systems?

One possibility may be to move to a more dimensional system, where aggressive behaviors are characterized not as belonging to discrete groups but as varying along one or more continuous dimensions. One kind of continuous dimensional model was proposed long ago by Lea Pulkinnen in her doctoral dissertation (described by Pitkanen, 1969, cited in Tremblay, 2000). As Figure 10.1 shows, this model includes vectors for intensity, indirect versus direct, and defensive versus offensive. This model includes dimensions that fit with subcategories proposed in recent research (indirect vs. direct aggression, and offensive vs. defensive aggression may reflect some features of proactive vs. reactive aggression). Although categorical systems have proved the easier path for research purposes, as research on social aggression advances, we may be wise to revisit the possibility of continuous dimensional models.

Continuous dimensional models may be particularly helpful for understanding social aggression because the boundaries for this category may be much less clear than for physical fighting. As Archer

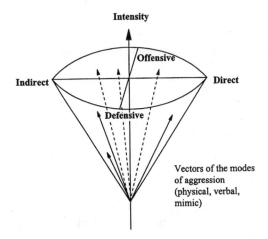

FIGURE 10.1. A descriptive model of aggression. Described by Pitkanen (1969, cited in Tremblay, 2000). From Tremblay (2000). Copyright 2000 by The International Society for the Study of Behavioral Development. Reprinted by permission.

(2001) cogently argued for the indirect forms of relational aggression, "there is a difficult dividing line between the overt use of a strategy to hurt someone and its covert use, for example, as a way of advancing oneself in an organizational setting. Is giving an unfavorable evaluation to a potential rival for promotion indirect relational aggression?" (p. 268). As another example, negative information about a third party may be shared for the purpose of malicious gossip or for enlisting aid or problem solving, and more than one of these goals may be achieved by a single interchange. Interestingly, psychologists in other areas of our field, especially psychopathology, have long argued that human behavior may not sort itself well into neat categories with precise boundaries and that continuous dimensional systems may be a better reflection of human difficulties as they occur in nature (R. C. Carson, 1996). Dimensional and multidimensional models may be enormously helpful in making subtle but important distinctions between forms of social aggression.

A second alternative might be to preserve some categorical features but, instead of designating aggressive behaviors as belonging to one of a single set of categories, behaviors could be characterized using several different categories or continuous dimensions. An example of this is the multiaxial approach to diagnosis of mental disorders described in detail in the DSM-IV (American Psychiatric Association, 1994). The DSM-IV approach requires that psychological difficulties be diagnosed on five axes, some of which are categorical and some of which are continuous: clinical disorders (categorical), personality disorders and mental retardation (categorical), general medical conditions (categorical), psychosocial and environmental problems (categorical), and global assessment of functioning (continuous).

A multiaxial approach to defining and classifying types of aggressive behavior might similarly include a blend of categorical and continuous dimensional axes. One could imagine a multiaxial system in which an aggressive behavior might be described with research to each of the following (presented in no particular order):

- Observable form of behavior—physical or not?
- Intensity
- Perpetrator's intent to harm
- Victim's perception of harm
- Type of harm inflicted—friendships, social standing, self-esteem, physical, property damage
- Direct versus indirect
- Reactive versus proactive
- Impulsive, "hot," angry versus deliberate, "cool"

An important advantage of a multiaxial approach is that it permits some components to be categorical and some to be continuous, according to which conceptualization makes most sense for the particular feature. For example, judging whether an aggressive behavior is physical or not seems by nature to be a categorical decision, whereas intensity or intention to harm could easily be conceived of as dimensional. A multiaxial system would preserve some of the categories that have proved generative and practically useful for researchers but also would force us to consider features of aggression that may truly be continuous dimensions.

Here it is important to note that if you consider social and physical aggression along more than one dimension, the fire and ice analogy quickly breaks down. Physical aggression may be reactive and fueled by anger (fiery) or may be more proactive and deliberate (in a manner that could seem icy). Similarly, social aggression may involve behaviors that indeed seem cool and deliberate and icy (giving someone the "cold shoulder"; carefully and meticulously spreading a rumor to undermine another's friendships and enhance one's own status), but social aggression could also take more fiery forms (reacting to a perceived slight by impulsively firing off a nasty rumor about someone to 150 people simultaneously via Instant Messenger). A clear advantage of a multiaxial system is that it will force us to appreciate the complexity of different forms of aggression by systematically considering them on several dimensions.

A third, more radical alternative to a strictly categorical system is conceiving of subtypes of aggression as prototypes. Prototypes are sets of associated features, some of which are core features shared by all members of the set and some of which are more peripheral and characteristic of only some category members. Conceiving of subtypes of aggression as prototypes makes sense because it conforms to our intuition that there are central defining features but also more borderline characteristics that may be shared by different subtypes. As R. C. Carson (1991) argued in discussing why prototypes might make sense for classifying psychopathology, "To anticipate that the outcomes of these multiple, complexly interwoven, and, one must assume, highly idiosyncratic antecedent processes (Meehl, 1978) will fall out naturally into neat, digital packages of the kind envisaged by a monothetic system of diagnosis is to strain the limits of credulity" (p. 303). Similarly, aggressive behavior may well be complex enough to require a prototypal approach.

Pursuing a prototypal approach for understanding social aggression would require theorizing as to what the core features might be, which could be augmented by careful analysis of accounts of perpetrating and being victimized by social aggression. A similar approach has been used to construct prototypes of basic emotions (see Shaver, Schwartz, Kirson, & O'Connor, 1987). Participants might be asked to describe both personal and typical experiences of social aggression, and accounts might be coded for specific features. Statistical analyses might examine which features seem core to the construct and which seem less central (techniques might include factor analyses, cluster analyses, or discriminant function analyses). For example, one good candidate for a core feature of social aggression might be harm to relationships. Other emergent but not always present features might be anger, jealousy, or desire for dominance. Building prototypes in this way could be helpful in determining features and subtypes of social aggression, while acknowledging the complexity of the phenomenon and that boundaries are not always firm.

Is Aggression the Only Framework for Understanding These Behaviors?

Note that the tendency to liken friendship manipulation and social exclusion to physical aggression began decades ago, when these behaviors were referred to as *indirect aggression* (A. H. Buss, 1961; Feshbach, 1969) and, more recently, *social aggression* (Cairns, Cairns, Neckerman, et al., 1989; Galen & Underwood, 1997) and *relational aggression* (Crick & Grotpeter, 1995; Crick et al., 1999). Without a doubt, scholars have offered strong arguments for referring to social exclusion and friendship manipulation as forms of aggression, namely, that these behaviors are intended to harm others and perceived as intensely hurtful by victims (Galen & Underwood, 1997).

However, it is important to acknowledge that other choices of terms were and still are conceivable, and using other terms may illuminate new possibilities. For example, some have studied social exclusion, malicious gossip, and friendship manipulation as forms of indirect bullying (e.g., Craig et al., 2000). Studying these behaviors within the framework of bullying invites attention to the dyad and to the larger social group involved, which could be very profitable for understanding these behaviors that are so intimately bound up with group processes.

Social Aggression as Harassment

Others have proposed that it might be enormously useful to conceive of hurtful behaviors among peers as forms of harassment, defined as follows:

victimization that entails face-to-face confrontation (e.g., physical aggression, verbal abuse, and nonverbal gesturing) or social manipulation through a third party (e.g. social ostracism, spreading rumors). . . .
The crucial element that distinguishes peer harassment from other
types of negative encounters, such as conflict, is that there is an imbalance of power between perpetrator and target. (Juvonen & Graham,
2001, p. xiii)

These authors argue that the term "harassment" is preferable to "victimization" because harassment encompasses a wide range of behaviors
and fits conceptually with difficulties that occur among adults and are
often addressed by policies in employment and educational settings.
Conceiving of social exclusion, malicious gossip, and friendship manipulation as harassment might be helpful because it alerts us to the issues
of power imbalances and chronicity that may make social aggression
particularly painful.

Social Aggression as Peer Rejection

Another possibility is that social aggression could be understood as one
of the many ways in which peers reject one another. Although a wealth
of research has investigated characteristics and correlates of children
who are sociometrically rejected, many fewer studies have examined
the specific social processes by which peer rejection occurs (Asher et
al., 2001). Some of these processes may include social aggression.

To learn more about specific rejecting behaviors, Asher and colleagues (2001) used wireless microphones for remote audiovisual recording of 35 focal children at school (13 who had developmental dis-
abilities and 22 who did not; half of the "typical" group had average
peer status and half was sociometrically rejected). Focal children were
observed at school for 6 hours per child, at school during lunch, recess,
and physical education class. On the basis of these rich observational
data, Asher and colleagues proposed a typology of peer rejection that
included 6 major categories and 32 subcategories. The major categories were excluding and terminating interaction, denial of access, aggression, dominance, moral disapproval, and involving a third party
(pp. 127–130).

None of these categories corresponds perfectly to social aggression. Socially aggressive behaviors are well represented in the category
for excluding and terminating interactions (e.g., leaving, expressing dislike or nonrelationship), but also in denial of access (denial of access to
self). Friendship manipulation may correspond to the "involving third

parties" category (e.g., relaying negative messages). Elements of malicious gossip are evident in the aggression category (insulting friends and reminiscing/repeating), but also in the "involving third parties" category (relaying negative messages).

Advantages of conceiving of social aggression as peer rejection are that it encourages thinking in terms of social interactions and processes, and reminds us of how these behaviors serve the purpose of rejecting others. Disadvantages may be that it takes the focus off of behaviors that may specifically undermine friendships and social status, a category that may be particularly meaningful for girls. Some of the specific processes of rejection seem to bear little resemblance to social aggression—for example, taking objects away, damaging possessions, aversive noises, flicking and throwing, and physical aggression (Asher et al., 2001). Another potential disadvantage is that research on peer rejection has focused mostly on correlates and lacks an integrative theory (but see Coie, 1990, for a discussion of theory). However, as I soon discuss (in the next major section), research on indirect/relational/social aggression may also lack an overarching theoretical framework to guide hypotheses and integrate findings. Studies of the process of peer rejection might provide helpful support for developing theories of social aggression.

Social Aggression as Relational Devaluation

Social psychologists studying adult relationships have investigated slightly broader processes that may be related to social aggression: interpersonal rejection (Leary, 2001) and ostracism (K. D. Williams, 2001). These approaches have the potential to inform research on social aggression in children because they illuminate possible processes and functions served by these behaviors.

Research and theory on interpersonal rejection begins with the premise that "human beings are an exceptionally social species with a strong need to belong and an even stronger aversion to being rejected" (Leary, 2001, p. 3). Social acceptance and social rejection exist on a continuum of relational evaluation, referred to as "the Inclusionary Status Continuum" (Leary, 2001, p. 5). Relational evaluation is defined as the extent to which a person views his or her relationship with another as significant, valuable, or close. The continuum of relational evaluation is proposed as a unifying framework for diverse types of experiences of rejection. Relational devaluation means believing that someone does not value his or her relationship with you as much as he or she used to and leads to feelings of rejection. Within this framework, interpersonal rejection is viewed as an unavoidable consequence of social life, because all of us have limited time and energy for relation-ships.

Some advantages of this model are that it provides a continuum on which relational harm can be evaluated and it acknowledges that some features of relational evaluation may be adaptive. This framework also connects nicely with social psychology research on ingroups, outgroups, and stigmatization. The constructs of interpersonal rejec-tion and relational evaluation remind of us children's needs to belong, and our understanding of children's social aggression might well be en-hanced by studying more systematically how they seek, maintain, and restore relational evaluation.

Social Aggression as Ostracism

A related but perhaps more narrow phenomenon is ostracism, defined as "the act of individuals or groups excluding or ignoring other groups or individuals" (K. D. Williams & Zadrow, 2001, p. 21). Ostracism can range from subtle inattention to extreme behaviors such as banish-ment, and it is described as beginning in preschool and extending into adulthood. In a survey study, 67% of adults reported using the silent treatment to convey contempt and disdain to another adult. Investiga-tors studying ostracism among adults have used a variety of question-naires and clever experimental methods, and they find no consistent gender differences (see K. D. Williams, 2001, for a review). On the ba-sis of these studies, they propose a comprehensive model of ostracism that includes the following: taxonomic dimensions (visibility, motive, quantity, and causal clarity), antecedents (individual differences, role or relational differences, and situational demands), moderators (attri-butions, individual differences), threatened needs (belonging, self-esteem, control, fear of death), and reactions (immediate, short-term, and long-term) (see K. D. Williams & Zadrow, 2001, p. 29, for a de-tailed presentation of this model). Each feature of this rich framework suggests many testable hypotheses for understanding ostracism among adults and perhaps also social aggression among children.

TOWARD A THEORETICAL FRAMEWORK FOR UNDERSTANDING DEVELOPMENTAL ORIGINS AND POSSIBLE OUTCOMES OF SOCIAL AGGRESSION: SOCIAL AGGRESSION AS DISPARAGEMENT

Research to date on social and relational aggression has suffered from the lack of an overarching theoretical framework. Because social aggression is by definition an interpersonal phenomenon and often seems motivated by developmental needs for peer acceptance and the desire to protect or further one's own social status, components of Harry Stack Sullivan's Interpersonal Theory of Psychiatry (1953) may be helpful in understanding these behaviors. Sullivan argued that individuals' personalities and relationships are formed around social needs, qualities we desire in our relationships with others, including warmth, companionship, acceptance, and intimacy (Buhrmester, 1996). These social needs expand with development: infants most desire tenderness from caregivers; preschool children also need play partners; children in the early elementary years (referred to as the "juvenile period" by Sullivan) need to feel a sense of belonging and acceptance as well; preadolescents additionally desire an intimate relationship with a same-sex peer ("chumships"); and adolescents wish also for sexual involvement. Sullivan argued that our character and our personality difficulties result from the ways in which we manage to meet these needs—or to defend ourselves when we become anxious because we cannot meet them (Buhrmester, 1996; Sullivan, 1953). When we feel anxious, we engage in defensive attempts, called security operations, to avoid or ameliorate the anxiety. These security operations may help us reduce immediate anxiety, but they can create serious problems in our relationships.

One security operation described by Sullivan is disparagement, and this phenomenon resembles social aggression. Disparagement is speaking derogatorily of those to whom we feel compared. According to Sullivan, when some youths feel a strong need to be liked by everyone and superior in every way, they cope with the inevitable disappointment resulting from another's success by disparaging the other, by maligning that person's other characteristics or abilities, and by "pulling down the social standing of others" (Sullivan, 1953, p. 242). Many features of social aggression resemble Sullivan's description of disparagement. Relationship manipulation and social exclusion are certainly ways of trying to disrupt others' friendships and reduce their social standing, and the content of gossip is often disparaging rumors. For all of these reasons, Sullivan's theory concerning disparagement may be helpful in guiding research on social aggression: its functions, its origins, and its outcomes.

Developmental Precursors of Social Aggression

This is a parental morbidity of security operations, such that the juvenile is taught to disparage others—a common phenomenon on the

American scene. It may be the way, for instance, that the significant figure in the home handles a juvenile "misfortune," such as being average instead of superior. It may occur because the parental figure has always disparaged all people who made her or him uncomfortable. It may occur because one or both parents feel threatened by the revealing nature of juvenile communication and so disparage teachers and all others with whom they feel compared. (Sullivan, 1953, p. 242)

Sullivan's (1953) theory suggests that children learn disparagement both by observing their parents disparage other adults and by a parent responding to his or her child's disappointment at other children's superiority by the parent maligning the child's peers. This premise fits well with social learning theory, which suggests that children may learn social aggression by observing their parents resolve conflicts in ways that harm relationships: giving one another the silent treatment when angry; enlisting other family members or friends to support their point of view in an argument; threatening to end the relationship; withdrawing love or affection; and, in particular, involving the child in arguments or conflicts. Preliminary evidence suggests that divorced parents' triangulation of children in conflicts mediates the relation between postdivorce conflict and relational aggression in daughters (Kerig et al., 2001).

Sullivan (1953) repeatedly emphasized that disparaging others undermines the child's sense of self-worth and security, because "one is encouraged to feel incapable of knowing what is good" (p. 243). Although Sullivan proposed that children learn disparagement from parents and may generalize this security operation to their friendships, he also acknowledged that friendships offer youth the opportunity to overcome security operations learned from parents. Sullivan argued that the intimacy of "chumships" provides the type of mutual validation of self-worth that could reduce tendencies toward disparagement.

Sullivan's (1953) theory suggests interesting possibilities for how exposure to parents' conflicts and observing parents coping with disappointment might contribute to disparagement and social aggression. Exposure to marital conflict is associated with insecure parental attachment, perhaps because parents in conflicted marriages are more negative in their parenting styles, less involved and emotionally available, and more likely to rely on their children for emotional support (see Cummings & Davies, 1994, for a review). Attachment theory suggests that, on the basis of early relationships with parents, children with insecure attachments develop working models that might lead them to expect to be rejected and excluded by others (Downey et al., 1998). Rejection sensitivity is "the disposition to defensively (i.e., anxiously or angrily) expect, readily perceive, or overreact to social rejection" (Downey et al., 1998, p. 1074). Rejection sensitivity might lead children to engage in social aggression as a defensive tactic or even as a preemptive strike when they feel that their friendships and/or social status are threatened.

Most research on the effects of rejection sensitivity on relationships has focused on romantic relations in adolescence (Downey et al., 1999; Purdie & Downey, 2000) and adulthood (Ayduk et al., 1999; Downey & Feldman, 1996). This body of work demonstrates that rejection-sensitive people overattribute rejection when their partners behave insensitively; they feel chronically threatened and behave in ways so as to undermine the quality of the relationship (Downey et al., 1999). Specifically, adult women who are rejection sensitive engage in more conflict with partners and make more hostile, spiteful remarks during conflicts, which results in decreases in partners' satisfaction with and commitment to the relationship (Downey & Feldman, 1996). Recently, Downey and colleagues (1998) developed a measure of rejection sensitivity for children's expectations of and responses to peers and teachers, and found that for a sample of fifth- through seventh-grade children rejection sensitivity predicted self-reported and teacher-rated aggression 1 year later (the measure of aggression included items to assess physical and verbal, but not social, aggression). Because one important function of social aggression may be to protect one's own social standing and reputation (Paquette & Underwood, 1999; Xie et al., in press-a), rejection-sensitive children may be more likely to perceive social slights and more likely to respond by harming others by social exclusion, relationship manipulation, and spreading rumors.

Is Social Aggression Developmentally Normative or Maladaptive?

> One of the feeblest props for an inadequate self-system is the attitude of disparaging others, which I once boiled down to the doctrine that if you are a molehill, by God, there shall be no mountains. (Sullivan, 1953, p. 309)

> If you have to maintain self-esteem by pulling down the standing of others, you are extraordinarily unfortunate in a variety of ways. (Sullivan, 1953, p. 242)

> This disparaging business is really like the dust of the streets—it settles everywhere. It is perhaps not so disastrous in the juvenile era as is it from then on; but it is very disastrous at any time. (Sullivan, 1953, p. 242)

One of the most challenging features of Sullivan's theory is that the security operations, including but not limited to disparagement, arise from our efforts to meet the social needs characteristic of developmental stages and to contain our anxiety when our efforts are unsuccessful. Therefore, following Sullivan's argument, security operations are both normative and adaptive in that we engage in them in response to frustrated efforts to meet our developmental needs, but they are also maladaptive in that they serve only to contain our immediate anxiety and in the long run create persistent difficulties in interpersonal relationships. Sullivan proposed that some children develop tendencies toward disparagement as a way of coping with the disappointment of others being superior in various ways and that disparagement provides immediate relief from the anxiety of not being as good as someone else. However, if disparagement persists, it undermines the individual's sense of self-worth because no accomplishments, one's own or those of others, can be viewed as worthwhile and the person becomes just as disparaging of herself as she is of others. In Sullivan's words (1953), "Since you have to protect your feeling of personal worth by noting how unworthy everyone around you is, you are not provided with any data that are convincing evidence of your having personal worth, so it gradually evolves into 'I am not as bad as the other swine' " (p. 242).

Just as Sullivan noted both the adaptive and the maladaptive features of security operations such as disparagement, so more contemporary researchers disagree as to whether social aggression is developmentally normative, frequent, and engaged in and directed toward many children (Cairns, Cairns, Neckerman, et al., 1989; Paquette & Underwood, 1999) or whether these behaviors, in a manner similar to those of physical aggression, are highly salient and engaged in by a small proportion of youths (Crick et al., 1999). In future research, it will be important to continue to study the normative development of social aggression, to understand the functions it might serve at different developmental periods. Research should examine several types of negative outcomes possibly associated with social aggression: outcomes that have been linked to physical aggression, disorders whose symptoms resemble social aggression (e.g., borderline personality), and syndromes more common among women than men (e.g., eating disorders and depression) (Crick et al., 1999). However, true to Sullivan's theory and a developmental psychopathology approach, it will also be important to investigate whether social aggression is developmentally normative at some points in the lifespan and whether it might serve some adaptive functions.

TOP 10 HOPES FOR FUTURE
RESEARCH ON SOCIAL AGGRESSION

In summary, the models and theories outlined above are presented not as the last word on any of these complex issues but as beginning frameworks for moving beyond likening social aggression to physical aggression and beyond excessive focus on gender differences. Whether or not girls are more socially aggressive than boys, social aggression and other forms of aggression among girls are important to understand in their own right and for their own sake.

Research to date has been tremendously valuable in demonstrating beyond the shadow of a doubt that girls are capable of hurting one another in many ways and that social aggression hurts children, perhaps especially girls. For those of us who believe that girls may have been slighted in previous research on aggression, it is deeply gratifying to see such a strong and flourishing body of current scholarship on aggression among girls.

Clearly, though we have learned much about girls' anger and aggression, this remains fertile ground for different approaches, new questions and models, and well-designed longitudinal studies. Further understanding aggression among girls, especially social aggression, will demand much of researchers.

However, reviewing the research to date inspires a great deal of hope, a general hope that a richer understanding of social aggression is possible and specific hopes for how we may continue to move forward. The following are ideas and principles that might guide future work.

1. Social aggression merits new models and theories. Testing applications of existing theories to social aggression (e.g., Sullivan's ideas) might be productive, but so might theory building on the basis of the massive amount of new research on indirect/relational/social aggression and research on related phenomena (peer rejection, interpersonal devaluation, and ostracism). It is no longer accurate to say that research on social aggression is in its infancy. It is time to build a theory.

2. We need to continue to refine constructs for the more subtle forms of aggression, to clarify definitions, to test empirically which behaviors tend to occur together and have similar developmental origins and outcomes, and to seek to come to some kind of consensus so that individual studies can build on each other. In the meanwhile, it will continue to be important to define and explain whatever term we choose to use, and to cite research broadly related to the question under investigation, whether it used the same term or not.

3. Although testing of gender differences remains important, we

need to move beyond focusing on these exclusively to examine what these behaviors mean for boys and for girls, and how they relate to psychological adjustment for each gender group. Whether or not boys and girls differ on their average levels of social aggression, such aggression probably means something very different for girls and for boys, and may relate differently to developmental origins and outcomes.

4. Understanding the role of emotions in social aggression may be helpful in illuminating its developmental origins and outcomes. Most investigations of social aggression have proceeded independently of research on emotions, and this seems unfortunate. Emotions are almost certainly involved in some forms of social aggression—anger, but also jealousy, shame, and embarrassment. Some forms of social aggression may be less closely related to emotions and deployed for instrumental purposes, and making this distinction may clarify when social aggression may be maladaptive and when it may not. It could also be fruitful to investigate whether refraining from social aggression might be related to moral engagement, prosocial motives, and specific types of positive affect (e.g., optimism).

5. Though we have learned much about social aggression by using peer nominations and questionnaires, if we seek to understand the social processes involved, we will need to use more diverse methods. Observational studies could be enormously helpful in allowing close analysis of how social aggression unfolds, but observing such subtle behaviors will likely be challenging (and expensive). Another way to analyze the social processes involved in social aggression might be to elicit detailed accounts of experiences of being victimized and maybe even perpetrating social aggression.

6. As we work to understand social aggression and how episodes unfold, it will be important also to study physical aggression among girls for several reasons. First, some girls do fight, and it is important to understand more about why and to intervene to try to reduce the myriad negative outcomes associated with childhood physical aggression for girls. It would be unfortunate indeed if focusing on social aggression led to the perception that it is no longer important to continue to study girls' physical aggression. Research on physical aggression will also be important for our understanding of social aggression because, in the rare events where girls become violent, social aggression is likely involved. This may be true for boys as well.

7. Research with both normal and clinical samples will be needed to examine whether these behaviors might be developmentally normal in milder forms and pathological in more extreme forms. Both are possible. To understand possible normative developmental functions, normal samples will be needed. To understand some of the more extreme

negative outcomes of social aggression, it will be useful to study clinical samples (meaning either samples of youth with related disorders or samples of youth selected as being high on social aggression).

8. For the fullest possible understanding of what social aggression means for girls, it will be important to acknowledge that it might serve some developmental functions that are not altogether negative, such as identity development, moral negotiation, and maintaining group boundaries. To say that social aggression might be deployed in the service of developmental goals or even of girls' social ascendancy does not mean that social aggression still does not hurt. Both are possible, and unless we acknowledge that this behavior may serve some self-advancing functions, we risk seriously underestimating girls as well as boys.

9. As we investigate developmental outcomes associated with social aggression, it might be especially fruitful to study not only what extreme social aggression portends for a girl's psychological adjustment but also what it means for her future social relationships. Thus far, the few studies that have examined outcomes associated with social aggression have focused on individual qualities or disorders (but see Linder et al., 2002, for a study that examined links between relational aggression and romantic relationship quality). If a girl perpetrates social aggression frequently or is intensely victimized, it seems highly likely that the developmental consequences might be especially evident in her relationships. What does engaging in or experiencing social aggression predict for a young woman's ability to form adult friendships, to get along with colleagues at work, to form an intimate romantic partnership, and to parent a child from infancy through adolescence?

Taken together, the large body of research on physical aggression suggests strongly that such antisocial behavior represents an underlying tendency that manifests in somewhat different but still related ways at different points in the lifespan. From an extensive longitudinal study of men's antisocial behavior over the life course, Sampson and Laub (1993) found that antisocial behavior was related not only to crime but also to drug and alcohol use, job instability, and poor attachment to the spouse and divorce. They concluded: "Overall, the evidence suggests that delinquent behavior is relatively stable across stages of the life course and that antisocial behavior in childhood predicts a wide range of troublesome adult outcomes" (p. 125).

Are extreme tendencies for perpetrating social aggression similar to antisocial behavior in that an underlying consistent tendency may be expressed in different ways at different developmental stages? Do preschool girls who frequently announce to peers, "You can't come to my birthday party!" become school-age girls who spread nasty rumors as revenge and subsequently young women who give romantic partners the silent treatment or threaten to withdraw from the relationship when angry? Do these same young women go on to engage in malicious gossip or relationship manipulation with work colleagues? Do they model social backbiting for their young children, and teach them to exclude others as a way of expressing anger or asserting status? To understand how social aggression influences girls' and women's relationships at different developmental periods, longitudinal studies are badly needed. Ideally, these studies will involve both normal and clinical samples to examine how social aggression unfolds across development for both typical and high-risk girls.

10. As important as it is to understand that girls can be extraordinarily mean, we should not forget girls' tremendous strengths. In acknowledging that girls can hurt one another in ways more subtle than hitting, it takes mental discipline not to race to assume that all girls are engaging in this behavior all of the time. That some girls sometime engage in social aggression some of the time must be balanced against the considerable evidence that girls have many qualities that make them outstanding relationship partners. Girls are capable of self-disclosure, intimate friendships, and empathy for others' plights—indeed, a wide range of prosocial behavior, perhaps especially defending victims of peer maltreatment. Girls are also human beings who at times feel anger and pursue their social goals, all the while trying to balance the goals of being open and honest but still being nice. We might be wise to study how girls resolve this vexing dilemma with our eyes wide open to their strengths as well as their vulnerabilities.

Many women who study aggression do so in part because we feel that girls have been misrepresented as not aggressive by research focusing exclusively on physical fighting. We study social aggression out of concern for girls' pain and because we want to understand more about what contributes to girls' psychological adjustment. However, if we insist that only girls are socially aggressive and that social aggression is always bad, we risk seriously misunderstanding both genders. I hope that we will continue to study social aggression in ways that will allow us to appreciate its power to harm as well as its possible other developmental functions and consequences, in honor of girls and their amazing capabilities:

> **"Growing Up"**
> We are girls, and we're proud.
> We make mistakes when we're
> Growing—maybe tears, maybe not.
> We have dreams because we're girls.
> (Wendy Garrett, grade 4, in Lyne, 1996, p. 27)

Girls indeed often hurt one another in their struggle to cope with their anger and to advance their social goals while trying to be nice. However, their social aggression is also likely related to girls' and women's hopes and dreams—that somehow it is possible to express emotions including anger, to achieve and succeed, but still be liked and develop close, loving relationships.

References

Adams, R., & Laursen, B. (2001). The organization and dynamics of adolescent conflict with parents and friends. *Journal of Marriage and the Family, 63,* 97–110.

Adler, P. A., & Adler, P. (1995). Dynamics of inclusion and exclusion in preadolescent cliques. *Social Psychology Quarterly, 58*(3), 145–162.

Alfieri, T., Ruble, D. N., & Higgins, E. T. (1996). Gender stereotypes during adolescence: Developmental changes and the transition to junior high school. *Developmental Psychology, 32,* 1129–1137.

American Psychiatric Association. (1987). *Diagnostic and statistical manual of mental disorders* (3rd ed., rev.). Washington, DC: Author.

American Psychiatric Association. (1994). *Diagnostic and statistical manual of mental disorders* (4th ed.). Washington, DC: Author.

Andrews, J. A., Foster, S. L., Capaldi, D., & Hops, H. (2000). Adolescent and family predictors of physical aggression, communication, and satisfaction in young adult couples: A prospective analysis. *Journal of Consulting and Clinical Psychology, 68,* 195–208.

Archer, J. (2001). A strategic approach to aggression: Commentary on Underwood, Galen, and Paquette. *Social Development, 10,* 267–271.

Archer, J., Pearson, N. A., & Westeman, K. E. (1988). Aggressive behavior of children aged 6–11: Gender differences and their magnitude. *British Journal of Social Psychology, 27,* 371–384.

Armsden, G. C., & Greenberg, M. T. (1987). The Inventory of Parent and Peer Attachment: Individual differences and their relationship to psychological well-being in adolescence. *Journal of Youth and Adolescence, 16,* 427–454.

Arnett, J. J. (1999). Adolescent storm and stress, reconsidered. *American Psychologist, 54,* 317–326.

Arnold, D. H., Hanrock, S., Ortiz, C., & Stove, R. M. (1999). Direct observation of peer rejection acts and their temporal relation with aggressive acts. *Early Childhood Research Quarterly, 14,* 183–196.

Arnold, D. H., McWilliams, L., & Harvey-Arnold, E. (1998). Teacher discipline and child misbehavior in daycare: Untangling causality with correlational data. *Developmental Psychology, 34*, 276–287.

Aronson, E., Blaney, N., Stephin, C., Sikes, J., & Snapp, M. (1978). *The jigsaw classroom.* Beverly Hills, CA: Sage.

Aronson, E., & Patnoe, S. (1997). *The jigsaw classroom: Building cooperation in the classroom* (2nd ed.). New York: Addison-Wesley-Longman.

Arsenio, W. F., & Killen, M. (1996). Conflict-related emotions during peer disputes. *Early Education and Development, 7*, 43–57.

Arsenio, W. F., & Lover, A. (1997). Emotions, conflicts, and aggression during preschoolers' free play. *British Journal of Developmental Psychology, 15*, 531–542.

Ashby Plant, E. A., Hyde, J. S., Keltner, D., & Devine, P. G. (2000). The gender stereotyping of emotions. *Psychology of Women Quarterly, 24*, 81–92.

Asher, S. R., & Rose, A. J. (1997). Promoting children's social-emotional adjustment with peers. In P. Salovey & D. Sluyter (Eds.), *Emotional development and intelligence: Educational implications* (pp. 196–230). New York: Basic Books.

Asher, S. R., Rose, A. J., & Gabriel, S. W. (2001). Peer rejection in everyday life. In M. R. Leary (Ed.), *Interpersonal rejection* (pp. 105–142). New York: Oxford University Press.

Asher, S. R., Singleton, L. C., Tinsley, B. R., & Hymel, S. (1979). A reliable sociometric measure for preschool children. *Developmental Psychology, 15*, 443–444.

Averill, J. R. (1982). *Anger and aggression: An essay on emotion.* New York: Springer-Verlag.

Ayduk, O., Downey, G., Testa, A., Yen, Y., & Shoda, Y. (1999). Does rejection elicit hostility in rejection sensitive women? *Social Cognition, 17*, 245–271.

Bagwell, C. L., Coie, J. D., Terry, R. A., & Lochman, J. E. (2000). Peer clique participation and social status in preadolescence. *Merrill-Palmer Quarterly, 46*(2), 280–305.

Baker, L. A., Mack, W., Moffitt, T. E., & Mednick, S. (1989). Sex differences in property crime in a Danish adoption cohort. *Behavior Genetics, 19*, 355–370.

Bandura, A. (1999). Moral disengagement in the perception of inhumanities. *Personality and Social Psychology Review, 3*, 193–209.

Bandura, A., Barbaranelli, C., Caprara, C. V., & Pastorelli, C. (1996). Mechanisms of moral disengagement in the exercise of moral agency. *Journal of Personality and Social Psychology, 71*, 364–374.

Bandura, A., Caprara, C. V., Barbaranelli, C., Pastorelli, C., & Regalia, C. (2001). Sociocognitive self-regulatory mechanisms governing transgressive behavior. *Journal of Personality and Social Psychology, 80*, 125–135.

Bandura, A., Ross, D., & Ross, S. A. (1961). Transmission of aggression through imitation of aggressive models. *Journal of Abnormal and Social Psychology, 63*, 757–582.

Bardone, A. M., Moffitt, T. E., Caspi, A., Dickson, N., & Silva, P. A. (1996). Adult mental health and social outcomes of adolescent girls with depression and conduct disorder. *Development and Psychopathology, 8*, 811–829.

Basow, S. A., & Rubin, L. R. (1999). Gender influences on adolescent development. In N. G. Johnson, M. C. Roberts, & J. Worell (Eds.), *Beyond appearance:*

A new look at adolescent girls (pp. 25–52). Washington, DC: American Psychological Association.

Bates, J. E. (1989). Concepts and measures of temperament. In G. A. Kohnstamm, J. E. Bates, & M. K. Rothbart (Eds.), *Temperament in childhood* (pp. 3–26). Chichester, UK: Wiley.

Bem, S. L. (1993). *The lenses of gender: Transforming the debate on sexual inequality.* New Haven, CT: Yale University Press.

Benenson, J. F. (1994). Ages four to six years: Changes in the structure of play networks of girls and boys. *Merrill-Palmer Quarterly, 40,* 478–487.

Benenson, J. F., Apostoleris, N. H., & Parnass, J. (1997). Age and sex differences in dyadic and group interaction. *Developmental Psychology, 33,* 538–543.

Benenson, J. F., & Benarroch, D. (1998). Gender differences in response to friends' hypothetical greater success. *Journal of Early Adolescence, 18,* 192–201.

Benenson, J. F., Morash, D., & Petrakos, H. (1998). Gender differences in emotional closeness between preschool children and their mothers. *Sex Roles, 38,* 975–985.

Benenson, J. F., Roy, R., Waite, A., Goldbaum, S., Linders, L., & Simpson, A. (2002). Greater discomfort as a proximate cause of sex differences in competition. *Merrill-Palmer Quarterly, 48,* 225–247.

Benton, D. (1992). Hormones and human aggression. In K. Bjorkqvist & P. Niemela (Eds.), *Of mice and women: Aspects of female aggression* (pp. 37–48). San Diego, CA: Academic Press.

Berndt, T. J. (1981). Relations between social cognition, nonsocial cognition, and social behavior: The case of friendship. In J. H. Flavell & L. D. Ross (Eds.), *Social cognitive development: Frontiers and possible futures* (pp. 176–199). Cambridge, UK: Cambridge University Press.

Berndt, T. J. (1982). The features and effects of friendship in early adolescence. *Child Development, 53,* 447–1460.

Berndt, T. J., Hawkins, J. A., & Jiao, Z. (1999). Influences of friends and friendships on adjustment to junior high school. *Merrill-Palmer Quarterly, 45,* 13–41.

Bers, S. A., & Rodin, J. (1984). Social-comparison jealousy: A developmental and motivational study. *Journal of Personality and Social Psychology, 47,* 766–799.

Besag, V. (1989). Management strategies with vulnerable children. In E. Munthe & E. Roland (Eds.), *Bullying: An international perspective* (pp. 81–90). London: Routledge.

Bjorkqvist, K. (1994). Sex differences in physical, verbal, and indirect aggression: A review of recent research. *Sex Roles, 30,* 177–188.

Bjorkqvist, K. (2001). Different names, same issue. *Social Development, 10,* 272–274.

Bjorkqvist, K., Lagerspetz, K., & Kaukiainen, A. (1992). Do girls manipulate and do boys fight? Developmental trends in regard to direct and indirect aggression. *Aggressive Behavior, 18,* 117–127.

Bjorkqvist, K., Lagerspetz, K., & Osterman, K. (1992). *The direct and indirect aggression scales.* Vasa, Finland: Abo Akademi University, Department of Social Sciences.

Bjorkqvist, K., & Niemela, P. (1992a). New trends in the study of female aggression. In K. Bjorkqvist & P. Niemela (Eds.), *Of mice and women: Aspects of female aggression* (pp. 3–16). San Diego, CA: Academic Press.

Bjorkqvist, K., & Niemela, P. (Eds.). (1992b). *Of mice and women: Aspects of female aggression.* San Diego, CA: Academic Press.

Bjorkqvist, K., Osterman, K., & Kaukiainen, A. (1992). The development of direct and indirect aggressive strategies in males and females. In K. Bjorkqvist & P. Niemela (Eds.), *Of mice and women: Aspects of female aggression* (pp. 51–64). San Diego, CA: Academic Press.

Bjorkqvist, K., Osterman, K., & Lagerspetz, K. M. J. (1994). Sex differences in covert aggression among adults. *Aggressive Behavior, 20,* 27–33.

Block, J. H. (1983). Differential premises arising from differential socialization of the genders: Some conjectures. *Child Development, 54,* 1335–1354.

Blurton-Jones, N. G. (1967). An ethological study of some aspects of social behavior of children in nursery school. In D. Morris (Ed.), *Primate ethology* (pp. 347–368). London: Weidenfeld & Nicolson.

Blurton-Jones, N. G., & Konner, M. J. (1973). Sex differences in the behavior of London and Bushmen children. In R. P. Michael & J. H. Crook (Eds.), *Comparative ecology and behavior of primates* (pp. 689–749). London: Academic Press.

Blyth, D. A., & Foster-Clark, F. S. (1987). Gender differences in perceived intimacy with different members of adolescents' social networks. *Sex Roles, 17,* 689–718.

Borja-Alvarez, T., Zarbatany, L., & Pepper, S. (1991). Contributions of male and female guests and hosts to peer group entry. *Child Development, 62,* 1079–1090.

Boulton, M. J. (1993). Proximate causes of aggressive fighting in middle school children. *British Journal of Educational Psychology, 63,* 231–244.

Boulton, M. J. (1994). Understanding and preventing bullying in the junior high school playground. In P. K. Smith & S. Sharp (Eds.), *School bullying: Insights and perspectives* (pp. 132–159). New York: Routledge.

Boulton, M. J. (1996). A comparison of 8- and 11-year-old girls' and boys' participation in specific types of rough-and-tumble play and aggressive fighting: Implications for functional hypotheses. *Aggressive Behavior, 22,* 271–287.

Boulton, M. J. (1999). Concurrent and longitudinal relations between children's playground behavior and social preference, victimization, and bullying. *Child Development, 70,* 944–954.

Bowlby, J. (1969). *Attachment and loss: Vol. 1. Attachment.* Harmondsworth, UK: Penguin.

Boyum, L. A., & Parke, R. D. (1995). The role of family emotional expressiveness in the development of children's social competence. *Journal of Marriage and the Family, 57,* 593–603.

Brain, P. F., & Susman, E. J. (1997). Hormonal aspects of aggression and violence. In D. M. Stoff, J. Breiling, & J. D. Maser (Eds.), *Handbook of antisocial behavior* (pp. 314–323). New York: Wiley.

Brendgen, M., Markiewicz, D., Doyle, A. B., & Bukowski, W. (2001). The relations between friendship quality, ranked friendship preference, and adolescents' behavior with their friends. *Merrill-Palmer Quarterly, 47,* 395–315.

Brody, L. R. (1993). On understanding gender differences in the expression of emotion: Gender roles, socialization, and language. In S. Ablon, D. Brown, E. Khantzian, & J. Mack (Eds.), *Human feelings: Explorations in affect development and meaning* (pp. 89–121). Hillsdale, NJ: Analytic Press.

Brody, L. R. (1997). Beyond stereotypes: Gender and emotion. *Journal of Social Issues, 53,* 369–394.

Brody, L. R. (1999). *Gender, emotion, and the family.* Cambridge, MA: Harvard University Press.

Brody, L. R. (2000). The socialization of gender differences in emotional expression: Display rules, infant temperament, and differentiation. In A. H. Fischer (Ed.), *Gender and emotion: Social psychological perspectives* (pp. 24–47). Cambridge, UK: Cambridge University Press.

Brown, L. M. (1998). *Raising their voices: The politics of girls' anger.* Cambridge, MA: Harvard University Press.

Brown, L. M., Way, N., & Duff, J. L. (1999). The others in my I: Adolescent girls' friendships and peer relations. In N. G. Johnson, M. C. Roberts, & J. Worrell (Eds.), *Beyond appearance: A new look at adolescent girls* (pp. 205–225). Washington, DC: American Psychological Association.

Buchanan, C. M., Eccles, J. S., Flanagan, C., Midgley, C., Feldlaufer, H., & Harold, R. D. (1990). Parents' and teachers' beliefs about adolescents: Effects of sex and experience. *Journal of Youth and Adolescence, 19,* 363–394.

Bugental, D. B., & Goodnow, J. J. (1998). Socialization processes. In N. Eisenberg (Ed.), *Handbook of child psychology: Vol. 3. Social, emotional, and personality development* (5th ed., pp. 389–462). New York: Wiley.

Buhrmester, D. P. (1996). Need fulfillment, interpersonal competence, and the developmental contexts of early adolescent friendship. In W. M. Bukowski, A. F. Newcomb, & W. W. Hartup (Eds.), *The company they keep: Friendship in childhood and early adolescence* (pp. 159–185). New York: Cambridge University Press.

Buhrmester, D. P., & Prager, K. (1995). Patterns and functions of self-disclosure during childhood and adolescence. In K. K. Rotenberg (Ed.), *Disclosure processes in children and adolescents* (pp. 10–56). New York: Cambridge University Press.

Bukowski, W. M., Sippola, L. K., & Newcomb, A. F. (2000). Variability in patterns of attraction to same- and other-sex peers during early adolescence. *Developmental Psychology, 36,* 147–154.

Buss, A. H. (1961). *The psychology of aggression.* New York: Wiley.

Buss, K. A., & Goldsmith, H. H. (1998). Fear and anger regulation in infancy: Effects on the temporal dynamics of affective expression. *Child Development, 69,* 359–374.

Bussey, K., & Bandura, A. (1992). Self-regulatory mechanisms governing gender development. *Child Development, 63,* 1236–1250.

Cairns, R. B., Cadwallader, T. W., Estell, D., & Neckerman, H. J. (1997). Groups to gangs: Developmental and criminological perspectives and relevance for prevention. In D. M. Stoff, J. Breiling, & J. D. Maser (Eds.), *Handbook of antisocial behavior* (pp. 194–204). New York: Wiley.

Cairns, R. B., & Cairns, B. D. (1984). Predicting aggressive patterns in girls and boys: A developmental study. *Aggressive Behavior, 11,* 227–242.

Cairns, R. B., & Cairns, B. D. (1994). *Lifelines and risks: Pathways of youth in our time.* New York: Cambridge University Press.

Cairns, R. B., Cairns, B. D., & Neckerman, H. J. (1989). Early school dropout: Configurations and determinants. *Child Development, 60,* 1437–1452.

Cairns, R. B., Cairns, B. D., Neckerman, H. J., Ferguson, L. L., & Gariepy, J. (1989). Growth and aggression: 1. Childhood to early adolescence. *Developmental Psychology, 25,* 320–330.

Cairns, R. B., Cairns, B. D., Neckerman, H. J., Gest, S., & Gariepy, J. (1988). Social networks and aggressive behavior: Peer support or peer rejection? *Developmental Psychology, 24,* 815–823.

Cairns, R. B., Leung, M. C., & Cairns, B. D. (1995). Social networks over time and space in adolescence. In L. J. Crockett & A. C. Crouter (Eds.), *Pathways through adolescence: Individual development in relation to social contexts* (pp. 35–56). Mahwah, NJ: Erlbaum.

Cairns, R. B., Perrin, J. E., & Cairns, B. D. (1985). Social structure and social cognition in early adolescence: Affiliative patterns. *Journal of Early Adolescence, 5,* 339–355.

Cairns, R. B., Peterson, G., & Neckerman, H. J. (1988). Suicidal behavior in aggressive adolescents. *Journal of Clinical Child Psychology, 17,* 298–309.

Campos, J. J., Kermoian, R., & Zumbahlen, M. R. (1992). Socioemotional transformations in the family system following infant crawling onset. In N. Eisenberg & R. Fabes (Eds.), Emotion and its regulation in early development. *New Directions in Child Development, 55,* 25–40.

Cantos, A. L., Neidig, P. H., & O'Leary, K. D. (1994). Injuries of women and men in a treatment program for domestic violence. *Journal of Family Violence, 9,* 113–124.

Capaldi, D. M., & Crosby, L. (1997). Observed and reported psychological and physical aggression in young at-risk couples. *Social Development, 6,* 184–206.

Capaldi, D. M., & Owen, L. D. (2001). Physical aggression in a community sample of at-risk young couples: Gender comparisons for high frequency injury, and fear. *Journal of Family Psychology, 15,* 425–440.

Caplan, M., Vespo, J., Pederson, J., & Hay, D. F. (1991). Conflict and its resolution in small groups of one- and two-year-olds. *Child Development, 62,* 1513–1524.

Carson, R. C. (1991). Dilemmas in the pathway of DSM-IV. *Journal of Abnormal Psychology, 100,* 302–307.

Carson, R. C. (1996). Aristotle, Galileo, and the DSM Taxonomy: The case of schizophrenia. *Journal of Consulting and Clinical Psychology, 64,* 1133–1139.

Caspi, A., Begg, D., Dickson, J., Harrington, H., Langley, J., Moffitt, T. E., & Silva, P. A. (1997). Personality differences predict health-risk behaviors in young adulthood: Evidence from a longitudinal study. *Journal of Personality and Social Psychology, 73,* 1052–1063.

Caspi, A., & Moffitt, T. E. (1991). Individual differences are accentuated during periods of social change: The sample case of girls at puberty. *Journal of Personality and Social Psychology, 61*, 157–168.

Cassidy, J., Parke, R. D., Butkovsky, L., & Braungart, J. M. (1992). Family–peer connections: The roles of emotional expressiveness within the family and children's understanding of emotions. *Child Development, 63*, 603–618.

Chamberlain, P., & Moore, K. J. (in press). Chaos and trauma in the lives of adolescent females with antisocial behavior and delinquency. In R. Geffner (Series Ed.) & R. Greenwald (Vol. Ed.), *Trauma and juvenile delinquency: Theory, research, and interventions*. New York: Haworth Press.

Chamberlain, P., & Reid, J. B. (1994). Differences in risk factors and adjustment for male and female delinquents in Treatment Foster Care. *Journal of Child and Family Studies, 3*, 23–39.

Chang, J. (1996). A comparative study of female gang and non-gang members in Chicago. *Journal of Gang Research, 4*, 9–18.

Charlesworth, W. R., & Dzur, C. (1987). Gender comparisons of preschoolers' behavior and resource utilization in group problem-solving. *Child Development, 58*, 191–200.

Chen, X., Rubin, K. H., & Li, Z. (1995). Social functioning and adjustment in Chinese children: A longitudinal study. *Developmental Psychology, 31*, 531–539.

Chen, X., Rubin, K. H., & Li, D. (1997). Relation between academic achievement and social adjustment: Evidence from Chinese children. *Developmental Psychology, 33*, 518–525.

Chesney-Lind, M. (1986). Women and crime: The female offender. *Signs: Journal of Women in Culture and Society, 12*, 78–98.

Chesney-Lind, M. (1988). Girls in jail. *Crime and Delinquency, 34*, 150–168.

Chesney-Lind, M. (1989). Girls' crime and woman's place: Toward a feminist model of female delinquency. *Crime and Delinquency, 35*, 5–29.

Chesney-Lind, M. (2001). Girls, violence, and delinquency: Popular myths and persistent problems. In S. O. White (Ed.), *Handbook of youth and justice* (pp. 135–158). New York: Kluwer Academic.

Chess, S., & Thomas, A. (1984). *Origins and evolution of behavior disorders*. New York: Brunner/Mazel.

Chung, T. Y., & Asher, S. R. (1996). Children's goals and strategies in peer conflict situations. *Merrill-Palmer Quarterly, 42*, 125–147.

Cicchetti, D., & Olsen, K. (1990). The developmental psychopathology of child maltreatment. In M. Lewis & S. M. Miller (Eds.), *Handbook of developmental psychopathology* (pp. 261–279). New York: Plenum Press.

Clanton, G., & Kosins, D. J. (1991). Developmental correlates of jealousy. In P. Salovey (Ed.), *The psychology of jealousy and envy* (pp. 132–147). New York: Guilford Press.

Cohen, J. (1988). *Statistical power analysis for the behavioral sciences*. Hillsdale, NJ: Erlbaum.

Coie, J. D. (1990). Toward a theory of peer rejection. In S. R. Asher & J. D. Coie (Eds.), *Peer rejection in childhood* (pp. 365–401). New York: Cambridge University Press.

Coie, J. D., Belding, M., & Underwood, M. K. (1988). Aggression and peer rejection in childhood. In B. B. Lahey & A. Kazdin (Eds.), *Advances in clinical child psychology* (Vol. 11, pp. 125–158). New York: Plenum Press.

Coie, J. D., Cillessen, A. H. N., Dodge, K. A., Hubbard, J. A., Schwartz, D., Lemerise, E. A., & Bateman, H. (1999). It takes two to fight: A test of relational factors and a method for assessing aggressive dyads. *Developmental Psychology, 35,* 1179–1188.

Coie, J. D., & Dodge, K. A. (1998). Aggression and antisocial behavior. In N. Eisenberg (Ed.), *Handbook of child psychology* (5th ed., Vol. 3, pp. 779–862). New York: Wiley.

Coie, J. D., Dodge, K. A., & Coppotelli, H. (1982). Dimensions and types of social status. *Developmental Psychology, 18,* 557–570.

Coie, J. D., Dodge, K. A., Terry, R., & Wright, V. (1991). The role of aggression in peer relations: An analysis of aggression episodes in boys' play groups. *Child Development, 62,* 812–826.

Coie, J. D., & Kupersmidt, J. B. (1983). A behavioral analysis of emerging social status in boys' groups. *Child Development, 54,* 1400–1416.

Coie, J. D., Terry, R., Zakriski, A., & Lochman, J. E. (1995). Early adolescent social influences on delinquent behavior. In J. McCord (Ed.), *Coercion and punishment in long-term perspectives* (pp. 229–244). New York: Cambridge University Press.

Cole, P. M. (1986). Children's spontaneous control of facial expression. *Child Development, 57,* 1309–1321.

Collins, W. A., & Laursen, B. (1992). Conflict and relationships during adolescence. In C. U. Shantz & W. W. Hartup (Eds.), *Conflict in child and adolescent development* (pp. 216–241). New York: Cambridge University Press.

Condry, J. C., & Ross, D. F. (1985). Sex and aggression: The influence of gender and label on the perception of aggression in children. *Child Development, 56,* 225–233.

Conduct Problems Prevention Research Group. (1992). A developmental and clinical model for the prevention of conduct disorder: The FAST Track Program. *Development and Psychopathology, 4*(4), 509–527.

Connellan, J., Baron-Cohen, S., Wheelwright, S., Batki, A., & Ahulwalia, J. (2000). Sex differences in human neonatal social perception. *Infant Behavior and Development, 23,* 113–118.

Connolly, J., Craig, W., Goldberg, A., & Pepler, D. (1999). Conceptions of cross-sex friendships and romantic relationships in early adolescence. *Journal of Youth and Adolescence, 28,* 481–494.

Connolly, J., Furman, W., & Konarski, R. (2000). The role of peers in the emergence of heterosexual romantic relationships in adolescence. *Child Development, 71,* 1395–1408.

Connolly, J., Pepler, D., Craig, W., & Taradash, A. (2000). Dating experiences of bullies in early adolescence. *Child Maltreatment, 5,* 299–310.

Cooper, M. L., Shaver, P. R., & Collins, N. L. (1998). Attachment styles, emotion regulation, and adjustment in adolescence. *Journal of Personality and Social Psychology, 74,* 1380–1397.

Cornell, D. G., & Loper, A. B. (1998). Assessment of violence and other high-risk behaviors with a school survey. *School Psychology Review, 27,* 317–330.

Cote, S., Zoccolillo, M., Tremblay, R. E., Nagin, D., & Vitaro, F. (2001). Predicting girls' conduct disorder in adolescence from childhood trajectories of disruptive behaviors. *Journal of the American Academy of Child and Adolescent Psychiatry, 40,* 678–688.

Cowie, H., & Sharp, S. (1994). Tackling bullying through the curriculum. In P. K. Smith & S. Sharp (Eds.), *School bullying: Insights and perspectives* (pp. 84–107). New York: Routledge.

Cowie, H., & Sharp, S. (Eds.). (1996). *Peer counseling in schools: A time to listen.* London: Fulton.

Craig, W. M. (1998). The relationship among bullying, victimization, depression, anxiety, and aggression in elementary school children. *Personality and Individual Differences, 24,* 123–130.

Craig, W. M., Pepler, D., & Atlas, R. (2000). Observations of bullying in the playground and in the classroom. *School Psychology International, 21,* 22–36.

Craig, W. M., Pepler, D. J., & Connolly, J. (2002, August). Continuity of physical and verbal victimization and three-year psychosocial consequences. In J. LeBlanc (Chair), *Aggression in the school setting.* Symposium presented at the International Meeting of the Society for Research on Aggression, Montreal, Ontario, Canada.

Craig, W. M., Pepler, D., Connolly, J., & Henderson, K. (2001). Developmental context of peer harassment in early adolescence: The role of puberty and the peer group. In J. Juvonen & S. Graham (Eds.), *Peer harassment in school: The plight of the vulnerable and the victimized* (pp. 242–261). New York: Guilford Press.

Crick, N. R. (1995). Relational aggression: The role of intent attributions, feelings of distress, and provocation type. *Development and Psychopathology, 7,* 313–322.

Crick, N. R. (1996). The role of overt aggression, relational aggression, and prosocial behavior in the prediction of children's future social adjustment. *Child Development, 67,* 2317–2327.

Crick, N. R. (1997). Engagement in gender normative versus gender non-normative forms of aggression: Links to social-psychological adjustment. *Developmental Psychology, 33,* 610–617.

Crick, N. R., Bigbee, M. A., & Howes, C. (1996). Gender differences in children's normative beliefs about aggression: How do I hurt thee? Let me count the ways. *Child Development, 67,* 1003–1014.

Crick, N. R., Casas, J. F., & Mosher, M. (1997). Relational and overt aggression in preschool. *Developmental Psychology, 33*(4), 589–600.

Crick, N. R., Casas, J. F., & Werner, N. E. (1997). *The social adjustment of children with eating disorders.* Manuscript forthcoming.

Crick, N. R., & Dodge, K. A. (1994). A review and reformulation of social-information mechanisms in children's social adjustment. *Psychological Bulletin, 115,* 74–101.

Crick, N. R., & Grotpeter, J. K. (1995). Relational aggression, gender, and social-psychological adjustment. *Child Development, 66,* 710–722.

Crick, N. R., & Grotpeter, J. K. (1996). Children's treatment by peers: Victims of relational and overt aggression. *Development and Psychopathology, 8,* 367–380.

Crick, N. R., Grotpeter, J. K., & Bigbee, M. A. (2002). Relationally and physically aggressive children's intent attributions and feelings of distress for relational and instrumental provocations. *Child Development, 73,* 1134–1142.

Crick, N. R., & Ladd, G. (1990). Children's perceptions of the outcomes of social strategies: Do the ends justify being mean? *Developmental Psychology, 26,* 612–626.

Crick, N. R., Wellman, N. E., Casas, J. F., O'Brien, M. A., Nelson, D. A., Grotpeter, J. K., & Markon, K. (1999). Childhood aggression and gender: A new look at an old problem. In D. Bernstein (Ed.), *Nebraska Symposium on Motivation* (pp. 75–140). Lincoln: University of Nebraska Press.

Crick, N. R., & Werner, N. E. (1999). Response decision processes in relational and overt aggression. *Child Development, 69,* 1630–1639.

Crick, N. R., Werner, N. E., & Rockhill, C. M. (1997). *A gender-balanced approach to the study of aggression and its consequences.* Manuscript forthcoming.

Crockenberg, S., & Laurie, A. (1996). Parents' conflict strategies with children and children's conflict strategies with peers. *Merrill-Palmer Quarterly, 42,* 495–518.

Crombie, G., & DesJardins, M. (1993, April). *Predictors of gender: The relative importance of children's play, games, and personality characteristics.* Paper presented at the biennial meeting of the Society for Research in Child Development, New Orleans, LA.

Cross, S. E., & Madson, L. (1997). Models of the self: Self-construals and gender. *Psychological Bulletin, 122,* 5–37.

Cummings, E. M., & Davies, P. (1994). *Children and marital conflict: The impact of family dispute and resolution.* New York: Guilford Press.

Cummings, E. M., Iannotti, R. J., & Zahn-Waxler, C. (1989). Aggression between peers in early childhood: Individual continuity and developmental change. *Child Development, 60,* 897–895.

Cunningham, C. E., Cunningham, L. J., Martorelli, V., Tran, A., Young, J., & Zacharias, R. (1998). The effects of primary division, student-mediated conflict resolution programs on playground aggression. *Journal of Child Psychology and Psychiatry, 39,* 653–662.

Curry, G. D., Fox, R. J., Ball, R. A., & Stone, D. (1992). *National assessment of law enforcement anti-gang information resources. Draft 1992 final report.* Morgantown: West Virginia University, National Assessment Survey.

Daniels-Beirness, T. (1989). Measuring peer status in boys and girls: A problem of apples and oranges? In B. H. Schneider, G. Attili, J. Nadel, & R. P. Weissberg (Eds.), *Social competence in developmental perspective* (pp. 107–120). Dordrecht, The Netherlands: Kluwer Academic.

David, C. F., & Kistner, J. A. (2000). Do positive self-perceptions have a "dark side"? Examination of the link between perceptual bias and aggression. *Journal of Abnormal Child Psychology, 28,* 327–337.

David, C. F., Steele, R., Forehand, R., & Armistead, L. (1996). The role of family context and marital conflict in adolescent functioning. *Journal of Family Violence, 11,* 81–91.

Davies, P. T., & Windle, M. (1997). Gender-specific pathways between maternal depressive symptoms, family discord, and adolescent adjustment. *Developmental Psychology, 33*, 657–668.

Davis, T. L. (1995). Gender differences in masking negative emotions: Ability or motivation? *Developmental Psychology, 31*, 660–667.

Dawe, H. C. (1934). An analysis of two hundred quarrels of preschool children. *Child Development, 5*, 139–156.

Deaux, K. (2000). Gender and emotion: Notes from a grateful tourist. In A. H. Fischer (Ed.), *Gender and emotion: Social psychological perspectives* (pp. 301–318). Cambridge, UK: Cambridge University Press.

Delveaux, K. D., & Daniels, T. (2000). Children's social cognitions: Physically and relationally aggression strategies and children's goals in peer conflict situations. *Merrill-Palmer Quarterly, 46*, 672–692.

Degirmencioglu, S. M., Urberg, K. A., Tolson, J. M., & Richard, R. (1998). Adolescent friendship networks: Continuity and change over the school year. *Merrill-Palmer Quarterly, 44*, 313–337.

Denham, S. A. (1998). *Emotional development in young children.* New York: Guilford Press.

Denham, S. A., Mitchell-Copeland, J., Strandberg, K., Auerbach, S., & Blair, K. (1997). Parental contributors to preschoolers' emotional competence: Direct and indirect effects. *Motivation and Emotion, 27*, 65–86.

Denham, S. A., von Salisch, M., Olthof, T., Kochanoff, A., & Caverty, S. (2002). Emotions and social development in childhood. In P. K. Smith & C. Hart (Eds.), *The handbook of social development* (pp. 307–328). London: Blackwell.

Denham, S. A., Workman, E., Cole, P. M., Weissbrod, C., Kendziora, K. T., & Zahn-Waxler, C. (2000). Prediction of externalizing behavior problems from early to middle childhood: The role of parental socialization and emotion expression. *Development and Psychopathology, 12*, 23–45.

Denton, K., & Zarbatany, L. (1996). Age differences in support processes in conversations between friends. *Child Development, 67*, 1360–1373.

Dettling, A. C., Gunnar, M. R., & Donzella, B. (1999). Cortisol levels of young children in full-day childcare centers: Relations with age and temperament. *Psychoendoneurocrinology, 24*, 519–536.

DiPietro, J. A. (1981). Rough-and-tumble play: A function of gender. *Developmental Psychology, 17*, 50–58.

Dodge, K. A. (1983). Behavioral antecedents of peer social status. *Child Development, 54*, 1386–1399.

Dodge, K. A., & Coie, J. D. (1987). Social information processing factors in reactive and proactive aggression in children's peer groups. *Journal of Personality and Social Psychology, 53*, 1146–1158.

Dodge, K. A., Pettit, G. S., McClaskey, C. L., & Brown, M. M. (1986). Social competence in children. *Monographs of the Society for Research in Child Development, 51*(2, Serial No. 213).

Dodge, K. A., & Somberg, D. R. (1987). Hostile attribution biases among aggressive boys are exacerbated under conditions of threats to the self. *Child Development, 58*, 213–224.

Dolgin, K. G., & Kim, S. (1994). Adolescents' disclosure to best and good friends: The effects of gender and topic intimacy. *Social Development, 3*, 146–157.

Dollard, J., Doob, L. W., Miller, N. E., Mowrer, O. H., & Sears, R. R. (1939). *Frustration and aggression*. New Haven, CT: Yale University Press.

Dorn, L. D., Nottelmann, E. D., Susman, E. J., Inoff-Germain, G., Cutler, G. B., Jr., & Chrousos, G. P. (1999). Variability in hormone concentrations and self-reported menstrual histories in young adolescents: Menarche as an integral part of a developmental process. *Journal of Youth and Adolescence, 28*, 283–297.

Downey, G., Bonica, C., & Rincon, C. (1999). Rejection sensitivity and adolescent romantic relationships. In W. Furman, B. B. Brown, & C. Feiring (Eds.), *The development of romantic relationships in adolescence* (pp. 148–174). New York: Cambridge University Press.

Downey, G., & Feldman, S. I. (1996). Implications of rejection sensitivity for intimate relationships. *Journal of Personality and Social Psychology, 70*, 1327–1343.

Downey, G., Lebolt, A., Rincon, C., & Freitas, A. L. (1998). Rejection sensitivity and children's interpersonal difficulties. *Child Development, 69*, 1074–1091.

Dunn, J. (2001). The development of children's conflict and prosocial behavior: Lessons from research on social aggression and gender. In J. Hill & B. Maughan (Eds.), *Conduct disorders in childhood and adolescence* (pp. 49–66). New York: Cambridge University Press.

Dunn, J., & Hughes, C. (1998). Young children's understanding of emotions within close relationships. *Cognition and Emotion, 12*, 171–190.

Dunn, J., & Munn, P. (1987). Development of justification in disputes with mother and sibling. *Developmental Psychology, 23*, 791–798.

Dunphy, D. (1963). The social structure of urban adolescent peer groups. *Sociometry, 26*, 230–246.

Eaton, W., & Ennis, L. (1986). Sex differences in human motor activity level. *Psychological Bulletin, 100*, 19–28.

Eckert, P. (1990). Cooperative competition in adolescent "girl talk." *Discourse Processes, 13*, 91–122.

Eder, D. (1985). The cycle of popularity: Interpersonal relations among female adolescents. *Sociology of Education, 58*, 154–165.

Eder, D. (1990). Serious and playful disputes: Variation in conflict talk about female adolescents. In A. D. Grimshaw (Ed.), *Conflict talk: Investigations of arguments in conversation* (pp. 67–84). Cambridge, UK: Cambridge University Press.

Eder, D., & Enke, J. L. (1991). The structure of gossip: Opportunities and constraints on collective expression among adolescents. *American Sociological Review, 56*, 494–508.

Eder, D., Evans, C. C., & Parker, S. (1995). *School talk: Gender and adolescent culture*. New Brunswick, NJ: Rutgers University Press.

Edwards, D. A. (1969). Early androgen stimulation and aggressive behavior in male and female mice. *Physiology and Behavior, 4*, 333–338.

Edwards, D. A., & Herndon, J. (1970). Neonatal estrogen stimulation and aggressive behavior in female mice. *Physiology and Behavior, 4*, 993–995.

Eisenberg, N., Fabes, R. A., Murphy, B. C., Shepard, S., Guthrie, I. K, Mazsk, P., Poulin, R., & Jones, S. (1999). Prediction of elementary school children's socially appropriate and problem behavior from anger reactions at 4–6 years. *Journal of Applied Developmental Psychology, 20,* 119–142.

Eisenberg, N., Fabes, R. A., Shepard, S. A., Guthrie, I. K., Murphy, B. C., & Rieser, M. (1999). Parental reactions to children's negative emotions: Longitudinal relations to quality of children's social functioning. *Child Development, 70,* 513–534.

Elkind, D. (1967). Egocentrism in adolescence. *Child Development, 38,* 1025–1034.

Elkind, D., & Bowen, R. (1979). Imaginary audience behavior in children and adolescents. *Developmental Psychology, 15,* 38–44.

Elliott, D. S. (1994). Serious violent offenders: Onset, developmental course, and termination. The American Society for Criminology 1993 Presidential Address. *Criminology, 32,* 1–21.

Eme, R. F. (1992). Selective female affliction in the developmental disorders of childhood: A literature review. *Journal of Clinical Child Psychology, 21,* 354–364.

Emery, R. E. (1982). Interparental conflict and the children of discord and divorce. *Psychological Bulletin, 92,* 310–330.

Eslea, M., & Smith, P. K. (1998). The long-term effects of anti-bullying work in primary schools. *Educational Research, 40,* 203–218.

Fabes, R. A. (1994). Physiological, emotional, and behavioral correlates of gender segregation. In C. Leaper (Ed.), Childhood gender segregation: Causes and consequences. *New Directions in Child Development, 65,* 19–34.

Fabes, R. A., & Eisenberg, N. (1992). Young children's coping with interpersonal anger. *Child Development, 63,* 116–128.

Fabes, R. A., Eisenberg, N., Smith, M. C., & Murphy, B. C. (1996). Getting angry at peers: Associations with liking of the provocateur. *Child Development, 67,* 942–956.

Fabes, R. A., Shepard, S. A., Guthrie, I. K., & Martin, C. L. (1997). Roles of temperamental arousal and gender-segregated play in young children's social adjustment. *Developmental Psychology, 33,* 693–702.

Fagot, B. I. (1984). The consequents of problem behavior in toddler children. *Journal of Abnormal Child Psychology, 12,* 385–396.

Fagot, B. I. (1985). Beyond the reinforcement principle: Another step toward understanding sex role development. *Developmental Psychology, 21,* 1097–1104.

Fagot, B. I. (1994). Peer relations and the development of competence in boys and girls. In C. Leaper (Ed.), Childhood gender segregation: Causes and consequences. *New Directions in Child Development, 65,* 53–66.

Fagot, B. I., & Hagan, R. (1985). Aggression in toddlers: Responses to the assertive acts of boys and girls. *Sex Roles, 12,* 341–351.

Fagot, B. I., & Leinbach, M. D. (1993). Gender role development in young children: From discrimination to labeling. *Developmental Review, 13,* 205–224.

Fagot, B. I., Leinbach, M. D., & Hagan, R. (1986). Gender labeling and the adoption of sex-typed behaviors. *Developmental Psychology, 22,* 440–443.

Fagot, B. I., Leinbach, M. D., & O'Boyle, C. (1992). Gender labeling, gender stereotyping, and parenting behaviors. *Developmental Psychology, 28*(2), 225–230.

Farver, J. M. (1996). Aggressive behavior in preschoolers' social networks: Do birds of a feather flock together? *Early Childhood Research Quarterly, 11,* 333–350.

Feiring, C. (1996). Concepts of romance in 15-year-old adolescents. *Journal of Research on Adolescence, 6,* 181–200.

Feiring, C., & Lewis, M. (1987). The child's social network: Sex differences from three to six years. *Sex Roles, 17,* 621–636.

Feshbach, N. D. (1964). The function of aggression and the regulation of aggressive drive. *Psychological Review, 71,* 257–272.

Feshbach, N. D. (1969). Gender differences in children's modes of aggressive responses toward outsiders. *Merrill-Palmer Quarterly, 15,* 249–258.

Feshbach, N. D., & Feshbach, S. (1969). The relationship between empathy and aggression in two age groups. *Developmental Psychology, 1,* 102–107.

Feshbach, N. D., & Sones, G. (1971). Sex differences in adolescent reactions toward newcomers. *Developmental Psychology, 4,* 381–386.

Fine, G. A. (1986). The social organization of adolescent gossip. In J. Cook-Gumperz, W. Corsara, & J. Streek (Eds.), *Children's worlds and children's language* (pp. 405–423). Berlin: Mouton.

Fivush, R. (1991). Gender and emotion in mother–child conversations about the past. *Journal of Narrative and Life History, 1,* 325–341.

Follingstad, D. R., Rutledge, L. I., Berg, B. J., Hause, E. S., & Polek, D. S. (1990). The role of emotional abuse in physically abusive relationships. *Journal of Family Violence, 5,* 107–120.

Foster, S. L., DeLawyer, D. D., & Guevrement, D. C. (1986). A critical incidents analysis of liked and disliked peer behaviors and their situational parameters in childhood and adolescence. *Behavioral Assessment, 8,* 115–133.

French, D. C., Jansen, E. A., & Pidada, S. (2002). US and Indonesian children's and adolescent's reports of relational aggression by disliked peers. *Child Development, 73,* 1143–1150.

Frodi, A., Macaulay, J., & Thome, P. (1977). Are women always less aggressive than men? A review of the experimental literature. *Psychological Bulletin, 84,* 635–657.

Frost, R. (1949). Fire and ice. In *Complete poems of Robert Frost* (p. 268). New York: Holt.

Fry, D. P., & Gabriel, A. H. (1994). Preface: The cultural construction of gender and aggression. *Sex Roles, 30,* 177–188.

Furman, W., & Simon, V. A. (1998). Advice from youth: Some lessons from the study of adolescent relationships. *Journal of Social and Personal Relationships, 15,* 723–739.

Galambos, N. L., Almeida, D. M., & Petersen, A. C. (1990). Masculinity, femininity, and sex role attitudes in early adolescence: Exploring gender intensification. *Child Development, 61,* 1905–1914.

Galen, B. R., & Luthar, S. (2000). *Peer maltreatment: Overt and indirect/relational/social victimization and adolescent developmental difficulties.* Manuscript under review.

Galen, B. R., & Underwood, M. K. (1997). A developmental investigation of social aggression among children. *Developmental Psychology, 33,* 589–600.

Garner, P. W., & Spears, F. M. (2000). Emotion regulation in low-income preschoolers. *Social Development, 9,* 246–264.

Gavin, L. A., & Furman, W. (1989). Age differences in adolescents' perceptions of their peer groups. *Developmental Psychology, 25,* 827–834.

Ge, X., Conger, R. D., & Elder, G. H. (1996). Coming of age too early: Pubertal influences on girls' vulnerability to psychological distress. *Child Development, 67,* 3386–3400.

Geiger, T. C., & Crick, N. R. (2001). A developmental psychopathology perspective on vulnerability to personality disorders. In R. E. Ingram & J. M. Price (Eds.), *Vulnerability to psychopathology: Risk across the lifespan* (pp. 57–102). New York: Guilford Press.

Gelb, R., & Jacobson, J. L. (1988). Popular and unpopular children's interactions during cooperative and competitive peer group activities. *Journal of Abnormal Child Psychology, 16,* 247–261.

Gibbs, J. (2001). TRIBES: A new way of learning and being together. New York: Center Source.

Gilligan, C. (1982). *In a different voice.* Cambridge, MA: Harvard University Press.

Giordano, P. C., Cernkovich, S. A., & DeMaris, A. (1993). The family and peer relations of Black adolescents. *Journal of Marriage and the Family, 55,* 277–287.

Giordano, P. C., Mulhollen, T. J., Cernkovich, S. A., Pugh, M. D., & Rudolph, J. L. (1999). Delinquency, identity, and women's involvement in relationship violence. *Criminology, 37,* 17–40.

Goldmsith, H., Buss, K., & Lemery, K. (1997). Toddler and child temperament: Expanded context, stronger genetic evidence, new evidence for the importance of environment. *Developmental Psychology, 33,* 891–905.

Goldstein, S. E., Tisak, M. S., & Boxer, P. (2002). Preschoolers' normative and prescriptive judgments about relational and overt aggression. *Early Education and Development, 13,* 23–39.

Goodenough, F. L. (1931). *Anger in young children.* Minneapolis: University of Minnesota Press.

Gossens, L. (1984). Imaginary audience behavior as a function of age, sex, and formal operational thinking. *International Journal of Behavioral Development, 7,* 77–93.

Gottman, J. M. (1986). The world of coordinated play: Same- and cross-sex friendship in young children. In J. M. Gottman & J. G. Parker (Eds.), *Conversations with friends: Speculations about affective development* (pp. 139–191). New York: Cambridge University Press.

Gottman, J. M., Gonso, J., & Rasmussen, B. (1975). Social interaction, social competence, and friendship in children. *Child Development, 46,* 709–718.

Gottman, J. M., & Mettetal, G. (1986). Speculations about social and affective development: Friendship and acquaintanceship through adolescence. In J. M. Gottman & J. G. Parker (Eds.), *Conversations with friends: Speculations on affective development* (pp. 192–237). New York: Cambridge University Press.

Gouze, K. R. (1987). Attention and social problem solving as correlates of aggression in preschool males. *Journal of Abnormal Child Psychology, 15,* 181–197.

Graber, J. A., Lewinsohn, P. M., Seeley, J. R., & Brooks-Gunn, J. (1997). Is psychopathology associated with the timing of pubertal development? *Journal of the American Academy of Child and Adolescent Psychiatry, 36*, 1768–1776.

Gray, J. (1992). *Men are from Mars, women are from Venus: A practical guide for improving communication and getting what you want in relationships.* New York: HarperCollins.

Green, L. R., Richardson, D. R., & Lago, T. (1996). How do friendship, indirect, and direct aggression relate? *Aggressive Behavior, 22*, 81–86.

Grotpeter, J. K., & Crick, N. R. (1996). Relational aggression, overt aggression, and friendship. *Child Development, 67*, 2328–2338.

Grych, J. H., & Fincham, F. D. (1990). Marital conflict and children's adjustment: A cognitive-contextual framework. *Psychological Bulletin, 108*, 267–290.

Guerin, D. W., & Gottfried, A. W. (1994). Developmental stability and change in parent reports of temperament: A ten-year longitudinal study from infancy through preadolescence. *Merrill-Palmer Quarterly, 40*, 334–355.

Guerra, N. G., & Slaby, R. G. (1989). Evaluative factors in social problem solving by aggressive boys. *Journal of Abnormal Child Psychology, 17*, 277–289.

Gunnar, M., & Donahue, M. (1980). Sex differences in social responsiveness between six months and twelve months. *Child Development, 51*, 262–265.

Halberstadt, A. G., Crisp, V. W., & Eaton, K. L. (1999). Family expressiveness: A retrospective and new directions for research. In P. Philippot, R. S. Feldman, & E. J. Coats (Eds.), *The social context of nonverbal behavior* (pp. 109–155). New York: Cambridge University Press.

Hall, G. S. (1904). *Adolescence: Its psychology and its relations to physiology, anthropology, sociology, sex, crime, religion, and education* (Vols. 1 & 2). New York: Appleton.

Hallinan, M. T. (1980). Patterns of cliquing among youth. In H. C. Foot, A. J. Chapman, & J. R. Smith (Eds.), *Friendship and social relations in children* (pp. 321–342). Chichester, UK: Wiley.

Harold, G. T., & Conger, R. D. (1997). Marital conflict and adolescent distress: The role of adolescent awareness. *Child Development, 68*, 333–350.

Harré, R., & Lamb, R. (1983). *The encyclopedic dictionary of psychology.* London: Blackwell.

Hart, C. H., Nelson, D.A., Robinson, C. C., Olsen, S. F., & McNeilly-Choque, M. K. (1998). Overt and relational aggression in Russian nursery-school-age children: Parenting style and marital linkages. *Developmental Psychology, 34*, 687–697.

Hart, C. H., Yang, C., Nelson, D. A., Jun, S., Bazarskaya, N., Nelson, L., Wu, X., & Wu, P. (2001). Peer contact patterns, parenting practices, and preschoolers' social competence in China, Russia, and the U.S. In P. T. Slee & K. Rigby (Eds.), *Children's peer relations* (pp. 3–30). New York: Routledge.

Hartup, W. W. (1999). Constraints on peer socialization: Let me count the ways. *Merrill-Palmer Quarterly, 45*, 172–183.

Hartup, W. W., & deWit, J. (1974). The development of aggression: Problems and perspectives. In J. deWit & W. W. Hartup (Eds.), *Determinants and origins of aggressive behavior* (pp. 595–615). The Hague: Mouton.

Hartup, W. W., French, D. C., Laursen, B., Johnston, M. K., & Ogawa, J. R. (1993).

Conflict and friendship patterns in middle childhood: Behavior in a closed field situation. *Child Development, 64,* 445–454.

Hartup, W. W., Glazer, J. A., & Charlesworth, R. (1967). Peer reinforcement and sociometric status. *Child Development, 38,* 1012–1024.

Haviland, J. M., Malatesta, C. Z., & Levlivica, M. L. (1984). Emotional communication in early infancy. *Infant Mental Health Journal, 5,* 135–147.

Hawley, P. H. (2001, April). Coercive strategies of resource control in pre-adolescents: Maladaptation versus Machiavellianism. In P. H. Hawley (Chair), *Aggression and adaptive functioning: The bright side to bad behavior.* Symposium presented at the biennial meeting of the Society for Research in Child Development, Minneapolis, MN.

Henington, C., Hughes, J. N., Cavell, T. A., & Thompson, B. (1998). The role of relational aggression in identifying boys and girls. *Journal of School Psychology, 36,* 457–477.

Hill, J. P., & Lynch, M. E. (1983). The intensification of gender-related role expectations during early adolescence. In J. Brooks-Gunn & A. C. Petersen (Eds.), *Girls at puberty: Biological and psychosocial perspectives* (pp. 201–228). New York: Plenum Press.

Hines, N. J., & Fry, D. P. (1994). Indirect modes of aggression among women of Buenos Aires, Argentina. *Sex Roles, 30,* 213–224.

Holmbeck, G. N., & Hill, J. P. (1991). Conflictive engagement, positive affect, and menarche in families with seventh-grade girls. *Child Development, 62,* 1030–1048.

Holmbeck, G. N., Paikoff, R. L., & Brooks-Gunn, J. (1995). Parenting adolescents. In M. H. Bornstein (Ed.), *Handbook of parenting: Vol. 1. Children and parenting* (pp. 91–118). Mahwah, NJ: Erlbaum.

Hubbard, J. A. (2001). Emotion expression processes in children's peer interaction: The role of peer rejection, aggression, and gender. *Child Development, 72,* 1426–1438.

Hubbard, J. A., Smithmyer, C. M., Ramsden, S. R., Parker, E. H., Flanagan, K. D., Dearing, K. F., Relyea, N., & Simons, R. F. (2002). Observational, physiological, and self-report measures of children's anger: Relations to reactive versus proactive aggression. *Child Development, 73,* 1101–1118.

Hughes, C., White, A., Sharpen, J., & Dunn, J. (2000). Antisocial, angry, and unsympathetic: "Hard-to-manage" preschoolers peer problems and possible cognitive influences. *Journal of Child and Adolescent Psychiatry, 41,* 169–179.

Humphreys, A. P., & Smith, P. K. (1987). Rough-and-tumble play, friendship, and dominance in school children: Evidence for continuity and change with age. *Child Development, 58,* 201–212.

Huston, A. C., Wright, J. C., Marquis, J., & Green, S. B. (1999). How young children spend their time: Television and other activities. *Developmental Psychology, 35*(4), 912–925.

Hyde, J. S. (1984). How large are gender differences in aggression? A developmental meta-analysis. *Developmental Psychology, 20*(4), 722–736.

Hymel, S., Bonanno, R. A., Henderson, N. R., & McCreith, T. (2002, July). Moral disengagement and school bullying: An investigation of student attitudes and beliefs. In J. LeBlanc (Chair), *Aggression in school.* Symposium conducted at the International Society for Research on Aggression, Montreal, Quebec, Canada.

Izard, C. E. (1979). *The maximally discriminative facial movement coding system (MAX)*. Newark: University of Delaware Instructional Resources Center.

Izard, C. E., Hembree, E. A., & Huebner, R. R. (1987). Infants' emotion expressions to acute pain: Developmental change and stability of individual differences. *Developmental Psychology, 23,* 105–113.

Jenkins, J. M. (2000). Marital conflict and children's emotions: The development of an anger organization. *Journal of Marriage and the Family, 62,* 723–736.

Jenkins, J. M., & Ball, S. (2000). Distinguishing between negative emotions: Children's understanding of the social-regulatory aspects of emotion. *Cognition and Emotion, 14,* 261–282.

Jenkins, J. M., Franco, L., Dokins, F., & Sevell, A. (1995). Toddlers' reactions to negative emotional displays: Forming models of relationships. *Infant Behavior and Development, 18,* 273–281.

Jessor, R., & Jessor, S. L. (1977). *Problem behavior and psychosocial development: A longitudinal study of youth.* New York: Academic Press.

Joe, K. A., & Chesney-Lind, M. (1995). "Just every mother's angel": An analysis of gender and ethnic variations in youth gang membership. *Gender and Society, 9,* 408–431.

Jones, D. C., Abbey, B. B., & Cumberland, A. (1998). The development of display rule knowledge: Linkages with family expressiveness and social competence. *Child Development, 69,* 1209–1222.

Jones, D. C., & Coston, S. E. (1995). Friendship quality during preadolescence and adolescence: The contributions of relationship orientations, instrumentality, and expressivity. *Merrill-Palmer Quarterly, 41,* 517–535.

Juvonen, J., & Graham, S. (Eds.). (2001). *Peer harassment in school: The plight of the vulnerable and the victimized.* New York: Guilford Press.

Karniol, R., & Heiman, T. (1987). Situational antecedents of children's anger experiences and subsequent responses to adult versus peer provocateurs. *Aggressive Behavior, 13,* 109–118.

Kashani, J. H., & Shepperd, J. A. (1990). Aggression in adolescents: The role of social support and personality. *Canadian Journal of Psychiatry, 35,* 311–315.

Katz, P. A., & Ksansnak, K. R. (1994). Developmental aspects of gender role flexibility and traditionality in middle childhood and adolescence. *Developmental Psychology, 30,* 272–282.

Kaukiainen, A., Bjorkqvist, K., Lagerspetz, K., Osterman, K., Salmivalli, C., Rothberg, S., & Ahlbo, A. (1999). The relationships between social intelligence, empathy, and three types of aggression. *Aggressive Behavior, 25,* 81–89.

Kavanaugh, K., & Hops, H. (1994). Good girls? Bad boys?: Gender and development as contexts for diagnosis and treatment. *Advances in Child Clinical Psychology, 16,* 45–79.

Kawaguchi, M. C., Welsh, D. P., Powers, S. I., & Rostosky, S. S. (1998). Mothers, fathers, sons, and daughters: Temperament, gender, and adolescent–parent relationships. *Merrill-Palmer Quarterly, 44,* 77–96.

Kazdin, A. E. (1987). Treatment of antisocial behavior in children: Current status and future directions. *Psychological Bulletin, 102,* 187–203.

Keenan, K., Loeber, R., & Green, S. (1999). Conduct disorder in girls: A review of the literatures. *Clinical Child and Family Psychology Review, 2,* 3–19.

Keenan, K., & Shaw, D. S. (1994). The development of aggression in toddlers: A study of low-income families. *Journal of Abnormal Child Psychology, 22,* 53–77.

Keenan, K., & Shaw, D. (1997). Developmental and social influences on young girls' early problem behavior. *Psychological Bulletin, 121,* 95–113.

Keiley, M. K., Bates, J. E., Dodge, K. A., & Pettit, G. S. (2000). A cross-domain growth analysis: Externalizing and internalizing behaviors during eight years of childhood. *Journal of Abnormal Child Psychology, 28,* 161–179.

Keltner, D., Young, R. C., Heery, E. A., Oenig, C., & Monarch, N. D. (1998). Teasing in hierarchical and intimate relations. *Journal of Personality and Social Psychology, 75,* 1231–1247.

Kerig, P. K., Brown, C., & Patenaude, R. (2001, April). Ties that bind: Coparenting, parent-child relations, and triangulation in post-divorce interpersonal conflicts. In M. El-Shiekh (Chair), *Marital conflict and child outcomes: Processes, risk variables, and protective factors.* Symposium presented at the biennial meeting of the Society for Research in Child Development, Minneapolis, MN.

Kerig, P. K., Cowan, P. A., & Cowan, C. P. (1993). Marital quality and gender differences in parent–child interactions. *Developmental Psychology, 29,* 931–939.

Kessler, R. C. (1990). The national comorbidity survey. *DIS Newsletter, 7,* 1–2.

Kindermann, T. A. (1993). Natural peer groups as contexts for individual development: The case of children's motivation in school. *Developmental Psychology, 29,* 970–977.

Kingston, L., & Prior, M. (1995). The development of patterns of stable, transient, and school-age onset of aggressive behavior in young children. *Journal of the American Academy of Child and Adolescent Psychiatry, 34,* 348–358.

Knight, G. P., Fabes, R. A., & Higgins, D. A. (1996). Concerns about drawing inferences from meta-analyses: An example in the study of gender differences in aggression. *Psychological Bulletin, 119,* 410–421.

Kochanska, G., Coy, K. C., Tjebkes, T. L., & Husarek, S. J. (1998). Individual differences in emotionality in infancy. *Child Development, 64,* 375–390.

Kohlberg, L. (1976). Moral stages and moralization: The cognitive-developmental approach. In T. Lickona (Ed.), *Moral development and behavior* (pp. 31–53). New York: Holt, Rinehart, & Winston.

Kohlberg, L., LaCrosse, I., & Ricks, D. (1972). The predictability of adult mental health from childhood behavior. In B. B. Wolman (Ed.), *Manual of child psychopathology* (pp. 1217–1284). New York: McGraw-Hill.

Kratzer, L., & Hodgins, S. (1999). A typology of offenders: A test of Moffitt's theory among males and females from childhood to age 30. *Criminal Behavior and Mental Health, 9,* 57–73.

Kring, A. M. (2000). Gender and anger. In A. H. Fischer (Ed.), *Gender and emotion: Social psychological perspectives* (pp. 211–231). Cambridge, UK: Cambridge University Press.

Krueger, R. F., Moffitt, T. E., Caspi, A., Bleske, A., & Silva, P. A. (1998). Assortative mating for antisocial behavior: Developmental and methodological implications. *Behavior Genetics, 28,* 173–186.

Kuebli, J., Butler, S., & Fivush, R. (1995). Mother–child talk about past emotions: Relations of maternal language and child gender over time. *Cognition and Emotion, 9,* 265–283.

Kupersmidt, J. B., Bryant, D., & Willoughby, M. (2000). Prevalence of aggressive behaviors in Head Start and community child care programs. *Behavior Disorders, 26,* 42–52.

Kupersmidt, J. B., & Coie, J. D. (1990). Preadolescent peer status, aggression, and school adjustment as predictors of externalizing problems in adolescence. *Child Development, 61,* 1350–1362.

Ladd, G. W. (1983). Social networks of popular, average, and rejected children in school settings. *Merrill-Palmer Quarterly, 29,* 283–307.

Ladd, G. W., & Pettit, G. S. (2002). Parenting and the development of children's peer relationships. In M. H. Bornstein (Ed.), *Handbook of parenting: Vol. 5. Practical issues in parenting* (2nd ed., pp. 269–309). Mahwah, NJ: Erlbaum.

Lagerspetz, K. M. J., Bjorkqvist, K., & Peltonen, T. (1988). Is indirect aggression typical of females? Gender differences in aggressiveness in 11- to 12-year-old children. *Aggressive Behavior, 14,* 403–414.

Lahey, B. B., Schwab-Stone, M., Goodman, S. H., Waldman, I. D., Canino, G., Rathouz, P. J., Miller, T. L., Dennis, K. D., Bird, H., & Jensen, P. S. (2000). Age and gender differences in oppositional behavior and conduct problems: A cross-sectional household study of middle childhood and adolescence. *Journal of Abnormal Psychology, 109,* 488–503.

Lancelotta, G. X., & Vaughn, S. (1989). Relation between types of aggression and sociometric status: Peer and teacher perceptions. *Journal of Educational Psychology, 81,* 86–90.

Lansford, J. E., & Parker, J. G. (1999). Children's interactions in triads: Behavioral profiles and effects of gender and patterns of friendship among members. *Developmental Psychology, 35,* 80–93.

Larson, R. (2001). How U.S. children and adolescents spend time: What it does (and doesn't) tell us about their development. *Current Directions in Psychological Science, 10,* 160–164.

Larson, R., & Asmussen, L. (1991). Anger, worry, and hurt in early adolescence: An enlarging world of negative emotions. In M. E. Colton & S. Gore (Eds.), *Adolescent stress: Causes and consequences* (pp. 21–41). New York: Aldine de Gruyter.

Larson, R., & Richards, M. H. (1994). *Divergent realities: The emotional lives of mothers, fathers, and adolescents.* New York: Basic Books.

Larson, R., Richards, M. H., Moneta, G., Holmbeck, G., & Duckett, E. (1996). Changes in adolescents' daily interactions with their families from ages 10 to 18: Disengagement and transformation. *Developmental Psychology, 32,* 744–754.

Larson, R. W., & Verma, S. (1999). How children and adolescents spend time across the world: Work, play, and developmental opportunities. *Psychological Bulletin, 125,* 701–736.

Larson, R. W., Wilson, S., Brown, B. B., Furstenberg, F. F., & Verma, S. (2002). Changes in adolescents' interpersonal competence: Are they being prepared for adult relationships in the 21st century? *Journal of Research on Adolescence, 12,* 31–68.

Laursen, B. (1993). The perceived impact of conflict on adolescent relationships. *Merrill-Palmer Quarterly, 39,* 535–550.

Laursen, B. (1995). Conflict and social interaction in adolescent relationships. *Journal of Research on Adolescence, 5,* 55–70.

Laursen, B. (1996). Closeness and conflict in adolescent peer relationships: Interdependence with friends and romantic partners. In W. M. Bukowski, A. F. Newcomh, & W. W. Hartup (Eds.), *The company they keep: Friendship in childhood and adolescence* (pp. 186–210). New York: Cambridge University Press.

Laursen, B., & Hartup, W. W. (1989). The dynamics of preschool children's conflicts. *Merrill-Palmer Quarterly, 35,* 281–297.

Laursen, B., Hartup, W. W., & Koplas, A. L. (1996). Towards understanding peer conflict. *Merrill-Palmer Quarterly, 42,* 536–553.

Laursen, B., & Koplas, A.L. (1995). What's important about important conflicts? Adolescents' perceptions of daily disagreements. *Merrill-Palmer Quarterly, 41,* 536–553.

Leadbeater, B. J., Kuperminc, G. P., Blatt, S. J., & Hertzog, C. (1999). A multivariate model of gender differences in adolescents' internalizing and externalizing problems. *Developmental Psychology, 35,* 1268–1282.

Leaper, C. (1994). Exploring the consequences of gender segregation on social relationships. In C. Leaper (Ed.), Childhood gender segregation: Causes and consequences. *New Directions in Child Development, 65,* 67–86.

Leaper, C., Anderson, K. J., & Sanders, P. (1998). Moderators of gender effects on parents' talk to their children: A meta-analysis. *Developmental Psychology, 34,* 3–27.

Leaper, C., Tenenbaum, H. R., & Schaffer, T. G. (1999). Communication patterns of African American girls and boys from low-income, urban backgrounds. *Child Development, 70*(6), 1489–1503.

Leary, M. R. (2001). Toward a conceptualization of interpersonal rejection. In M. R. Leary (Ed.), *Interpersonal rejection* (pp. 3–20). New York: Oxford University Press.

Leckie, B. A. (1999, April). Girls' perceptions of two subtypes of aggression: Are there differences and does sociometric status play a mediating role? In D. S. J. Hawker & N. H. Bartlett (Co-Chairs), *Subtypes of peer aggression and victimization: Current issues and controversies.* Symposium presented at the biennial meeting of the Society for Research in Child Development, Albuquerque, NM.

Lefever, H. (1981). Playing the dozens: A mechanism of social control. *Phylon, 42,* 73–85.

Legault, F., & Strayer, F. F. (1990). The emergence of gender-segregation in preschool peer groups. In F. F. Strayer (Ed.), *Social interaction and behavioral development during early childhood.* Annual research report, Université de Québec à Montréal, Laboratoire d'Éthologie Humaine, Département de Psychologie.

Leinbach, M. D., & Hort, B. E. (1995, April). *Do young children sex type emotions?* Paper presented at the biennial meeting of the Society for Research in Child Development, Indianapolis, IN.

Leinbach, M. D., Hort, B. E., & Fagot, B. I. (1997). Bears are for boys: Metaphorical associations in young children's gender stereotypes. *Cognitive Development, 12*, 107–130.

Lemerise, E. A., & Dodge, K. A. (2000). The development of anger and hostile interactions. In M. Lewis & J. M. Haviland-Jones (Eds.), *Handbook of emotions* (2nd ed., pp. 594–606). New York: Guilford Press.

Lempers, J. D., & Clark-Lempers, D. S. (1992). Young, middle, and late adolescents comparisons of the functional importance of 5 significant relationships. *Journal of Youth and Adolescence, 21*, 53–96.

Leve, L. D., & Chamberlain, P. (in press). Girls in the juvenile justice system: Risk factors and clinical implications. To appear in D. J. Pepler, K. Madsen, C. Webster, & K. Levene (Eds.), *The development and treatment of girlhood aggression.* Mahwah, NJ: Erlbaum.

Lever, J. (1976). Sex differences in the games children play. *Social Problems, 23*, 478–487.

Levy, S. R., Ayduk, O., & Downey, G. (2001). The role of rejection sensitivity in people's relationships with significant others and significant social groups. In M. R. Leary (Ed.), *Interpersonal rejection* (pp. 251–290). New York: Oxford University Press.

Lewis, M. (1993). Basic psychological processes in emotion. In M. Lewis & J. M. Haviland (Eds.), *Handbook of emotions* (pp. 223–236). New York: Guilford Press.

Lewis, M., Alessandri, S. M., & Sullivan, M. W. (1992). Differences in shame and pride as a function of children's gender and task difficulty. *Child Development, 63*, 630–638.

Lightner, R. M., Bollmer, J. M., Harris, M. J., Milich, R., & Scrambler, D. J. (2000). What do you say to teasers?: Parent and child evaluations of responses to teasing. *Journal of Applied Developmental Psychology, 24*, 403–427.

Linder, J. R., Crick, N. R., & Collins, W. A. (2002). Relational aggression and victimization in young adults' romantic relationships: Associations with perceptions of parent, peer, and romantic relationship quality. *Social Development, 11*, 69–86.

Lochman, J. E., Coie, J. D., Underwood, M. K., & Terry, R. (1993). Effectiveness of a social relations intervention program for aggressive-rejected children. *Journal of Consulting and Clinical Psychology, 61*(6), 1053–1058.

Loeber, R. (1982). The stability of antisocial and delinquent child behavior: A review. *Child Development, 53*, 1431–1446.

Loeber, R., & Hay, D. (1997). Key issues in the development of aggression and violence from childhood to early adulthood. *Annual Review of Psychology, 48*, 371–410.

Loeber, R., & Stouthamer-Loeber, M. (1998). Development of juvenile aggression and violence: Some common misconceptions and controversies. *American Psychologist, 53*, 242–259.

Lutz, C. A. (1990). Engendered emotion: Gender, power, and the rhetoric of emotional control in American discourse. In C. A. Lutz & L. Abu-Lughod (Eds.), *Language and the politics of emotion* (pp. 69–92). Cambridge, UK: Cambridge University Press.

Lyne, S. (1996). *Ten-second rainshowers: Poems by young people.* New York: Simon & Schuster.

Lytton, H., & Romney, D. M. (1991). Parents' differential socialization of boys and girls: A meta-analysis. *Psychological Bulletin, 109,* 267–296.

Maccoby, E. E. (1966). *The development of sex differences.* Stanford, CA: Stanford University Press.

Maccoby, E. E. (1980). *Social development: Psychological growth and the parent–child relationship.* New York: Harcourt Brace.

Maccoby, E. E. (1990). Gender and relationships: A developmental account. *American Psychologist, 45,* 513–520.

Maccoby, E. E. (1998). *The two sexes: Growing up apart, coming together.* Cambridge, MA: Belknap Press of Harvard University Press.

Maccoby, E. E., & Jacklin, C. N. (1974). *The psychology of gender differences.* Stanford, CA: Stanford University Press.

Maccoby, E. E., & Jacklin, C. N. (1987). Gender segregation in childhood. In H. Reese (Ed.), *Advances in child behavior and development* (pp. 239–287). New York: Academic Press.

MacDonald, C. D., & O'Laughlin, E. M. (1997, April). *Relational aggression and risk behaviors in middle school students.* Poster presented at the biennial meeting of the Society for Research in Child Development, Washington, DC.

Madsen, C. (1968). Nurturance and modeling in preschoolers. *Child Development, 39,* 221–236.

Magdol, L., Moffitt, T. E., Caspi, A., Newman, D. L., Fagan, J., & Silva, P. A. (1997). Gender differences in partner violence in a birth cohort of 20-year-olds: Bridging the gap between clinical and epidemiological approaches. *Journal of Consulting and Clinical Psychology, 65,* 68–78.

Magdol, L., Moffitt, T. E., Caspi, A., & Silva, P. A. (1998). Developmental antecedents of partner abuse: A prospective-longitudinal study. *Journal of Abnormal Psychology, 107,* 375–389.

Main, M. (1991). Metacognitive knowledge, metacognitive monitoring and singular (coherent) versus multiple (incoherent) model of attachment: Findings and directions for future research. In C. M. Parkes, J. Stevenson-Hinde, & P. Marris (Eds.), *Attachment across the life cycle* (pp. 127–159). New York: Tavistock/Routledge.

Maines, B., & Robinson, G. (1992). *The no-blame approach.* Bristol, UK: LameDuck.

Malatesta, C. Z., Culver, C., Tesman, J. R., & Shepard, B. (1989). The development of emotion expression during the first two years of life. *Monographs of the Society for Research in Child Development, 54* (1-2), 1–104.

Malatesta, C. Z., & Haviland, J. (1982). Learning display rules: The socialization of emotion expression in infancy. *Child Development, 53,* 991–1003.

Malatesta-Magai, C., Leak, S., Tesman, J., Shepard, B., Culver, C., & Smaggia, B.

(1994). Profiles of emotional development: Individual differences in facial and vocal expression of emotion during the second and third year of life. *International Journal of Social and Behavioral Development, 17,* 239–269.

Maltz, D. N., & Borker, R. A. (1982). A cultural approach to male–female miscommunication. In J. J. Gumperz (Ed.), *Language and social identity* (pp. 195–216). New York: Cambridge University Press.

Markovits, H., Benenson, J., & Dolensky, E. (2001). Evidence that children and adolescents have internal models of peer interactions that are gender differentiated. *Child Development, 72,* 879–886.

Martin, C.L. (1994). Cognitive influences on the development and maintenance of gender segregation. In C. Leaper (Ed.), Childhood gender segregation: Causes and consequences. *New Directions in Child Development, 65,* 35–52.

Martin, R. P., Wisenbaker, J., Baker, J., & Huttenen, M. O. (1997). Gender differences in temperament at 6 months and 5 years. *Infant Behavior and Development, 20,* 339–357.

Masciuch, S., & Kienapple, K. (1993). The emergence of jealousy in children 4 months to 7 years of age. *Journal of Social and Personal Relationships, 10,* 421–435.

Mazerolle, P., Brame, P., Paternoster, R., Piquero, A., & Dean, C. (2000). Onset age, persistence, and offending versatility: Comparisons across gender. *Criminology, 38,* 1143–1172.

McCabe, A., & Lipscomb, T. J. (1988). Sex differences in children's verbal aggression. *Merrill-Palmer Quarterly, 34,* 389–401.

McDowell, D. J., O'Neil, R., & Parke, R. D. (2000). Display rule application in a disappointing situation and children's emotional reactivity. *Merrill-Palmer Quarterly, 46,* 306–324.

McDowell, D. J., & Parke, R. D. (2000). Differential knowledge of display rules for positive and negative emotions: Influences from parents, influences on peers. *Social Development, 9,* 415–432.

McHale, S. M., Crowter, A. C., & Tucker, C. J. (1999). Family context and gender role socialization in middle childhood: Comparing girls to boys and sisters to brothers. *Child Development, 70,* 990–1004.

McNeilly-Choque, M.K., Hart, C. H., Robinson, C.C., Nelson, L. J., & Olsen, S. F. (1996). Overt and relational aggression on the playground: Correspondence among different informants. *Journal of Research in Childhood Education, 11,* 47–67.

McNelles, L. R., & Connolly, J. A. (1999). Intimacy between adolescent friends: Age and gender differences in intimate affect and intimate behaviors. *Journal of Research on Adolescence, 9,* 143–159.

Meehl, P. E. (1978). Theoretical risks and tabular asterisks: Sir Karl, Sir Ronald, and the slow progress of soft psychology. *Journal of Consulting and Clinical Psychology, 46,* 806–834.

Merten, D. E. (1997). The meaning of meanness: Popularity, competition, and conflict among junior high school girls. *Sociology of Education, 40,* 175–191.

Miller, P. M., Danaher, D. L., & Forbes, D. (1986). Sex-related strategies for coping of interpersonal conflict in children ages 5 to 7. *Developmental Psychology, 22,* 543–548.

Miller, P. M., & Sperry, L. L. (1987). The socialization of anger and aggression. *Merrill-Palmer Quarterly, 33*, 1–31.

Miller, W. B. (1980). The molls. In S. K. Datesman & F. R. Scarpitti (Eds.), *Women, crime, and justice* (pp. 238–248). New York: Oxford University Press.

Miller-Johnson, S., Winn, D. M., Coie, J., Maumary-Gremaud, A., Hyman, C., Terry, R., & Lochman, J. (1999). Motherhood during the teen years: A developmental perspective on risk factors for childbearing. *Development and Psychopathology, 11*, 85–100.

Mills, R. S. L., & Rubin, K. H. (1992). A longitudinal study of maternal beliefs about children's social behaviors. *Merrill-Palmer Quarterly, 38*, 494–512.

Moffitt, T. E. (1993). "Life-course-persistent" and "adolescent-limited" antisocial behavior: A developmental taxonomy. *Psychological Review, 100*, 674–701.

Moffitt, T. E. (1994). Natural histories of delinquency. In E. G. M. Weitekamp & H.-J. Kerner (Eds.), *Cross-national longitudinal research on human development and criminal behavior* (pp. 3–61). Dordrecht, The Netherlands: Kluwer Academic.

Moffitt, T. E., & Caspi, A. (2001). Childhood predictors differentiate life-course persistent and adolescent-limited antisocial pathways among males and females. *Development and Psychopathology, 13*, 355–375.

Moore, J. (1991). *Going down to the barrio: Homeboys and homegirls in change.* Philadelphia: Temple University Press.

Moran, P. B., & Eckenrode, J. (1991). Gender differences in the costs and benefits of peer relationships during adolescence. *Journal of Adolescent Research, 6*, 396–409.

Moretti, M. M., Holland, R., & McKay, S. (2001). Self–other representations and relational and overt aggression in adolescent girls and boys. *Behavioral Sciences and the Law, 19*, 109–126.

Morgan, R. (1970). Introduction: The women's revolution. In R. Morgan (Ed.), *Sisterhood is powerful: An anthology of writings from the women's liberation movement* (pp. xv–xivi). New York: Vintage.

Murphy, B., & Eisenberg, N. (1996). Provoked by a peer: Children's anger-related responses and their relation to social functioning. *Merrill-Palmer Quarterly, 42*, 103–124.

Murphy, B., Eisenberg, N., Fabes, R. A., Shepard, S. A., & Guthrie, I. K. (1999). Consistency and change in children's emotionality and regulation: A longitudinal study. *Merrill-Palmer Quarterly, 45*, 413–444.

Musante, L., & Treiber, F. A. (2000). The relationship between anger-coping styles and lifestyle behaviors in teenagers. *Journal of Adolescent Health, 27*, 63–68.

Newcomb, A. F., & Bagwell, C. L. (1995). Children's friendship relations: A meta-analytic review. *Psychological Bulletin, 117*, 306–347.

Newcomb, A. F., Bukowski, W. M., & Pattee, L. (1993). Children's peer relations: A meta-analytic review of popular, rejected, neglected, controversial, and average status. *Psychological Bulletin, 113*, 99–128.

Nolen-Hoeksema, S. (1994). An interactive model for the emergence of gender differences in depression in adolescence. *Journal of Research on Adolescence, 4*, 519–534.

Nolen-Hoeksema, S., Morrow, J., & Fredrickson, B. L. (1993). Response styles and the duration of depressed mood. *Journal of Abnormal Psychology, 102,* 20–28.

Obeidallah, D. A., & Earls, F. J. (1999, July). Adolescent girls: The role of depression in the development of delinquency. *National Institute of Justice Research Preview.*

O'Connell, P., Pepler, D., & Craig, W. (1999). Peer involvement in bullying: Insights and challenges. *Journal of Adolescence, 22,* 437–452.

Olweus, D. (1996). Bully/victim problems at school: Facts and effective intervention. *Journal of Emotional and Behavioral Problems, 5,* 15–22.

Osterman, K., Bjorkqvist, K., & Lagerspetz, K. M. J. (1997). Sex differences in styles of conflict resolution: A developmental and cross-cultural study with data from Finland, Israel, Italy, and Poland. In D. P. Fry & K. Bjorkqvist (Eds.), *Cultural variation in conflict resolution: Alternatives to violence* (pp. 185–197). New York: Erlbaum.

Osterman, K., Bjorkqvist, K., Lagerspetz, K. M. J., Kaukiainen, A., Huesmann, L. R. , & Fraczek, A. (1994). Peer and self-estimated aggression and victimization in 8-year-old children from five ethnic groups. *Aggressive Behavior, 20,* 411–428.

Osterman, K., Bjorkqvist, K., Lagerspetz, K. M. J., Kaukiainen, A., Landau, S. F., Fraczek, A., & Caprara, G. (1998). Cross-cultural evidence of female indirect aggression. *Aggressive Behavior, 24,* 1–8.

Owens, L., Slee, P., & Shute, R. (2001). Victimization among teenage girls: What can be done about indirect harassment? In J. Juvonen & S. Graham (Eds.), *Peer harassment in school: The plight of the vulnerable and the victimized* (pp. 215–241). New York: Guilford Press.

Owens, L. D. (1996). Sticks and stones and sugar and spice: Girls' and boys' aggression in schools. *Australian Journal of Guidance and Counseling, 6,* 45–55.

Owens, L. D., Shute, R., & Slee, P. (2000a). "Guess what I just heard!": Indirect aggression among teenage girls in Australia. *Aggressive Behavior, 26,* 67–83.

Owens, L. D., Shute, R., & Slee, P. (2000b). "I'm in and your're out . . . ": Explanations for teenage girls' indirect aggression. *Psychology, Evolution, and Gender, 21,* 19–46.

Owens, L. D., Shute, R., & Slee, P. (2000c). "It hurts a hell of a lot . . . ": The effects of indirect aggression on teenage girls. *School Psychology International, 21,* 359–376.

Pajer, K. A. (1998). What happens to "bad girls"?: A review of the adult outcomes of antisocial adolescent girls. *American Journal of Psychiatry, 155,* 862–870.

Pakaslahti, L., & Keltigangas-Jarvinen, L. (2000). Comparison of peer, teacher, and self-assessments on adolescent direct and indirect aggression. *Educational Psychology, 20,* 177–190.

Paley, V. G. (1992). *You can't say you can't play.* Cambridge, MA: Harvard University Press.

Papini, D. R., Farmer, F. F., Clark, S. M., Micha, J. C., & Barnett, J. K. (1990). Early adolescent age and gender differences in patterns of emotional self-disclosure to parents and to friends. *Adolescence, 100,* 959–976.

Paquette, J. A., & Underwood, M. K. (1999). Young adolescents' experiences of peer victimization: Gender differences in accounts of social and physical aggression. *Merrill-Palmer Quarterly, 45,* 233–258.

Parke, R. D., & Buriel, R. (1998). Socialization in the family: Ethnic and ecological perspectives. In N. Eisenberg (Ed.), *Handbook of child psychology. Vol. 3: Social, emotional, and personality development* (5th ed., pp. 463–552). New York: Wiley.

Parke, R. D., & O'Neil, R. (1999). Social relationships across contexts: Family–peer linkages. In W. A. Collins & B. Laursen (Eds.), Relationships as developmental contexts. *Minnesota Symposium on Child Psychology, 30,* 211–239.

Parke, R. D., & Slaby, R. G. (1983). The development of aggression. In P. Mussen (Series Ed.) & E. M. Hetherington (Vol. Ed.), *Handbook of child psychology: Vol. 4. Socialization, personality, and social development* (pp. 547–641). New York: Wiley.

Parker, J. G., & Asher, S. R. (1987). Peer relations and later personal adjustment: Are low-accepted children at risk? *Psychological Bulletin, 102,* 357–389.

Parker, J. G., & Asher, S. R. (1993). Friendship and friendship quality on middle childhood: Links with peer group acceptance and feelings of loneliness and social dissatisfaction. *Developmental Psychology, 29,* 611–621.

Parker, J. G., & Low, C. M. (1999, April). Children's jealousy over their friends' friends: Personal and relational correlates in preadolescent and adolescent boys and girls. In J. G. Parker (Chair), *Vulnerabilities, sensitivities, and insecurities: Inquiry into the dark side of children's friendships and romantic relationships.* Symposium presented at the biennial meeting of the Society for Research in Child Development, Albuquerque, NM.

Parkhurst, J. T., & Hopmeyer, A. (1998). Sociometric popularity and peer-perceived popularity: Two distinct dimensions of peer status. *Journal of Early Adolescence, 18,* 125–144.

Patterson, G. R. (1982). *Coercive family process.* Eugene, OR: Castalia.

Patterson, G. R., Forgatch, M. S., Yoerger, K. L., & Stoolmiller, M. (1998). Variables that initiate and maintain an early-onset trajectory for juvenile offending. *Development and Psychopathology, 10,* 531–547.

Pellegrini, A. D. (1988). Elementary school children's rough-and-tumble play and social competence. *Developmental Psychology, 24,* 802–806.

Pellegrini, A. D. (1994). A longitudinal study of school peer networks and adjustment to middle school. *Educational Psychology, 14,* 403–412.

Pellegrini, A. D. (2001). A longitudinal study of heterosexual relationships, aggression, and sexual harassment during the transition from primary school through middle school. *Applied Developmental Psychology, 22,* 119–133.

Pellegrini, A. D., & Smith, P. K. (1998). Physical activity play: The nature and function of a neglected aspect of play. *Child Development, 69,* 577–598.

Pepler, D. J., & Craig, W. M. (1995). A peek behind the fence: Naturalistic observations of aggressive children with remote audiovisual recording. *Developmental Psychology, 31,* 357–389.

Pepler, D. J., Craig, W. M., & O'Connell, P. (1999). Understanding bullying from a dynamic systems perspective. In A. Slater & D. Muir (Eds.), *The Blackwell readers in developmental psychology* (pp. 440–451). London: Blackwell.

Pepler, D. J., Craig, W. M., & Roberts, W. L. (1998). Observations of aggressive and non-aggressive children on the school playground. *Merrill-Palmer Quarterly, 44,* 55–76.

Perry, D. G., Perry, L. C., & Rasmussen, P. (1986). Cognitive social learning mediators of aggression. *Child Development, 57,* 700–711.

Perry, D. G., Perry, L. C., & Weiss, R. J. (1989). Sex differences in the consequences that children anticipate for aggression. *Developmental Psychology, 25,* 312–319.

Peterson, K. L., & Roscoe, B. (1991). Imaginary audience behavior in older adolescent females. *Adolescence, 26,* 195–200.

Phelps, C. E. R. (2001). Children's responses to overt and relational aggression. *Journal of Clinical Child Psychology, 30,* 240–252.

Phillipsen, L. C., Deptula, D. P., & Cohen, R. (1999). Relating characteristics of children and their friends to overt and relational aggression. *Child Study Journal, 29,* 269–289.

Pikas, A. (1989). The Common Concern Method for the treatment of mobbing. In E. Munthe & E. Roland (Eds.), *Bullying: An international perspective* (pp. 81–90). London: Routledge.

Pilgrim, C., Luo, Q., & Urberg, K. A. (1999). Influence of peers, parents, and individual characteristics on adolescent drug use in two cultures. *Merrill-Palmer Quarterly, 45,* 85–107.

Pitkanen, L. (1969). *A descriptive model of aggression and nonaggression with applications to children's behavior* (Jyvaskyla Studies in Education, Psychology and Social Research, No. 19). Jyvaskyla: University of Jyvaskyla.

Poulin-Dubois, D., Serbin, L. A., Eichstedt, J. A., Sen, M. G., & Beissel, C. F. (2002). Men don't put on makeup: Toddlers' knowledge of the gender stereotyping of household activities. *Social Development, 11,* 166–181.

Price, J. M., & Dodge, K. A. (1989). Reactive and proactive aggression in childhood: Relations to peer status and social context dimensions. *Journal of Abnormal Child Psychology, 17,* 455–471.

Prinstein, M. J., Boergers, J.,& Vernberg, E. M. (2001). Overt and relational aggression in adolescents: Social-psychological adjustment of aggressors and victims. *Journal of Child Clinical Psychology, 30,* 479–491.

Prinstein, M. J., & Cohen, G. L. (2001, April). Adolescent peer crowd affiliation and overt, relational, and social aggression: Using aggression to protect one's status? In P. H. Hawley (Chair), *Aggression and adaptive functioning: The bright side to bad behavior.* Symposium presented at the biennial meeting of the Society for Research in Child Development, Minneapolis, MN.

Pulkkinen, L. (1992). The pathway to adulthood for aggressively inclined girls. In K. Bjorkqvist & P. Niemela (Eds.), *Of mice and women: Aspects of female aggression* (pp. 113–121). San Diego, CA: Academic Press.

Purdie, V., & Downey, G. (2000). Rejection sensitivity and adolescent girls' vulnerability to relationship-centered difficulties. *Child Maltreatment, 5*(4), 338–349.

Putallaz, M. (1983). Predicting children's sociometric status from their behavior. *Child Development, 54,* 1417–1426.

Putallaz, M., Costanzo, P. R., Grimes, C. L., & Sherman, D. M. (1998). Intergenerational continuities and their influences on children's social development. *Social Development, 7,* 389–427.

Putallaz, M., & Gottman, J. M. (1981). An interactional model of children's entry into peer groups. *Child Development, 52,* 986–994.

Putallaz, M., Hellstem, L., Sheppard, B. H., Grimes, C. L., & Glodis, K. A. (1995). Conflict, social competence, and gender: Maternal and peer contexts. *Early Education and Development, 6,* 433–447.

Putallaz, M., Klein, T. P., Costanzo, P. R., & Hodges, L. A. (1994). Relating mothers' social framing to their children's social competence with peers. *Social Development, 3,* 222–237.

Putallaz, M., & Sheppard, B. H. (1992). Conflict management and social competence. In C. U. Shantz & W. W. Hartup (Eds.), *Conflict in child and adolescent development* (pp. 330–355). New York: Cambridge University Press.

Radke-Yarrow, M., & Kochanska, G. (1990). Anger in young children. In N. L. Stein, B. Leventhal, & T. Trabasso (Eds.), *Psychological and behavioral approaches to emotion* (pp. 297–310). Hillsdale, NJ: Erlbaum.

Raffaelli, M., & Duckett, E. (1989). "We were just talking . . . ": Conversation in early adolescence. *Journal of Youth and Adolescence, 18,* 567–583.

Raine, A., Venables, P. H., & Mednick, S. A. (1997). Low resting heart rate at age 3 years predisposes to aggression at age 11 years: Evidence from the Mauritius Child Health Project. *Journal of the American Academy of Child and Adolescent Psychiatry, 36,* 1457–1454.

Rauste–von Wright, M. (1989). Physical and verbal aggression in peer groups among Finnish adolescent boys and girls. *International Journal of Behavioral Development, 12,* 473–484.

Rest, J. R. (1995). *Concerns for the social-psychological adjustment of youth and educational strategies: Report for the Kaufmann Foundation.* Minneapolis: University of Minnesota, Department of Educational Psychology.

Richards, M. H., Crowe, P. A., Larson, R., & Swarr, A. (1998). Developmental patterns and gender differences in the experience of peer companionship during adolescence. *Child Development, 69,* 154–163.

Rigby, K. (2001). Gender and bullying in schools. In P. T. Slee & K Rigby (Eds.), *Children's peer relations* (pp. 47–59). New York: Routledge.

Rigby, K., & Slee, P. (1999). Suicidal ideation among adolescent school children, involvement in bully–victim problems, and perceived social support. *Suicide and Life-Threatening Behavior, 29,* 119–130.

Robins, L. N. (1986). The consequences of conduct disorder in girls. In D. Olweus, J. Block, & M. Radke-Yarrow (Eds.), *Development of antisocial and prosocial behavior* (pp. 385–414). New York: Academic Press.

Rodkin, P. C., Farmer, T. W., Pearl, R., & Van Acker, R. (2000). Heterogeneity of popular boys: Antisocial and prosocial configurations. *Developmental Psychology, 36,* 14–24.

Roff, M., & Roff, L. (1940). An analysis of the variance of conflict behavior in preschool children. *Child Development, 11,* 43–60.

Rose, A. J. (2001, April). Co-rumination in the friendships of girls and boys. In K. D. Rudolph & A. J. Rosen (Co-Chairs), *Sex differences in relationship processes: Positive and negative contributions to adolescent adjustment.* Symposium presented at the biennial meeting of the Society for Research in Child Development, Minneapolis, MN.

Rose, A. J., & Asher, S. R. (1999). Children's goals and strategies in response to conflicts within a friendship. *Developmental Psychology, 35*, 69–79.

Rose, J. S., Chassin, L., Presson, C. C., & Sherman, S. J. (1999). Peer influences on adolescent cigarette smoking: A prospective sibling analysis. *Merrill-Palmer Quarterly, 45*, 62–84.

Rosen, W. D., Adamson, L. B., & Bakeman, R. (1992). An experimental investigation of infant social references: Mothers' messages and gender differences. *Developmental Psychology, 28*, 1172–1178.

Rosenbaum, J. L. (1996). A violent few: Gang girls in the California Youth Authority. *Journal of Gang Research, 3*, 17–23.

Rosenbaum, J. L., & Chesney-Lind, M. (1994). Appearance and delinquency: A research note. *Crime and Delinquency, 40*, 250–261.

Ross, H., Tesla, C., Kenyon, B., & Lollis, S. (1990). Maternal intervention in toddler peer conflict: The socialization of principles of justice. *Developmental Psychology, 26*, 994–1003.

Rothbart, M. K. (1986). Longitudinal observation of infant temperament. *Developmental Psychology, 22*, 356–365.

Rothbart, M. K., & Bates, J. E. (1998). Temperament. In N. Eisenberg (Ed.), *Handbook of child psychology* (pp. 105–176). New York: Wiley.

Rubin, K. H., Bukowski, W., & Parker, J. G. (1998). Peer interactions, relationships, and groups. In N. Eisenberg (Ed.), *Handbook of child psychology* (5th ed., Vol. 3, pp. 619–700). New York: Wiley.

Rubin, K. H., Hastings, P., Chen, X., Stewart, S., & McNichol, K. (1998). Intrapersonal and maternal correlates of aggression, conflict, and externalizing problems in toddlers. *Child Development, 69*, 1614–1629.

Rudolph, K. D. (2002). Gender differences in emotional responses to interpersonal stress during adolescence. *Journal of Adolescent Health, 30*(Suppl. 1), 3–13.

Russell, A., & Owens, L. D. (1999). Peer estimates of school-aged boys' and girls' aggression to same- and cross-gender targets. *Social Development, 8*, 364–379.

Rusting, C. L., & Nolen-Hoeksema, S. (1998). Regulating responses to anger: Effects of rumination and distraction on angry mood. *Journal of Personality and Social Psychology, 74*, 790–803.

Rys, G. S., & Bear, G. G. (1997). Relational aggression and peer relations: Gender and developmental issues. *Merrill-Palmer Quarterly, 43*, 87–106.

Saarni, C. (1984). An observational study of children's attempts to monitor their expressive behavior. *Child Development, 55*, 1504–1513.

Saarni, C. (1999). *The development of emotional competence.* New York: Guilford Press.

Saarni, C., & von Salisch, M. (1993). The socialization of emotional dissemblance. In M. Lewis & C. Saarni (Eds.), *Lying and deception in everyday life* (pp. 106–125). New York: Guilford Press.

Saarni, C., & Weber, H. (1999). Emotional displays and dissemblance in childhood: Implications for self-presentation. In P. Phillipot, R. S. Feldman, & E. J. Coats (Eds.), *The social context of non-verbal behavior* (pp. 71–105). New York: Cambridge University Press.

Sage, N. A., & Kindermann, T. A. (1999). Peer networks, behavior contingencies, and children's engagement in the classroom. *Merrill-Palmer Quarterly, 45,* 143–171.

Salmivalli, C. (1998). Intelligent, attractive, well-behaving, unhappy: The structure of adolescents' self-concept and its relation to their social behavior. *Journal of Research on Adolescence, 8,* 333–354.

Salmivalli, C., Kaukiainen, A., & Lagerspetz, K. (2000). Aggression and sociometric status among peers: Do gender and type of aggression matter? *Scandinavian Journal of Psychology, 41,* 17–24.

Salmivalli, C., Kaukiainen, A., & Lagerspetz, K. (2001). Aggression in the social relations of school-aged girls and boys. In P. T. Slee & K Rigby (Eds.), *Children's peer relations* (pp. 60–75). New York: Routledge.

Salmivalli, C., Lagerspetz, K., Bjorkqvist, K., Osterman, K., & Kaukiainen, A. (1996). Bullying as a group process: Participant roles and their relations to social status within the group. *Aggressive Behavior, 22,* 1–15.

Sampson, R. J., & Laub, J. H. (1993). *Crime in the making: Pathways and turning points through life.* Cambridge, MA: Harvard University Press.

Savin-Williams, R. C. (2001). A critique of research on sexual-minority youths. *Journal of Adolescence, 24,* 5–13.

Scaramella, L. V., Conger, R. D., & Simons, R. L. (1999). Parental protective influences and gender-specific increases in adolescent internalizing and externalizing problems. *Journal of Research on Adolescence, 9,* 111–141.

Schacter, R., Shore, E., Hodapp, R., Chaflin, S., & Bundy, C. (1978). Do girls talk earlier?: Mean length of utterance in toddlers. *Developmental Psychology, 14,* 388–392.

Scheff, T. J. (1984). The taboo on coarse emotions. In P. Shaver (Ed.), *Review of personality and social psychology: Emotions, relationships, and health* (Vol. 5, pp. 188–209). Beverly Hills, CA: Sage.

Schlossman, S., & Cairns, R. B. (1994). Problem girls: Observations on past and present. In G. H. Elder, Jr., J. Modell, & R. D. Parke (Eds.), *Children in time and place: Developmental and historical insights* (pp. 110–130). Cambridge, UK: Cambridge University Press.

Schneider, B. H., Atkinson, L., & Tardif, C. (2001). Child–parent attachment and children's peer relations: A quantitative review. *Developmental Psychology, 37,* 86–100.

Schneider, B. H., & Younger, A. J. (1996). Adolescent–parent attachment and adolescents' relations with their peers: A closer look. *Youth and Society, 28,* 95–108.

Schulenberg, J., Maggs, J. L., Dielman, T. E., Leech, S. L., Kloska, D. D., Shope, J. T., & Laetz, V. B. (1999). On peer influences to get drunk: A panel study of young adolescents. *Merrill-Palmer Quarterly, 45,* 108–141.

Schultz, D., Izard, C. E., & Ackerman, B. P. (2000). Children's anger attribution biases: Relations to family environment and social adjustment. *Social Development, 9,* 234–301.

Sears, R. R. (1961). Relation of early socialization experiences to aggression in middle childhood. *Journal of Abnormal Psychology, 63,* 466– 492.

Sears, R. R., Rau, L. L., & Alpert, R. (1965). *Identification and child rearing.* Stanford, CA: Stanford University Press.

Serbin, L. A., Cooperman, J. M., Peters, P. L., Lehoux, P. M., Stack, D. M., & Schwartzmen, A. E. (1998). Intergenerational transfer of psychosocial risk in women with childhood histories of aggression, withdrawal, or aggression and withdrawal. *Developmental Psychology, 34,* 1246–1262.

Serbin, L. A., Marchessault, K., McAffer, V., Peters, P., & Schwartzman, A. E. (1993). Patterns of social behavior on the playground in 9- to 11-year-old girls and boys: Relation to teacher perceptions and to peer ratings of aggression, withdrawal, and likeability. In C. H. Hart (Ed.), *Children on playgrounds: Research perspectives and applications* (pp. 162–183). Albany: State University of New York Press.

Serbin, L. A., Moller, L. C., Gulko, J., Powlishta, K. K., & Colbourne, K. A. (1994). The emergence of gender segregation in toddler playgroups. In C. Leaper (Ed.), Childhood gender segregation: Causes and consequences. *New Directions in Child Development, 65,* 7–18.

Serbin, L. A., Powlishta, K. K., & Gulko, J. (1993). The development of sex typing in middle childhood. *Monographs of the Society for Research in Child Development, 58*(2, Serial No. 232), pp. 1–75.

Shantz, C. U. (1987). Conflicts between children. *Child Development, 58,* 283–305.

Shantz, D.W. (1986). Conflict, aggression, and peer status. *Child Development, 57,* 1322–1332.

Sharabany, R., Gershoni, R., & Hofman, J. E. (1981). Girlfriend, boyfriend: Age and sex differences in intimate friendship. *Developmental Psychology, 17,* 800–808.

Sharp, S. (1995). How much does bullying hurt?: The effects of bullying on the personal well-being and educational progress of secondary aged students. *Educational and Child Psychology, 12,* 81–88.

Sharp, S., & Cowie, H. (1994). Empowering students to take action against bullying. In P. K. Smith & S. Sharp (Eds.), *School bullying: Insights and perspectives* (pp. 109–131). New York: Routledge.

Sharp, S., & Thompson, D. (1994). The role of whole-school policies in tackling bullying behavior in schools. In P. K. Smith & S. Sharp (Eds.), *School bullying: Insights and perspectives* (pp. 57–83). New York: Routledge.

Shaver, P., Schwartz, J., Kirson, D., & O'Connor, C. (1987). Emotion knowledge: Further exploration of a prototype approach. *Journal of Personality and Social Psychology, 52,* 1061–1086.

Shaw, D. S., Keenan, K., & Vondra, J. I. (1994). Developmental precursors or externalizing behavior: Ages 1 to 3. *Developmental Psychology, 30,* 355–364.

Shelden, R. G., & Chesney-Lind, M. (1993). Gender and race differences in delinquent careers. *Juvenile and Family Court Journal, 44,* 73–90.

Shields, S. A. (2000). Thinking about gender, thinking about theory: Gender and emotional experience. In A. H. Fischer (Ed.), *Gender and emotion: Social psychological perspectives* (pp. 3–23). Cambridge, UK: Cambridge University Press.

Shrum, W., & Cheek, N. H. (1987). Social structure during the school years: Onset of the degrouping process. *American Sociological Review, 52,* 218–223.

Shrum, W., Cheek, N. H., & Hunter, S. M. (1988). Friendship in school: Gender and racial homophily. *Sociology of Education, 61,* 227–239.

Shulman, S., & Scharf, M. (2000). Adolescent romantic behaviors and perceptions: Age and gender-related differences, and links with family and peer relationships. *Journal of Research on Adolescence, 10*, 99–118.

Sikes, G. (1997). *8 ball chicks: A year in the violent world of girl gangsters.* New York:
Anchor Books.

Silverthorn, P., & Frick, P. J. (1999). Developmental pathways to antisocial behavior: The delayed-onset pathway in girls. *Development and Psychopathology, 11*,
101–126.

Simmons, R. (2002). *Odd girl out: The hidden culture of aggression in girls.* New York:
Harcourt.

Sippola, L. K. (1999). Getting to know the "other": The characteristics and developmental significance of other-sex relationships in adolescence. *Journal of
Youth and Adolescence, 28*, 407–417.

Smetana, J. G. (1989). Toddlers' social interactions in the context of moral and
conventional transgressions in the home. *Developmental Psychology, 25*, 499–
508.

Smith, P. K., & Boulton, M. (1990). Rough and tumble play, aggression, and dominance: Perception and behavior in children's encounters. *Human Development, 33*, 271–282.

Smith, P. K., & Green, M. (1975). Aggressive behavior in English nurseries and
play groups: Sex differences and responses of adults. *Child Development, 46*,
211–214.

Smith, P. K., Morita, Y., Junger-Tas, J., Olweus, D., Catalano, R., & Slee, P. (Eds.).
(1998). *The nature of bullying: A cross-national perspective.* London: Routledge.

Smith, P. K., & Sharp, S. (Eds.). (1994). *School bullying: Insights and perspectives.*
New York: Routledge.

Snyder, H. N., & Sickmund, M. (1999). *OJJDP statistical briefing book.* Washington,
DC: U.S. Department of Justice, Office of Juvenile Justice and Delinquency
Prevention.

Snyder, J., Horsch, E., & Childs, J. (1997). Peer relationships of young children:
Affiliative choices and the shaping of aggressive behavior. *Journal of Child
Clinical Psychology, 26*, 145–156.

Stenberg, C. R., & Campos, J. J. (1990). The development of anger expressions in
infancy. In N. L. Stein, B. Leventhal, & T. Trabasso (Eds.), *Psychological and
biological approaches to emotion* (pp. 247–282). Hillsdale, NJ: Erlbaum.

Stenberg, C. R., Campos, J. J., & Emde, R. N. (1983). The facial expression of anger in seven-month-old infants. *Child Development, 54*, 178–184.

Stipek, D., Recchia, S., & McClintic, S. (1992). Self-evaluation in young children.
Monographs of the Society for Research in Child Development (Serial No. 226), *57*.

Stormshak, E. A., Bierman, K. L., Bruschi, C., Dodge, K. A., Coie, J. D., and the
Conduct Problems Prevention Research Group. (1999). The relation between behavior problems and peer preference in different classroom contexts. *Child Development, 70*, 169–182.

Straus, M. A. (1979). Measuring intrafamily conflict and violence: The Conflict
Tactics (CT) Scales. *Journal of Marriage and the Family, 41*, 75–88.

Sullivan, H. S. (1953). *The interpersonal theory of psychiatry.* New York: Norton.

Susman, E. J. (1997). Modeling developmental complexity in adolescence: Hormones and behavior in context. *Journal of Research on Adolescence, 7,* 283–306.

Talbott, E. (1997). Reflecting on antisocial girls and the study of their development: Researchers' view. *Exceptionality, 7,* 267–272.

Tangney, J. P., Hill-Barlow, D., Wagner, P. E., Marschall, D. E., Borenstein, J. K., Sanftner, J., Mohr, T., & Gramzow, R. (1996). Assessing individual differences in constructive versus destructive responses to anger across the lifespan. *Journal of Personality and Social Psychology, 70,* 780–796.

Tangney, J. P., Wagner, P. E., Hill-Barlow, D., Marschall, D. E., & Gramzow, R. (1996). Relation of shame and guilt to constructive and destructive anger across the lifespan. *Journal of Personality and Social Psychology, 70,* 797–809.

Taylor, G. (1996). Creating a circle of friends: A case study. In H. Cowie & S. Sharp (Eds.), *Peer counseling in schools: A time to listen* (pp. 73–86). London: Fulton.

Tavris, C. (2002, July 5). Are girls really as mean as the books say they are? *Chronicle of Higher Education, 48*(43), B7–B10.

Thompson, R. A. (1990). Vulnerability in research: A developmental perspective on research risk. *Child Development, 61,* 1–16.

Thorne, B. (1986). Girls and boys together but mostly apart: Gender arrangements in elementary schools. In W. W. Hartup & Z. Rubin (Eds.), *Relationships and development* (pp. 167–184). Hillsdale, NJ: Erlbaum.

Thorne, B. (1993). *Gender play: Girls and boys in school.* New Brunswick, NJ: Rutgers University Press.

Thorne, B., & Luria, Z. (1986). Sexuality and gender in children's daily worlds. *Social Problems, 33,* 176–190.

Tiet, Q. Q., Wasserman, G. A., Loeber, R., McReynolds, L. S., & Miller, L. S. (2001). Developmental and sex differences in types of conduct problems. *Journal of Child and Family Studies, 10,* 181–197.

Tomada, G., & Schneider, B. H. (1997). Relational aggression, gender, and peer acceptance: Invariance across culture, stability over time, and concordance among informants. *Developmental Psychology, 33,* 601–609.

Tremblay, R. E. (2000). The development of aggressive behavior during childhood: What have we learned in the past century? *International Journal of Behavioral Development, 24,* 129–141.

Tremblay, R. E. (2001). The development of physical aggression during childhood and the prediction of later dangerousness. In G. F. Pinard & L. Pagani (Eds.), *Clinical assessment of dangerousness: Empirical contributions* (pp. 47–65). New York: Cambridge University Press.

Tremblay, R. E., Japel, C., Perusse, D., McDuff, P., Boivin, M., Zoccolillo, M., & Montplaisir, J. (1999). The search for the age of "onset" of physical aggression: Rousseau and Bandura revisited. *Criminal Behavior and Mental Health, 9,* 8–23.

Underwood, M. K. (1997). Peer social status and children's choices about the expression and control of positive and negative emotions. *Merrill-Palmer Quarterly, 43,* 610–634.

Underwood, M. K. (in press). Gender and peer relations: Are the two gender cultures really all that different? In J. B. Kupersmidt & K. A. Dodge (Eds.),

Children's peer relations: From developmental science to intervention to policy. A Festschrift for John D. Coie. Washington, DC: American Psychological Association.

Underwood, M. K., & Bjornstad, G. J. (2001). Children's emotional experience of peer provocation: The relation among observed behavior and self-reports of emotions, expressions, and social goals. *International Journal of Behavioral Development, 25,* 320–330.

Underwood, M. K., Coie, J. D., & Herbsman, C. R. (1992). Display rules for anger and aggression in school-aged children. *Child Development, 63,* 366–380.

Underwood, M. K., Galen, B. R., & Paquette, J. A. (2001a). Admirations rather than hostilities: Response to Archer, Bjorkqvist, and Crick et al. *Social Development, 10,* 275–280.

Underwood, M. K., Galen, B. R., & Paquette, J. A. (2001b). Top ten challenges for understanding aggression and gender: Why can't we all just get along? *Social Development, 10,* 248–266.

Underwood, M. K., Hurley, J. C., Johanson, C. A., & Mosley, J. E. (1999). An Experimental, observational investigation of children's responses to peer provocation: Developmental and gender differences in middle childhood. *Child Development, 70,* 1428–1446.

Underwood, M. K., Kupersmidt, J. B., & Coie, J. D. (1996). Childhood peer sociometric status and aggression as predictors of adolescent childbearing. *Journal of Research on Adolescence, 6,* 201–223.

Underwood, M. K., Moore, B. M., Bjornstad, G. J., Sexton, A. E., & Galperin, M. (2002). *An experimental, observational study of social aggression: Gender and developmental differences.* Manuscript in preparation.

Updegraff, K. A., Moltale, S. M, & Crouter, A. C. (2000). Adolescents' sex-typed friendship experiences: Does having a sister or brother matter? *Child Development, 71,* 1597–1610.

Urberg, K. A., Degirmencioglu, S. M., Tolson, J. M., & Halliday-Scher, K. (1995). The structure of adolescent peer networks. *Developmental Psychology, 31,* 540–547.

van IJzendoorn, M. H. (1997). Attachment, emergent morality, and aggression: Toward a developmental, socioemotional model of antisocial behavior. *International Journal of Behavioral Development, 21,* 703–727.

Vaughn, B. E., Bost, K., & Vollenweider, M. (2001, April). Negative behavior and social competence in a sample of preschool children attending Head Start. In P. H. Hawley (Chair), *Aggression and adaptive functioning: The bright side to bad behavior.* Symposium presented at the biennial meeting of the Society for Research in Child Development, Minneapolis, MN.

Vaughn, B. E., Colvin, T. N., Azria, M. R., Caya, L., & Krzysik, L. (2001). Dyadic analyses of friendship in a sample of preschool-age children attending Head Start: Correspondence between measures and implications for social competence. *Child Development, 72*(3), 862–878.

Vespo, J. E., Pedersen, K., & Hay, D. F. (1995). Young children's conflicts with peers and siblings: Gender effects. *Child Study Journal, 25,* 189–214.

Vuchinich, S., Emery, P. E., & Cassidy, J. (1988). Family members as third parties in dyadic family conflict: Strategies, alliances, and outcomes. *Child Development*, *59*, 1293–1302.

Walters, R. H., & Parke, R. D. (1964). Social motivation, dependency, and susceptibility to social influence. In L. Berkowitz (Eds.), *Advances in experimental social psychology* (Vol. 1, pp. 231–276). New York: Academic Press.

Warren, A. R., & Tate, C. S. (1992). Egocentrism in children's telephone conversations. In R. M. Diaz & L. E. Bert (Eds.), *Private speech: From social interaction to self-regulation* (pp. 245–264). Hillsdale, NJ: Erlbaum.

Watkins, M. J. (1990). Mediationism and the obfuscation of memory. *American Psychologist*, *45*, 328–335.

Way, N. (1995). "Can't you see the courage, the strength I have?": Listening to urban adolescent girls speak about their relationships. *Psychology of Women Quarterly*, *19*, 107–128.

Weinberg, M. K., Tronick, E. Z., Cohn, J. F., & Olson, K. L. (1999). Gender differences in emotional expressivity and self-regulation during early infancy. *Developmental Psychology*, *35*, 175–188.

Werner, N. E., & Crick, N. R. (1999). Relational aggression and social-psychological adjustment in a college sample. *Journal of Abnormal Psychology*, *108*, 615–623.

White, G. L., & Mullen, P. E. (1989). *Jealousy: Theory, research, and clinical strategies*. New York: Guilford Press.

Whitesell, N. R., & Harter, S. (1996). The interpersonal context of emotion: Anger with close friends and classmates. *Child Development*, *67*,1345–1359.

Whiting, B. B., & Edwards, C. P. (1973). A cross-cultural analysis of sex differences in the behavior of children aged three through eleven. *Journal of Social Psychology*, *91*, 171–188.

Whiting, B. B., & Edwards, C. P. (1988). *Children of different worlds: The formation of social behavior*. Cambridge, MA: Harvard University Press.

Williams, J. H. (1977). *Psychology of women: Behavior in a biosocial context*. New York: Norton.

Williams, K. D. (2001). *Ostracism: The power of silence*. New York: Guilford Press.

Williams, K. D., & Zadro, L. (2001). Ostracism: On being ignored, excluded, and rejected. In M. Leary (Ed.), *Interpersonal rejection* (pp. 21–53). New York: Oxford University Press.

Williams, T. M., Joy, L. A., Kimball, M. M., & Zarback, M. L. (1983, April). *How is the sex difference in aggression distributed?* Paper presented at the biennial meeting of the Society for Research in Child Development, Detroit, MI.

Willoughby, J., Kupersmidt, J. B., & Bryant, D. (2001). Overt and covert dimensions of antisocial behavior. *Journal of Abnormal Child Psychology*, *29*, 177–187.

Windle, M. (1992). Revised dimensions of temperament survey (DOTS-R): Simultaneous group confirmatory factor analysis for adolescent gender groups. *Psychological Assessment*, *4*, 228–234.

Windle, M., & Lerner, R. M. (1986). Reassessing the dimensions of temperamental individuality across the lifespan: The Revised Dimensions of Temperament Survey (DOTS-R). *Journal of Adolescent Research*, *1*, 213–230.

Wiseman, R. (2002). *Queen bees and wannabes: Helping your daughter survive cliques, gossip, boyfriends, and other realities of adolescence*. New York: Crown.

Wright, J. C., Zakriski, A. L., & Drinkwater, M. (1999). Developmental psychopathology and the patterning of behavior and environment: Distinctive situational and behavioral signatures of internalizing, externalizing, and mixed-syndrome children. *Journal of Consulting and Clinical Psychology, 67,* 95–107.

Xie, H., Cairns, B. D., & Cairns, R. B. (in press). The development of aggressive behaviors among girls: Measurement issues, social functions, and differential trajectories. In D. J. Pepler, K. Madsen, C. Webster, & K. Levine (Eds.), *The development and treatment of girlhood aggression.* Mahwah, NJ: Erlbaum.

Xie, H., Cairns, R. B., & Cairns, B. D. (2002). The development of social and physical aggression: A narrative analysis of interpersonal conflicts. *Aggressive Behavior, 28,* 341–355.

Xie, H., Swift, D. J., Cairns, B. D., & Cairns, R. B. (2002). Aggressive behaviors in social interaction and developmental adaptation: A narrative analyses of interpersonal conflicts during early adolescence. *Social Development, 11,* 205–224.

Yussen, Y. R. (1977). Characteristics of moral dilemmas written by adolescents. *Developmental Psychology, 13,* 162–163.

Zahn-Waxler, C. (1993). Warriors and worriers: Gender and psychopathology. *Development and Psychopathology, 5,* 79–90.

Zahn-Waxler, C. (in press). The development of empathy, guilt, and internalization of distress. In R. Davidson (Ed.), *Anxiety, depression, and emotion: Wisconsin Symposium on Emotion* (Vol. 2, pp. 222–265). New York: Oxford University Press.

Zahn-Waxler, C., Iannotti, R. J., Cummings, E. M., & Denham, S. (1990). Antecedents of problems behaviors in children of depressed mothers. *Development and Psychopathology, 2,* 271–292.

Zahn-Waxler, C., Klimes-Dougan, B., & Kendziora, K. T. (1998). The study of emotion socialization: Conceptual, methodological, and developmental considerations. *Psychological Inquiry, 9,* 313–316.

Zahn-Waxler, C., Radke-Yarrow, M., Wagner, E., & Chapman, M. (1992). Development of concern for others. *Developmental Psychology, 28,* 126–136.

Zanarini, M. C., & Gunderson, J. G. (1997). Differential diagnosis of antisocial and borderline personality disorders. In D. M. Stoff, J. Breiling, & J. D. Maser (Eds.), *Handbook of antisocial behavior* (pp. 83–91). New York: Wiley.

Zarbatany, L., Hartmann, D. P., & Rankin, D. B. (1990). The psychological functions of preadolescent peer activities. *Child Development, 61,* 1067–1080.

Zarbatany, L., McDougall, P., & Hymel, S. (2000). Gender-differentiated experience in the peer culture: Links to intimacy in preadolescence. *Social Development, 9,* 62–79.

Zarbatany, L., Van Brunschot, M., Meadows, K., & Pepper, S. (1996). Effects of friendship and gender on peer group entry. *Child Development, 67,* 2287–2300.

Zeman, J., & Garber, J. (1996). Display rules for anger, sadness, and pain: It depends on who is watching. *Child Development, 67,* 957–973.

Zeman, J., & Penza, S. (1997). Preschoolers as functionalists: The impact of social context on emotion regulation. *Child Study Journal, 27,* 21–47.

Zeman, J., & Shipman, K. (1996). Children's expressions of negative affect: Reasons and methods. *Developmental Psychology, 32,* 842–849.

Zimmerman, P. (1999). Structure and functions of internal working models of attachment and their role for emotion regulation. *Attachment and Human Development, 1*, 291–306.

Zimmerman, P., Maier, M. A., Winter, M., & Grossman, K. E. (2001). Attachment and adolescents' emotion regulation during a joint problem-solving task with a friend. *International Journal of Social and Behavioral Development, 25*, 331–343.

Zoccolillo, M. (1993). Gender and the development of conduct disorder. *Development and Psychopathology, 5*, 65–78.

Zoccolillo, M., Tremblay, R., & Vitaro, F. (1996). DSM-III-R and DSM-III criteria for conduct disorder in adolescent girls: Specific but insensitive. *Journal of the American Academy of Child and Adolescent Psychiatry, 35*, 461–470.

Index